PLANT BASED
HEALTH BASICS

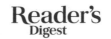

Reader's Digest

New York | Montreal

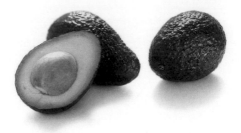

NOTE TO OUR READERS

The information in this book should not be substituted for, or used to alter, medical therapy without your doctor's advice. For a specific health problem, consult your physician for guidance.

contents

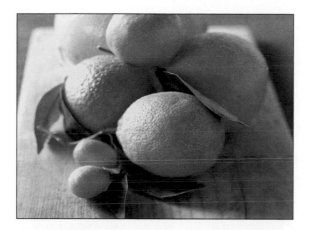
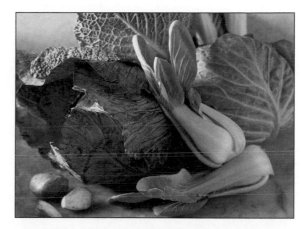
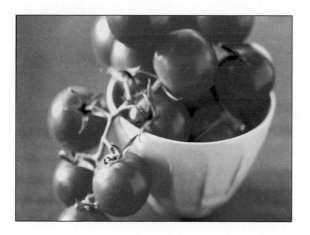
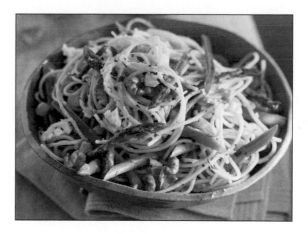

plant-based basics

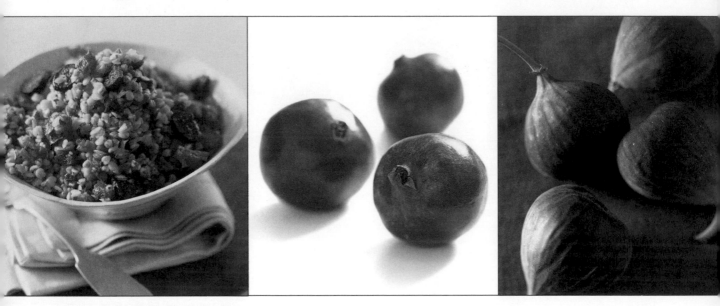

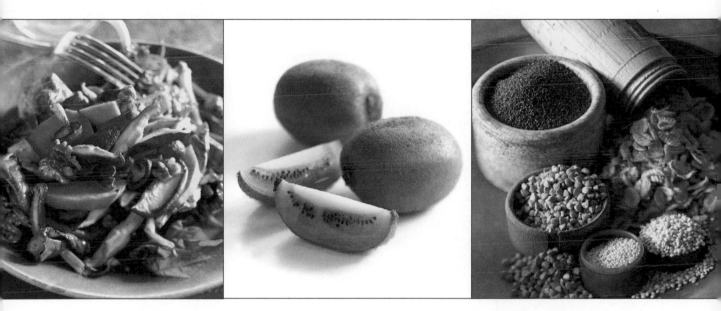

An A-to-Z Guide

to the Nutrients in a

Plant-Based Diet That Help

Reverse and Prevent Disease

plant-based basics

What do pickles, chia seeds, sweet potatoes, kidney beans, and bananas have in common? They're all superfoods—fruits, vegetables, and seeds that have been elevated to superstar status thanks to decades of scientific research culminating in a deeper understanding of their many health benefits. While superfood trends come and go, the real stars become staples in the

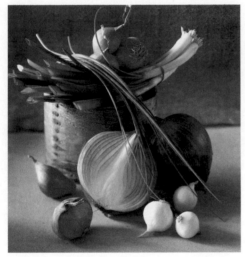

diets of all health-conscious Americans. Most vegetables, fruits, legumes (beans and lentils), whole grains, nuts, and seeds are superfoods in their own right. Together, they form the core of a whole food plant-based diet, earning a reputation as the healthiest diet of all.

A plant-based diet can take any of several forms. While a vegan diet is clearly plant-based, so are the different types of vegetarian diets, from the lacto-ovo, which includes some dairy in the diet, to pescatarian, which includes fish but avoids meat, poultry, and other animal products. The most common plant-based diet in America is probably an eating style that focuses mostly on vegetables, fruits, grains, legumes, and other plant foods, but also includes small amounts of animal foods from time to time. The bottom line: The fuller your diet is from plant foods, the more you have to gain from the many health benefits they provide, while you're young and as you age.

"Let medicine be your food, and food your medicine."
— Hippocrates

Those health benefits aren't just about the role of fruits, vegetables, grains, and other plant foods in preventing vitamin and mineral deficiencies, as they were thought to be when the science of nutrition first burst onto the research scene more than 150 years ago. Nor are they solely aimed at weight control, a public health problem of "over-nutrition" that came to light in early 20th-century America and has since risen to epidemiological proportions in this country. Although these are very important considerations when choosing the types and amount of food you eat on a regular basis, they are perhaps not the most intriguing aspects of the many connections between diet and health.

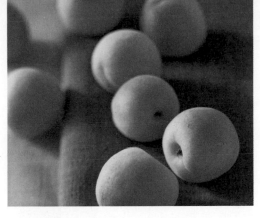

food as medicine

People of many different cultures have long been conscious of the relationship between food and health. Traditional Chinese healers prescribed particular foods to help invigorate the body's vital energy. And the ancient Indians, Egyptians, Greeks, and Romans were also keenly aware that medicinal and healing properties of certain foods could play a crucial role in human health. This sentiment was put into words over 2,500 years ago when the father of medicine, Hippocrates, wrote "Let medicine be your food, and food your medicine." The idea that food can function as medicine has come full circle. What the people of these ancient cultures believed about the therapeutic value of certain foods, modern nutritional science is now confirming.

the foundation

Over a century ago, scientists discovered the essential food substances—vitamins and minerals—that remedied common debilitating nutritional diseases and maintained good health. They found that if the body doesn't get enough of the proper nutrients, its normal functioning can become impaired. For example, it was discovered that a calcium deficiency could lead to osteoporosis, a lack of iron could cause anemia, and insufficient folate could result in birth defects. Along with this fundamental understanding of the relationship between nutrients and disease prevention came the realization that a broad array of nutrients and other healthful substances found in food is also required to energize all the body's cells, foster normal growth and development, and promote longevity.

Over the past few decades, nutrition databases have all but exploded with scientific studies on plant foods and plant-based diets and their positive effects on health. This research not only confirms much of what folk medicine has long suggested about the medicinal qualities of certain foods, but also reveals just how powerful plant foods are when it comes to keeping you healthy throughout every stage of your life and ensuring that you are able to live out your life to the fullest degree possible.

the new nutrition

Today, we are at the forefront of a new and exciting era in nutrition research. Scientists have moved beyond the vitamins and minerals we all know and have

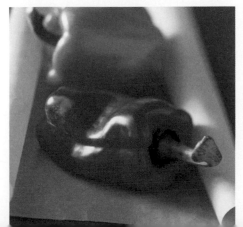

been able to identify an army of other compounds that appear to play an active role in preventing, reversing, and/or managing disease. One of the newer discoveries in modern nutrition is the existence and role of thousands of phytonutrients (plant nutrients), sometimes referred to as phytochemicals

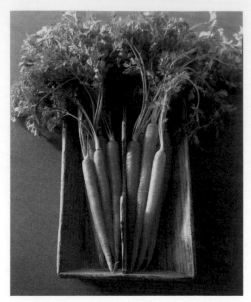

(plant chemicals). Phytonutrients are powerful substances that, while not technically nutrients, have been found to play a huge role in maintaining good health as well as longevity. Phytonutrients are thought to play a major role in fighting inflammation and oxidative stress (an imbalance of toxins that cause oxidation that damages cells and the antioxidants needed to fight and repair the damage). Both inflammation and oxidative stress appear to underlie numerous chronic diseases, including diabetes, cancer, cardiovascular disease, and neurological conditions. Research shows that a single plant food can contain hundreds of these disease-fighting substances that are also responsible for the brilliant color and distinct flavor and aroma of fruits, vegetables, legumes, nuts, seeds, and whole grains. Everyday foods—such as green peas, blueberries, sweet potatoes, and apples—contain phytonutrients that may help ward off chronic disease and disorders. Coffee, tea, and cocoa also contain beneficial phytonutrients.

Phytonutrients, in their native state, act as protective barriers, shielding plants against insects, bacteria, viruses, UV light, and other environmental threats. Fortunately, the benefits of phytonutrients extend beyond the botanical world: These potent plant compounds appear to guard the human body from disease in a variety of ways. According to research, many phytonutrients help the body to dispose of potentially hazardous substances, including carcinogens, and may protect DNA in cells from damage that can trigger a disease process. Numerous phytonutrients stimulate the body's immune cells and infection-fighting enzymes. Still other phytonutrients help to balance hormone levels, thus reducing the risk for hormone-related conditions and cancers, such as symptoms of menopause, and breast and prostate cancer. And a vast number of phytonutrients function as antioxidants, which neutralize the harmful free radicals (unstable oxygen molecules) that may play a role in the onset of degenerative diseases.

The difference between nutrients and phytonutrients is simple: Nutrients are absolutely essential for life, while phytonutrients enhance that life by fighting disease and supporting good health. Nutrients exist in all foods; phytonutrients are only found in plant foods. That's what makes a plant-based diet worth considering. The quality of your life, and the number of productive years you live, may depend on it.

Today's nutrition researchers also look closely at foods with probiotic and prebiotic qualities. Probiotic foods—kimchi, kombucha, fresh sauerkraut, pickled vegetables, miso, and others—contain beneficial bacteria that balance the natural microcosm of organisms found in the gastrointestinal tract. Poor eating habits, or a diet lacking in nutrients and phytonutrients, can throw off

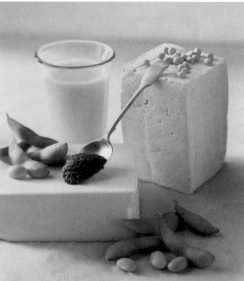

that balance and lead to overgrowth of harmful bacteria that can lead to illness. Prebiotic foods—apples, asparagus, onions, cocoa powder, and others—contain fibers that feed probiotic bacteria and help them thrive. Both appear to serve the digestive tract in ways that support many other aspects of physical, psychological, and neurological health. And both help support the healthfulness of a plant-based diet.

Another recently discovered role of the many nutrients and phytonutrients found in plant foods is the maintenance of good mental health. There is no longer any question about the health connection between your brain and the rest of your body—we know they work together to support all aspects of health and well-being. We also know that what happens to one affects what happens to the other.

While the specific cognitive and mental health benefits of a plant-based diet have yet to be fully explored, studies are beginning to show a positive association between mental and neurological health and prebiotic and probiotic foods. For instance, lab studies have shown a link between the health of the gut microbiome and brain metabolism. Another small, preclinical study found that probiotics slightly improved memory and reduced stress.

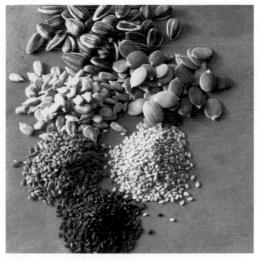

The benefits of omega-3 fatty acids—found in nuts, seeds, plant oils, and avocado—for physical health have been well established, especially for maintaining cardiovascular health and preventing heart disease. In addition, it is becoming clear that these polyunsaturated fats also play a role in good mental health. Early research appears to confirm that a deficiency of omega-3s in the diet is linked to increased risk of many different psychiatric disorders, including attention-deficit disorder, schizophrenia, autism, and dementia. Ongoing research focuses on the role of omega-3 fatty acids in the prevention and treatment of these conditions.

the importance of whole foods

Because phytonutrient research is an ever-emerging science, optimal as well as safe intakes of phytonutrients have not yet been established. The best way to get phytonutrients from your diet is by consuming a variety of plant foods, including the recommended 5 to 13 servings of fruits and vegetables each day. This is beneficial for several reasons: Just as phytonutrients in a particular food can team up to combat disease and enhance well-being, so do the phytonutrients from a wide range of foods work together to promote good health. It also seems that fiber, vitamins, minerals, and other substances in food may enhance, regulate, and be supported by the actions of phytonutrients.

what the future holds

Current research is now on the road to better understanding not only the healthful substances themselves but also how they work together and how phytonutrients behave in the human body. For example, scientists are exploring the bioavailability of phytonutrients in foods, the mechanism by which they fight off environmental toxins, and the effects of processing on their quality. Researchers are also hoping to discover how certain foods can influence complex aspects of human mental and physical health, including mood, memory, longevity, and immune responsiveness. We are also witnessing enormously promising innovations resulting from "functional food" research (see *Enhancing Foods for Health, page 20*).

With all these new and advanced discoveries, it would be easy to forget about the basics of good nutrition and simply focus on a few superfoods. But that's not the healthiest path to take. For optimal nutrition and good health, a plant-based diet should include a wide variety of foods from a variety of different food groups. You need a balance of macronutrients—complex carbohydrates, healthy fats, and quality protein—and micronutrients, the essential vitamins and minerals—along with enough different types of fiber and different phytonutrients to keep your body and mind working at their best. All of these are found in a plant-based diet and all work

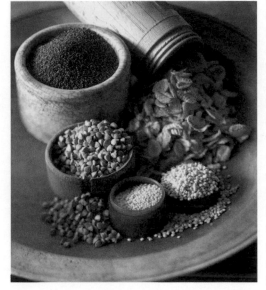

synergistically to regulate body functions and fight inflammation by enhancing absorption of nutrients, interacting with the microbiome, increasing the antioxidant capacity of foods, and targeting different cells and pathways that are susceptible to disease. While most health conditions can't be controlled by diet alone, nutrition plays a huge role in the state of your overall health. The better your health, the better your body is able to fight off the physical and mental changes that lead to everyday ailments as well as chronic disease.

Now, as the 21st century is upon us, the science of nutrition will allow us to understand how a food's chemical properties, its nutrient interaction with other foods (as well as medications), its organic compounds, phytonutrients, vitamins, and minerals all work together to avoid disease and enhance human health. Each year, researchers discover new interactions and beneficial effects of phytonutrients. Who knows what is yet to be discovered about healing plant compounds that will contribute to our arsenal of knowledge about foods that fight disease?

the plant-based pantry

In addition to the foods on your regular shopping list—the ones highlighted on pages 34 to 128—which should include fresh and dried fruits and vegetables; whole-grains and whole grain products; herbs and spices; baking supplies; plant-based dairy substitutes; and a variety of legumes, plant oils and vinegars, common nuts, including walnuts and almonds, and seeds such as pumpkin, sunflower, and sesame, you'll want to be sure to round out your pantry (and refrigerator) with some or all of these foods that also contribute important nutrients, phytonutrients, and probiotics to a whole food plant-based diet:

Chia seeds A handy way to sneak some healthful omega-3 fatty acids and extra calcium into your diet, chia seeds are used in smoothies, puddings, grain bowls, yogurt parfaits, and oatmeal and other hot cereals. When mixed with liquid, they swell slightly but retain their signature crunch.

Flaxseeds In order to be used by your body, flaxseeds need to be ground. If you have a grinder, keep whole flaxseeds on hand; if not, you can purchase them already ground. Be sure to choose opaque packaging because the nutrients in flaxseed can be destroyed by light and the oils in the seeds can easily go rancid.

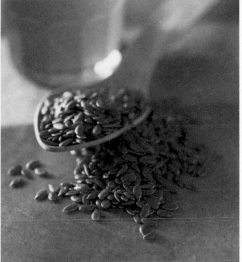

Storing in the freezer helps keep them fresh. Add ground flaxseed to hot or cold breakfast cereals; smoothies; yogurt; pancake, waffle, muffin, and quick bread batters; and condiments like mayonnaise or mustard. Use ground flaxseeds for a plant-based egg substitue to use in cooking and baking. For each egg called for in a recipe, add 3 tablespoons water to 1 tablespoon ground flaxseed and allow to stand for 5 minutes or until gelatinous. Add the mixture to recipes in place of the eggs.

Kimchi Available in Asian markets and in the refrigerated section of some supermarkets, fresh kimchi (like fresh sauerkraut) is a fermented vegetable condiment loaded with beneficial bacteria.

Kombucha A bubbly, refreshing, fermented, tea-based beverage loaded with probiotic potential.

Miso A fermented soybean paste added to many Japanese dishes, miso is a salty, savory seasoning used to make soups, spreads, sauces, and salad dressings. To maintain miso's probiotic benefits in cooked foods, stir it in at the end of cooking time. High or extended heat will destroy its beneficial bacteria.

Nori sheets A popular dried seaweed product, nori is used to wrap sushi and can be crumbled and sprinkled on stir-fries, stews, soups, and salads. Some Asian American restaurants even sprinkle finely crumbled nori over French fries!

Nutritional yeast Not to be confused with dry active baking yeast, nutritional yeast is a vegan seasoning product that gives a cheese-like flavor to dishes. It supplies protein and more than your daily requirement for the B vitamins niacin, thiamin, riboflavin, folic acid, B_6, and B_{12}. Nutritional yeast is the best source of plant-based vitamin B_{12}.

Tempeh This fermented soybean product is used as a meat substitute that supplies not only protein but also beneficial bacteria with probiotic qualities. Most large supermarkets carry tempeh and you may find brands of tempeh made with seeds, grains, and beans other than soy.

Tofu Mild-flavored tofu can be the base for many sauces or condiments, including homemade plant-based mayonnaise. It takes on the flavor of marinades and sauces, and works well as a meat substitute in stir-fries, kebabs, curries, and sandwiches to name a few. Look for tofu that has calcium in the ingredient list. Tofu that has been processed with calcium is a good source of the mineral in addi-

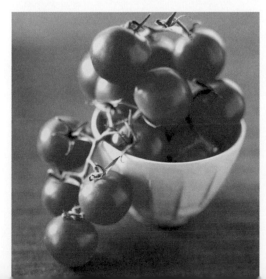

tion to protein and other nutrients as well as phytonutrients.

Tomato paste This is one of the most concentrated sources of the cancer-fighting phytonutrient lycopene. Although fresh foods are usually best, some phytonutrients actually benefit from processing. Lycopene in tomatoes is one of them.

guide to the new nutrition

The following compendium of nutrition terms and food substances demonstrates the complexity of nutrition, and the wealth of nutrients and phytonutrients that play important roles in our health.

For an overview of the most prominent vitamins, minerals, and phytonutrients, see *10 Top Vitamins & Minerals* (page 16) and *10 Top Phytonutrients* (page 26).

actinidin An enzyme found in kiwifruit, actinidin is believed to aid digestion. It may also be present in mangoes, pineapples, and papayas.

ajoenes These phytonutrients are found in garlic and may reduce LDL ("bad") cholesterol and may possess antithrombotic (anticlotting), anticancer, and antifungal activity. *See also* SULFUR COMPOUNDS.

allicin Responsible for garlic's pungent odor, allicin produces numerous SULFUR COMPOUNDS, with potenial antibacterial, anti-inflammatory, and anticancer properties.

allium compounds *See* SULFUR COMPOUNDS.

allyl isothiocyanate This ISOTHIOCYANATE compound may battle cancer, and its pungent nature can help clear congestion due to colds and flu. Sources: brussels sprouts, cabbage, horseradish, kale, brown mustard seeds.

allyl methyl trisulfide This SULFUR COMPOUND may stimulate the activity of glutathione S-transferase, an enzyme known to assist in the detoxification of carcinogens in the liver and colon. Sources: garlic, onions, leeks.

allyl sulfides These SULFUR COMPOUNDS, found in garlic, onions, leeks, scallions, and other members of the onion family, may help reduce the risk of stomach and colon cancers.

alpha-carotene Like BETA-CAROTENE, alpha-carotene is an antioxidant CAROTENOID and a precursor to VITAMIN A. Sources: apricots, carrots, pumpkins, sweet potatoes.

alpha-linolenic acid (ALA) Alpha-linolenic acid (ALA) is an ESSENTIAL FATTY ACID linked to a wide range of health benefits. Vital for many functions, alpha-linolenic acid cannot be made in the body and must therefore be obtained from foods. ALA is important for the maintenance of cell membranes and for creating regulatory substances in the body that protect against inflammation. ALA converts in the human body into two omega-3 fatty acids: EPA (EICOSAPENTAENOIC ACID) and DHA (DOCOSAHEXAENOIC ACID). Sources: canola oil, soybean oil, flaxseed, purslane, walnuts.

amino acids These are the building blocks of protein. Twenty amino acids are necessary for proper human growth and function. Many amino acids can be synthesized in the body when needed; these are called nonessential. Essential amino acids (such as LYSINE and TRYPTOPHAN to name two) cannot be synthesized in sufficient quantities and must be provided by diet. A varied plant-based diet can provide all the essential amino acids.

anthocyanins Responsible for the red and blue pigments found in certain fruits and vegetables, anthocyanins are FLAVONOIDS under review for their potential to suppress tumor cell growth, to lower LDL ("bad") cholesterol levels, and to prevent blood from forming too many clots. Sources: apples, acai, berries, red cabbage, cherries, red and purple grapes, plums, pomegranates.

antioxidants Found in a wide variety of plant-based foods, antioxidants are compounds that may have the potential to prevent numerous diseases. Serving as internal bodyguards, antioxidants roam through the body and scout out and destroy FREE RADICALS. By scavenging and destroying free radicals, antioxidants may protect against various types of cancer, improve cardiovascular health, enhance immunity, and protect against cataracts and macular degeneration. Some of the most potent disease-fighting powers attributed to certain phytonutrients, vitamins, and minerals (particularly VITAMIN E, VITAMIN C, CAROTENOIDS, SELENIUM, and FLAVONOIDS) are due to their antioxidant abilities. A natural synergy occurs when some of the antioxidants work together to disarm free radicals and protect cells from damage.

apigenin This compound is a FLAVONOID that may stop tumor growth as well as exert anti-inflammatory action. Sources: celery, parsley.

arginine This cardioprotective nonessential (essential only in childhood) amino acid is believed to enhance circulation and strengthen blood flow around the heart. For people who are prone to developing cold sores,

however, it may be a good idea to lower your intake of arginine-rich foods and increase your intake of LYSINE-rich foods if you are feeling run-down. Sources: soy foods, legumes, whole grains, brown rice, nuts, seeds.

beta-carotene One of the most studied of the CAROTENOIDS, beta-carotene is a potent antioxidant plentiful in red, orange, and yellow plant foods (as well as in dark green vegetables where its orange color is masked by CHLOROPHYLL). Beta-carotene is converted by the body into VITAMIN A. Sources: apricots, carrots, brussels sprouts, dark leafy greens, pumpkin, spinach, sweet potatoes, winter squash.

beta-cryptoxanthin This CAROTENOID may help to prevent colon and lung cancer. It may also protect against osteoporosis. Sources: apricots, oranges, tangerines.

beta-glucan Beta-glucan is a type of soluble dietary FIBER that helps to lower serum cholesterol levels. Sources: barley, brown rice bran, maitake, reishi, and shiitake mushrooms.

beta-sitosterol A PLANT STEROL similar in structure to cholesterol, beta-sitosterol may help to manage benign prostatic hyperplasia (BPH), as well as protect against high cholesterol. Sources: avocados, seeds, soy foods, wheat germ.

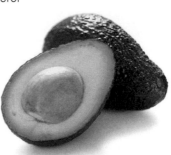

betacyanin A plant pigment, betacyanin gives beets their rich crimson color and is also linked with antioxidant activity in the body.

betaine This phytonutrient may be helpful in lowering HOMOCYSTEINE levels. Source: beets.

biotin This B vitamin is required for the metabolism of fatty acids, amino acids, and carbohydrates from food. Biotin also assists the body in the utilization of blood sugar (glucose), a major source of energy.

10 top vitamins & minerals

vitamin/mineral	may be helpful for	where to find it
calcium	osteoporosis, anxiety & stress, high blood pressure, hyperthyroidism, overweight, perimenopause & menopause, PMS, pregnancy	broccoli, fortified orange juice and non-dairy milk substitutes, tofu
folate	anemia, cancer, depression, heart disease, infertility & impotence, insomnia, osteoporosis, pregnancy, rheumatoid arthritis	asparagus, avocados, beans, beets, broccoli, cabbage family, citrus fruit, corn, dark leafy greens, lentils, peas, rice, spinach
iron	anemia, immune deficiency, memory loss, pregnancy	apricots, beans, figs, lentils, peas, quinoa, tofu
magnesium	allergies & asthma, anxiety & stress, chronic fatigue syndrome, constipation, diabetes, high blood pressure, kidney stones, migraine, PMS	avocados, nuts, rice, seeds, spinach, whole grains, winter squash
selenium	allergies & asthma, cancer, hypothyroidism, infertility & impotence, macular degeneration, prostate problems	mushrooms, nuts, rice, seeds, whole grains
vitamin B_6	acne, anemia, anxiety & stress, depression, heart disease, hypothyroidism, insomnia, memory loss, PMS, pregnancy	asparagus, bananas, figs, mushrooms, peas, potatoes, rice, sweet potatoes, winter squash
vitamin B_{12}	anemia, depression, heart disease, infertility & impotence	fortified cereals and dairy substitutes, nutritional yeast
vitamin C	allergies & asthma, anemia, bronchitis, cancer, cataracts, chronic fatigue syndrome, cold sores, colds & flu, diabetes, eczema, heart disease, hemorrhoids, infertility & impotence, high blood pressure, hyperthyroidism, immune deficiency, macular degeneration, osteoarthritis, osteoporosis, rheumatoid arthritis, sinusitis, sprains & strains	berries, cabbage family, citrus fruits, kiwifruit, melons, peas, peppers, pineapple, potatoes, salad greens, spinach, sweet potatoes, tomatoes, turnips, winter squash
vitamin E	bronchitis, cancer, cataracts, eczema, hyperthyroidism, immune deficiency, infertility & impotence, memory loss, macular degeneration, osteoarthritis, prostate problems, rheumatoid arthritis	avocados, nuts, olive oil, salad greens, seeds, whole grains
zinc	acne, bronchitis, chronic fatigue syndrome, colds & flu, cold sores, eczema, hemorrhoids, hypothyroidism, immunity, infertility & impotence, macular degeneration, rosacea, sinusitis	beans, fortified cereal, lentils, seeds, wheat germ, whole grains,

Sources: barley, legumes, cauliflower, corn, mushrooms, oats, peanut butter, rice, soy foods.

boron This bone-nourishing mineral is thought to enhance the body's ability to use CALCIUM, MAGNESIUM, and VITAMIN D. Sources: beans, nuts.

bromelain An enzyme derived from pineapples, bromelain is believed to have anti-inflammatory and pain-reducing properties.

caffeic acid This widely available PHENOLIC COMPOUND may have antioxidant and anti-inflammatory capabilities to block carcinogenic substances and protect brain health. Sources: apples, carrots, celery, coffee beans, grapes, onions, potatoes, soy foods, tomatoes, spinach.

calcium The most abundant and important mineral in the body, calcium is vital for maintaining the integrity of bones and teeth. Sources: broccoli, fortified dairy alternatives, tofu.

calcium pectate Responsible for the characteristic crunch of certain fruits and vegetables, calcium pectate is a PECTIN FIBER that may lower LDL ("bad") cholesterol levels. Sources: apples, cabbage, carrots, onions.

campesterol A PLANT STEROL, campesterol may be helpful in managing symptoms of benign prostatic hyperplasia (BPH) and high cholesterol. Sources: nuts, olive oil, peanuts, seeds, soybeans.

capsaicin This phytonutrient gives hot peppers their fiery taste. Along with easing congestion, capsaicin is currently being investigated for its antioxidant and disease-protective effects. Sources: chili peppers, cayenne pepper.

carbohydrates These energy-yielding nutrients are the most efficient fuel source for the body (PROTEIN and FATS also provide energy to the body). Carbohydrates are readily broken down into glucose, a simple sugar that rapidly and effectively feeds the body's tissues. Though there are different types of carbohydrates (including simple carbohydrates or simple sugars), the most nutritionally valuable are the COMPLEX CARBO-HYDRATES found in whole grains, legumes, vegetables, and fruits.

carnosol A substance that has anti-oxidant potential, carnosol may fight tumors by detoxifying cancerous chemicals. Sources: rosemary, sage.

carotenoids These pigments give certain produce like carrots, winter squash, tomatoes, and peppers their characteristic orange, yellow, and red colors. They may possess potent anti-oxidant power to fight heart disease, certain types of cancer, as well as degen-erative eye diseases such as cataracts and macular degeneration. To date, more than 600 carotenoids have been identified, and some, such as ALPHA-CAROTENE, BETA-CAROTENE, BETA-CRYPTOXANTHIN, LYCOPENE, LUTEIN, and ZEAXANTHIN, provide us with significant health benefits.

catechins This class of FLAVONOIDS appears predominantly in green tea and exhibits cardioprotective, chemo-protective, and antimicrobial properties. Other sources: black tea, dark chocolate, red grapes, red wine, pomegranates. *See also* EGCG (EPIGALLOCATECHIN GALLATE).

chlorogenic acid This antioxidant PHENOLIC COMPOUND may reduce high blood pressure. Sources: apples, citrus fruits, coffee, cocoa, pears, tea.

chlorophyll The green pigment of leaves and plants, chlorophyll not only helps to freshen breath but it may also help to prevent DNA damage to cells and provide other protective health benefits. Sources: dark leafy greens, herbs, kiwi-fruit, parsley, peas, peppers.

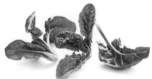

cholesterol This is a type of fat is present only in animal foods and is also synthesized by the body. Cholesterol is an important element of all cell membranes and serves as a precursor to VITAMIN D, hormones, and bile (for digestion). Excessive cholesterol circulating in the blood can build up on artery walls, leading to heart disease and stroke.

choline A vitamin-like substance required for cell membrane integrity, choline is also important for normal brain and liver function. Sources: cabbage, cauliflower, navy beans, soybeans, wheat germ.

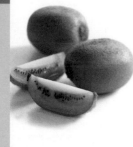

chromium This essential trace mineral is necessary for the manufacture of insulin and for the breakdown of MACRONUTRIENTS. Sources: nuts, potatoes, prunes, whole grains.

complex carbohydrates The starchy components of fruits, legumes, vegetables, and whole grains are complex carbohydrates. A diet rich in complex carbohydrates is also high in FIBER and can help protect against cardiovascular disease, improve blood sugar levels, and relieve constipation and other intestinal disorders.

copper This trace mineral is instrumental in bone formation, blood clotting, normal immune function, and skeletal mineralization. Sources: amaranth, avocados, mushrooms, potatoes, sunflower seeds.

balancing fats

Health professionals speculate that some chronic diseases in America may be due to an imbalance in the types of fats consumed in the average American diet. Over the past 100 years or so, due in part to advances in technology and the prevalence of processed foods, Americans are consuming disproportionately lower levels of the beneficial fats, such as MONOUNSATURATED FATS and OMEGA-3 FATTY ACIDS, and higher levels of SATURATED FATS, TRANS FATTY ACIDS, and OMEGA-6 FATTY ACIDS. For optimal health, it's best to try to shift this balance toward foods rich in omega-3 and monounsaturated fatty acids, since these healthful fats have been linked to the prevention of numerous diseases.

cruciferous vegetables A family of phytonutrient-rich vegetables named for their cross-shaped flowers, cruciferous vegetables are touted for their powerful healing compounds that exhibit cancer-fighting activity. Cruciferous vegetables include bok choy, broccoli, brussels sprouts, cabbage, cauliflower, kale, mustard greens, radishes, rutabaga, watercress.

curcumin A phytonutrient compound that lends yellow color to turmeric, curcumin appears to have anti-inflammatory properties that help relieve pain. Sources: curry powder, turmeric seasoning, turmeric tea, certain types of mustard with turmeric.

cyanidin A type of ANTHOCYANIN, cyanidin may reduce pain by blocking inflammatory enzymes in the body. Sources: berries, cherries.

cynarin Found in artichokes, cynarin may support liver health, lower harmful cholesterol, and combat environmental carcinogens. Cynarin also appears to lend a sweet aftertaste to other foods and drinks.

daidzein An ISOFLAVONE found in soy foods, daidzein is thought to inhibit the growth of cancer cells and the onset of osteoporosis, and may improve heart health. Daidzein's mild estrogenic attributes may relieve menopausal symptoms as well. *See also* PHYTOESTROGENS.

DHA An OMEGA-3 FATTY ACID, DHA (docosahexaenoic acid) is important for all phases of the human life cycle. A major building block of human brain tissue and the primary structural fatty acid in the gray matter of the brain and the retina, DHA is vital for brain and eye health. Studies indicate that DHA may have cardiovascular benefits as well as neurological benefits. The body can convert ALPHA-LINOLENIC ACID from foods like nuts and seeds into DHA. You can get DHA directly from seaweed and algae products.

diallyl sulfide A powerful SULFUR COMPOUND, diallyl sulfide may help fight stomach and lung cancer and may also have significant cholesterol-lowering properties. Sources: chives, garlic, leeks, onions, scallions, shallots.

diosmin A FLAVONOID found in citrus fruit and rosemary, diosmin is thought to bolster blood vessels and help prevent certain types of cancer.

dithiolthiones These phytonutrients are thought to activate enzymes in the body that detoxify carcinogens. Studies suggest that dithiolthiones may inhibit the development of tumors of the lung, colon, breast, and bladder. Sources: bok choy, broccoli, cabbage, cauliflower.

EGCG A CATECHIN in green tea, EGCG (epigallocatechin gallate) is part of the POLYPHENOL family. As an antioxidant, EGCG appears to destroy harmful free radicals, and may possess cardio-protective and anticancer attributes.

ellagic acid A PHENOLIC COMPOUND with potent antioxidant capabilities, ellagic acid is thought to fight cancer by inducing cancer cell death as well as by inhibiting carcinogens such as tobacco smoke or air pollution. This phytonutrient also helps protect against atherosclerosis and neurodegenerative disease. Sources: apples, apricots, berries, grapes, pomegranates, walnuts.

EPA An OMEGA-3 FATTY ACID, eicosapentaenoic acid (EPA) is linked to cardiovascular and anticancer benefits, and may help improve inflammatory conditions such as rheumatoid arthritis. The body can convert ALPHA-LINOLENIC ACID into EPA, and you can get EPA directly from marine algae products.

ergosterol Found in mushrooms, ergosterol is converted in the body into VITAMIN D.

eritadenine Preliminary laboratory studies suggest that eritadenine may reduce LDL ("bad") cholesterol levels in the blood. Source: shiitake mushrooms.

essential fatty acids (EFAs) The building blocks of necessary fats, EFAs must be obtained through food. They are involved in the manufacture of anti-inflammatory compounds, the transmission of nerve impulses, energy metabolism, and the promotion of cardiovascular and immune system health. Sources: canola oil, flaxseed oil, sunflower seeds, walnuts, wheat germ.

fats An important energy reserve for the body, fat also cushions organs, provides insulation, transports fat-soluble nutrients, and lends structure to cell membranes. The major type of fat in food and in the body is triglycerides. CHOLESTEROL is a fatlike substance produced by the liver. Your body normally produces as much cholesterol as you need. It is found only in animal products. Fatty acids are the building blocks of triglycerides, and the ESSENTIAL FATTY ACIDS (such as OMEGA-3S and OMEGA-6S) must be obtained from the diet, because they cannot be manufactured by the body. As the most dense source of food energy, fat serves up more than twice the amount of calories per gram as carbohydrates or protein. For optimal health, experts advise a diet rich in nourishing plant-based MONOUNSATURATED AND POLYUNSATURATED FATS, along with omega-3 fatty acids, in place of SATURATED FAT and TRANS FATS in your diet.

ferulic acid Research suggests that this phytonutrient may inhibit cancer-causing substances, such as nitrosamines. Sources: apples, pineapple.

enhancing foods for health

Research, technology, and widespread interest in nutrition have sparked an explosion of health-promoting foods. Supermarket shelves are filled with foods created to boost health and longevity: calcium-fortified orange juice, folate-fortified cereal, cholesterol-lowering margarine spreads, and many more. Through processing, growing methods, or biotechnology, a broad spectrum of foods is supplemented with ingredients designed to ward off disease.

The idea of adding ingredients to food is not new, of course: For example, at the beginning of the 20th century, iodine was first added to salt to help guard against goiter. But with current research, many products and foods are now being enhanced with more esoteric ingredients, such as phytonutrients and cardioprotective fats. To categorize an ever-evolving genre of health-promoting foods, a number of terms have been coined by the food industry.

enriched foods Many grain-based foods, such as bread, flour, and cereal, are commonly "enriched" with certain nutrients—riboflavin, thiamin, folate, and iron. These essential nutrients are lost during processing and are added back into the food in varying amounts after it has been processed. Note that whole-grain products generally possess superior nutrition to processed grains since enrichment does not replace all the nutrients, fiber, and phytonutrients lost during processing. One cup of whole-wheat flour, for example, contains higher levels of nutrients than 1 cup of "enriched" white flour.

fortified foods To boost protection against chronic disease or to help prevent a nutrient deficiency, certain foods are fortified with nutrients not present in the original food. Vitamin D-fortified plant-based dairy alternatives, iodized salt, folate-fortified wheat products, calcium-fortified orange juice, and cereal fortified with vitamin B_{12} are well-known fortified foods that help to prevent nutrient deficiencies.

functional food A loosely defined umbrella term, "functional food" refers to any food that promotes health beyond satisfying basic nutrition needs. The term reflects the growing number of enhanced foods available to us and does not carry scientific or legal meaning. Falling into the category of functional foods are "nutraceuticals," "pharmafoods," and "designer foods," all of which are promoted as imparting a particular health or medicinal benefit, including the prevention and treatment of disease. Genetically modified foods (see below) fall into the category of designer foods. Unenhanced foods with natural disease-fighting properties (such as garlic or tomatoes), as well as enriched and fortified foods, are also considered functional foods.

genetically modified foods These are foods whose genetic makeup is altered in an effort to produce a new plant with more desirable characteristics, such as increased resistance to spoilage or improved nutritional content. Considerable controversy surrounds genetically modified foods, as long-term health and environmental effects and ethical issues are not resolved.

organic foods Organic foods are grown and/or processed without the use of such synthetic chemicals as pesticides, herbicides, preservatives, growth hormones, and antibiotics. The health benefits of organic foods are not clear-cut. Organic fruits and vegetables may be more or less flavorful and colorful and their nutritional value has not been established as superior to nonorganic fruits and vegetables. Also, many organic foods tend to spoil faster and organically grown fruits and vegetables may harbor harmful microbes, such as *E. coli*, due to organic methods of fertilization and preservation.

fiber, insoluble Composed of indigestible plant parts, insoluble fiber adds bulk to stools, which eases elimination. Insoluble fiber may promote satiety as well. Sources: broccoli, cabbage, celery, flaxseed, salad greens, sweet potatoes, whole grains.

fiber, soluble Soluble fiber forms a gel-like mass around food particles, preventing cholesterol from being absorbed and promoting its excretion. PECTIN and BETA-GLUCAN are two types of soluble fiber that are particularly beneficial for lowering cholesterol levels. Soluble fiber also helps to manage diarrhea and may regulate levels of blood glucose as well. Sources: apples, apricots, legumes, berries, figs, oats, plums, prunes, pumpkin.

ficin Found in figs, ficin is an enzyme with mild laxative properties.

flavonoids Powerful antioxidants, flavonoids are phytonutrients linked to a reduced risk of cardiovascular disease and may impede the development of cancer. The free-radical scavenging properties of flavonoids are thought to reduce inflammation associated with rheumatoid arthritis, slow age-related decline in memory function, bolster blood vessels, and improve the potency of immune cells. Some important flavonoid compounds include CATECHINS, ELLAGIC ACID, KAEMPFEROL, QUERCETIN, and RUTIN. Sources: fruits, vegetables, whole grains, wine.

fluoride Known as a mineral that protects teeth against dental decay, fluoride is also involved in the maintenance of bone structure and is found primarily in bone tissue. Sources: fluoridated water.

folate This B vitamin is present mostly in green leafy vegetables. The synthetic form is called folic acid, which is found in most fortified cereal. Folate helps to prevent neural tube defects in newborns and may lower levels of the amino acid HOMOCYSTEINE. Sources: asparagus, avocado, beans, beets, broccoli, chicory, lentils, oranges, peas, salad greens, spinach.

free radicals Unstable, highly reactive oxygen molecules, free radicals are the by-products of metabolism and are also found in the environment: UV radiation from sunlight, smoke, and other forms of pollution. Free radicals contribute to oxidative stress, which is implicated in premature aging as well as the onset of many diseases.

fructooligosaccharides (FOS) Indigestible carbohydrate compounds, fructooligosaccharides (FOS) are thought to encourage the growth of friendly bacteria in the body and may reduce the amount of toxins produced by unfriendly flora in the colon. Sources: bananas, chicory, onion family.

genistein A potent ISOFLAVONE with estrogenlike activity, genistein may help balance hormones and may reduce the risk of hormone-related cancer, such as prostate cancer, as well as help prevent fibrocystic breasts and premenstrual syndrome. Sources: soy foods. *See also* PHYTOESTROGENS.

gingerol A phytonutrient in ginger, gingerol is believed to reduce swelling and tenderness of the joints. Ginger may help with nausea and vomiting as well.

glucosinolates A class of anticancer phytonutrients present in CRUCIFEROUS VEGETABLES, glucosinolates are metabolized into various beneficial compounds such as INDOLES, ISOTHIOCYANATES, and SULFORAPHANE.

glutathione An essential part of several antioxidant enzymes that naturally occur in the body, glutathione may detoxify carcinogenic compounds and enhance the immune system. Sources: apples, asparagus, avocados.

gluten Gluten is a protein in barley, rye, triticale (a cross between wheat and rye), and wheat. Certain people, particularly those with celiac disease, have an intolerance to gluten; they experience an adverse gastrointestinal reaction to gluten, so they must avoid foods made with these grains.

goitrogens When eaten in large quantities, goitrogens in uncooked foods have the potential to interfere with the absorption of IODINE and slow thyroid function. Small quantities of goitrogens are primarily found in cabbage, turnips, mustard greens, and radishes.

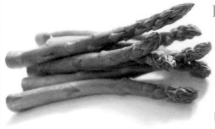

hesperidin A FLAVONOID found in the zest (or outer, colored portion of the peel) of citrus fruits, hesperidin may reduce inflammation, lower blood fats and cholesterol, and improve the integrity of capillary linings.

homocysteine A compound that results from the breakdown of methionine, an essential amino acid, homocysteine, at high levels in the blood, increases the risk for atherosclerosis, and possibly other conditions. Although the significance of homocysteine as a risk factor for cardiovascular disease and stroke is controversial, an estimated 20% to 40% of people with clogged arteries, or those who have suffered strokes or heart attacks, have abnormally high levels of homocysteine. Researchers have discovered that several B vitamins—FOLATE, VITAMIN B_6, and VITAMIN B_{12}—can help lower homocysteine levels.

hydroxytyrosol A PHENOLIC COMPOUND that contributes to the characteristic flavor and aroma of olives and olive oil, hydroxytyrosol may help protect against breast cancer, high blood pressure, heart disease, and stroke.

indole-3-carbinol A well-studied INDOLE compound and a member of the GLUCOSINOLATE phytonutrient family, indole-3-carbinol is particularly abundant in broccoli. Indole-3-carbinol may offer protection against hormone-dependent cancers, such as breast cancer. Sources: CRUCIFEROUS VEGETABLES.

indoles Partially responsible for the strong taste of broccoli and brussels sprouts, indoles are a class of GLUCOSINOLATE phytonutrients present in CRUCIFEROUS VEGETABLES that may stimulate cancer-fighting enzymes.

inulin An indigestible carbohydrate compound, inulin may help stabilize blood glucose levels, activate immune cells, reduce inflammation, and promote friendly intestinal bacteria. Sources: chicory, Jerusalem artichokes.

iodine Tiny amounts of this trace mineral are required for normal cell metabolism and thyroid function. Sources: iodized salt, seaweed.

iron This mineral is an essential component of hemoglobin, the oxygen-carrying pigment in red blood cells. Plant-based (nonheme) iron is found in amaranth, dried apricots, dried plums (prunes), figs, lentils, quinoa, and tofu.

isoflavones Found primarily in soy foods, isoflavones are a major class of PHYTOESTROGENS, which are plant chemicals with mild estrogen activity. GENISTEIN and DAIDZEIN are the most prominent isoflavones. Soy isoflavones may help ease menopause symptoms and protect against osteoporosis-related fractures, Alzheimer's disease, high cholesterol, and hormone-dependent cancers, such as breast and prostate cancer.

isothiocyanates Providing pungency to numerous CRUCIFEROUS VEGETABLES, isothiocyanates are potent cancer fighters. SULFORAPHANE in broccoli and phenethyliocyanate (PEITC) in watercress are two powerful isothiocyanates that may short-circuit enzymes that activate carcinogens as well as stimulate the production of natural anticancer enzymes.

kaempferol A FLAVONOID compound, kaempferol is converted in the liver into QUERCETIN. Kaempferol may lower the risk of mortality from heart disease and enhance the immune system. Sources: berries, cabbage, chives, green beans, horseradish, leeks, onions, radishes.

lecithin Found in legumes and soy products, lecithin is a fatty substance present in all cells and is involved with fat digestion in the intestines.

lentinan A polysaccharide (carbohydrate compound) extracted from shiitake mushrooms, lentinan may have the potential to enhance immunity and protect against cancer, high blood pressure, and high cholesterol.

lentinula edodes mycelium (LEM) Found in shiitake mushrooms, LEM is a polysaccharide compound that appears to have antiviral and cardiovascular benefits.

lignans These compounds are PHYTOESTROGENS with mild estrogenlike activity. They may have antitumor effects and antimicrobial benefits and provide relief from PMS and protection against osteoporosis. Sources: beans, flaxseeds (ground up), flaxseed oil, olive oil, soy foods, whole grains.

lignins Similar in chemical makeup to LIGNANS, lignins are a type of insoluble fiber that may be useful for relieving constipation. Sources: brown rice, fruits, legumes, seeds, vegetables, whole grains.

limonene This phytonutrient is known for its anti-inflammatory, anticancer, anti-diabetic, and antiviral effects. Sources: zest of citrus fruits.

lutein & zeaxanthin Found in foods that are bright yellow, orange, and green, lutein and zeaxanthin are pigments in the CAROTENOID family that are linked to a reduced risk for age-related macular degeneration and cataracts. Lutein is also being studied for its potential to inhibit artherosclerosis and reduce inflammation. Collard greens, spinach, and kale are especially high in lutein. Other sources: broccoli, corn, kiwifruit, mustard greens, oranges, peas, romaine lettuce, turnip greens, zucchini.

luteolin A FLAVONOID present in artichokes, luteolin is under review for its anti-inflammatory activity, potential to reduce heart disease risk, involvement in blocking the spread of cancer cells, and ability to block the release of histamine, a substance that triggers congestion.

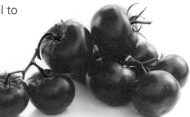

lycopene An antioxidant CAROTENOID that lends red color to numerous foods, lycopene is particularly abundant in red tomatoes. Lycopene may

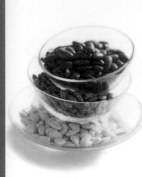

defend immune cells against oxidative damage and protect against macular degeneration, cardiovascular disease, prostate cancer, and male infertility. Sources: apricots, pink and red grapefruit, tomatoes, tomato paste, watermelon.

lysine This essential AMINO ACID must be obtained from dietary sources. Some experts advocate lysine to help prevent or reduce the severity of cold sores. Sources: amaranth, beans, potatoes.

macronutrients The food we eat provides two types of essential building blocks, or nutrients, known as macronutrients and MICRONUTRIENTS. The three primary macronutrients—CARBOHYDRATE, PROTEIN, and FAT—are vital energy-yielding nutrients that work in harmony with micronutrients to keep the body fit and functioning well. Although water provides no nutrients, it is sometimes referred to as a macronutrient because it is essential for life.

magnesium Required for hundreds of biochemical reactions, this mineral assists in maintaining normal enzyme, muscle, and nerve function. It also keeps bones and teeth strong and helps to regulate heart rhythm. Sources: amaranth, avocados, quinoa, brown rice, sunflower seeds, wheat bran, wheat germ.

manganese This trace mineral is important for bone and connective tissue formation, as well as for the actions of enzymes involved in carbohydrate metabolism. Sources: amaranth, blackberries, pineapples.

micronutrients Required in small amounts from the diet, VITAMINS and MINERALS are noncaloric essential nutrients known as micronutrients. They are critical for normal growth, development, and good health. Micronutrients promote and regulate chemical reactions vital for life and participate in all body processes,

such as deriving energy from MACRONUTRIENTS, transmitting nerve impulses, and battling infections.

minerals Naturally occurring nutrients in soil, water, and food, minerals are involved in a variety of specialized roles, such as maintaining skin health and building bone. Minerals also serve as cofactors—assistants to the body's many enzymes. Nutritional requirement for minerals is relatively small but exceedingly important. Minerals are classified as major or trace, according to the body's daily requirements. Major minerals are needed in higher quantities than trace minerals and include POTASSIUM, CALCIUM, and MAGNESIUM. Examples of trace minerals include IRON, ZINC, SELENIUM, and MANGANESE.

molybdenum Essential for normal growth and development, this trace mineral assists several enzymes and is needed to manufacture red blood cells. Sources: beans, lentils, nuts, peas, whole grains.

monoterpenes A family of phytonutrients that includes LIMONENE, PERILLYL ALCOHOL, and carvone, monoterpenes are under review for their ability to detoxify carcinogens, hinder cancer cell growth, and improve cholesterol levels. Sources: cherries, citrus fruits, caraway, dill, mint.

monounsaturated fat Plentiful in many high-fat plant foods, heart-healthy monounsaturated fat is not easily damaged by oxidation, so is less likely than SATURATED FAT and TRANS FATS to clog arteries. When consumed in place of saturated and trans fats, monounsaturated fat may protect against high blood pressure, high cholesterol, heart disease, and some cancers and may help control blood glucose levels. Sources: avocados, nuts, olives, olive oil.

naringin A FLAVONOID that gives white grapefruit its characteristic bitter flavor, naringin may suppress cancer-causing compounds, bolster blood vessels, and shield delicate lung tissue from environmental toxins. Naringin can interfere with the absorption and metabolism of certain drugs, causing elevated or diminished blood levels of the drug.

niacin An indispensable B vitamin, niacin is required for energy metabolism, as well as healthy skin and proper functioning of the digestive and nervous systems. Sources: nuts, whole grains.

nobiletin A FLAVONOID found in the flesh of oranges, nobiletin is known for its anti-inflammatory and anticancer activity and may help protect the brain against Alzheimer's disease.

oleic acid When consumed in place of saturated fat, this MONOUNSATURATED FAT is linked to healthier cholesterol levels. Sources: avocados, canola oil, olive oil.

oleuropein A POLYPHENOL with significant antioxidant power, oleuropein may team up with HYDROXYTYROSOL, a phytonutrient, to help protect against heart disease, high blood pressure, infertility, and infection-causing bacteria. Source: olive oil.

omega-3 fatty acids Omega-3s are ESSENTIAL FATTY ACIDS. Alpha-linolenic acid is the precursor to omega-3s and must be obtained from the diet. The body converts alpha-linolenic acid into EPA (EICOSAPENTAENOIC ACID) and DHA (DOCOSAHEXAENOIC ACID). Omega-3s are under review for their potential to improve cardiovascular health, suppress inflammatory compounds, as well as relieve depression. Sources: chia seeds, flaxseed, pumpkin seeds, soy foods, walnuts.

omega-6 fatty acids Omega-6s are ESSENTIAL FATTY ACIDS. They are important for cell membrane structure and are converted by the body into anti-inflammatory compounds, as well as some potentially harmful compounds, some of which are associated with cancer. Most experts advocate an increased intake of OMEGA-3S for better balance, since the American diet is typically excessive in omega-6 fatty acids. Sources: nuts, seeds, whole grains, vegetable oils.

oryzanol Also known as gamma oryzanol, oryzanol is a natural compound found in rice bran and rice bran oil. Oryzanol is touted for its anti-inflammatory, anticancer, antidiabetic, and cholesterol-lowering properties.

oxalates Found in the greatest quantities in green vegetables, oxalates are compounds that bind CALCIUM, IRON, and ZINC, blocking their absorption in the body. In addition, people prone to kidney stones should avoid foods high in oxalates since these compounds may fuel the formation of certain types of kidney stones. Sources: chocolate, coffee, cranberries, dark leafy greens, nuts, parsley, rhubarb, soy, tea, wheat bran.

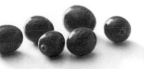

pantothenic acid This bountiful B vitamin is involved in many of the body's processes, including the release of energy from macronutrients, the transmission of nerve impulses, and the synthesis of cell membranes. Sources: avocados, broccoli, legumes, mushrooms.

pectin Pectin is a SOLUBLE FIBER that helps to lower artery-damaging LDL cholesterol. Pectin may also be useful for managing diarrhea and diabetes. Sources: apples, apricots, bananas, carrots, figs, kiwifruit, sweet potatoes.

perillyl alcohol This phytonutrient helps destroy tumor cells without harming healthy cells and may have the potential to treat brain tumors. Sources: cherries, peppermint, sage.

phenolic compounds Numerous types of phenolic compounds—CAFFEIC, CHLOROGENIC, ELLAGIC, and FERULIC ACIDS—

10 top phytonutrients

phytonutrient	may be helpful for	where to find it
anthocyanins	cancer	apples, beets, berries, cherries, grapes, plums & prunes, pomegranates, potatoes

carotenoids:
  beta-carotene
  lutein & zeaxanthin
  lycopene
	anemia, cancer, hyperthyroidism, immune deficiency, memory loss, eye diseases, skin conditions, prostate problems, heart disease, high cholesterol, infertility & impotence	**beta-carotene:** apricots, broccoli, carrots, melons, peppers, spinach, sweet potatoes
		lutein & zeaxanthin: cooking greens, corn, kiwifruit, peas, winter squash
		lycopene: apricots, red & pink grapefruit, tomatoes

catechins	cancer	green tea, pomegranates

flavonoids:
  kaempferol
  luteolin
  quercetin
  citrus flavonoids
	cancer, hemorrhoids, high cholesterol, infertility & impotence, memory loss, rheumatoid arthritis	apples, berries, citrus fruit, leeks, onions

glucosinolates:
  indoles
  isothiocyanates
  sulforaphane
	cancer; bacterial, fungal, and viral infections	broccoli, brussels sprouts, cabbage, kale

phenolic compounds:
  caffeic acid
  ellagic acid
  ferulic acid
  curcumin
	cancer	apples, berries, cereal grains, green tea, pomegranates

phytoestrogens:
  soy isoflavones
  (genistein & daidzein)
  lignans
	hormone-dependent cancers, colon cancer, heart disease, osteoporosis, hyperthyroidism	**soy isoflavones:** soy foods
		lignans: flaxseeds, grains, legumes, olive oil

resveratrol	cancer, stroke	peanuts, red and purple grapes, red wine

sulfur compounds:
  ajoenes
  allicin
  allyl sulfides
  diallyl sulfide
	cancer, high cholesterol	chives, garlic, leeks, onions, shallots

terpenes:
  limonene
  perillyl alcohol
	cancer, pain	**limonene:** caraway, cardamom, citrus zest (colored portion of peel), coriander, mint, thyme
		perillyl alcohol: cherries

may battle cancer by destroying free radicals and activating cancer-fighting enzymes that suppress tumors in early stages. Sources: apples, berries, green tea, lettuce, pomegranates, turmeric, whole grains.

phosphorus A constituent of every cell, this mineral is involved in almost all metabolic reactions and helps to build strong bones, teeth, and muscles. Sources: almonds, legumes.

phthalides (3-n-butyl phthalide) Present in celery, phthalide phytonutrients are thought to contribute to reduced blood pressure.

phytic acid Also known as inositol hexaphosphate, phytic acid binds to minerals (particularly IRON). This can be beneficial because excessive levels of iron generate harmful free radicals that can contribute to cancer. Phytic acids may also slow starch digestion and help to stabilize blood sugar levels. Sources: grains, soy foods.

phytoestrogens These compounds exhibit estrogen-like activity and may lower the risk of hormone-related cancers, as well as relieve fibrocystic breasts, osteoarthritis, and symptoms of perimenopause and menopause. The two major classes of phytoestrogens are ISOFLAVONES and LIGNANS. Sources: beans, flaxseed, pomegranates, soy foods.

plant sterols Structurally similar to cholesterol, plant sterols may protect against heart disease, cancer, and benign prostatic hyperplasia (BPH). Sources: figs, grains, lentils, nuts, pineapple, seeds, sweet potatoes.

polyphenols A class of ANTIOXIDANTS, polyphenol phytonutrients are under review for their potential to suppress tumor growth, detoxify carcinogens, interfere with the damaging effects of high estrogen levels, lower the risk of stroke, and prevent plaque buildup in the arteries. Sources: apples, berries, citrus fruits, figs, olives, wheat.

polysaccharides Polysaccharides are carbohydrate compounds (starch and glycogen) that may possess disease-fighting properties. LENTINAN in shiitake mushrooms is a type of polysaccharide. Other sources: fruits, grains, vegetables.

potassium We need this mineral for the regulation of blood pressure, muscle contraction, heartbeats, and insulin secretion. Potassium functions as an electrolyte to help maintain proper fluid balance in the body. Sources: apricots, avocados, bananas, citrus fruits, potatoes, quinoa.

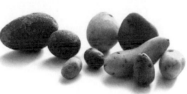

prebiotics These are specific types of fiber that feed and support probiotics, the beneficial bacteria found in the gut. Sources: artichokes, chicory, bananas, onions.

probiotics A group of beneficial bacteria and yeasts in the body that are also present in fermented food products such as kombucha and kimchi with live bacterial cultures. Consuming probiotics may improve immune responses against viruses and cancer cells, prevent antibiotic-associated diarrhea, treat gum disease, and promote remission of ulcerative colitis.

protease inhibitors Powerful anti-cancer compounds, protease inhibitors appear to short-circuit enzyme production in cancer cells, block the binding of hormones to cells, and inhibit malignant changes in healthy cells. Soy foods and other legumes, in particular, are rich in a unique cancer-fighting protease inhibitor known as the Bowman-Birk inhibitor. Sources: broccoli sprouts, legumes, potatoes, soy foods.

protein Protein is important for health, since AMINO ACIDS—the building blocks of protein—form muscles, hormones, genes, immune cells, brain chemicals, and countless other substances that we rely on daily. All plant foods contain some protein. Lentils, beans, and nuts are good plant sources of protein (especially soy beans and soy products). Grains high in protein include amaranth, buckwheat, and quinoa.

quercetin Red onions are the richest source of quercetin, a potent FLAVONOID linked to a reduced risk of cancer, cardiovascular disease, and cataracts. Quercetin may also prevent the release of histamine, an action essential for managing respiratory and inflammatory conditions. Sources: apples, berries, cherries, grapes, green tea, red onions, plums, wine.

resveratrol A phytonutrient particularly abundant in the skin of red grapes, resveratrol may help improve cholesterol levels, prevent atherosclerosis, reduce the risks for stroke and cancer, and benefit those with diabetes and neurological disorders. Sources: peanuts, red and purple grapes and grape juice, red wine.

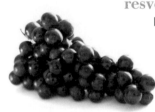

riboflavin Important for the release of energy from carbohydrates, riboflavin is a B vitamin instrumental in protecting the nervous system, building immunity, and maintaining normal metabolism. Sources: asparagus, broccoli, fortified cereals, mushrooms, quinoa.

rutin Preliminary research suggests that this FLAVONOID may inhibit the formation of cancer cells and improve osteoarthritis symptoms, as well as reduce blood pressure and levels of LDL ("bad") cholesterol. Buckwheat is a particularly good food source of this phytonutrient. Other sources: apples, cherries.

saponins Present in many vegetables and grains, saponins are phytonutrients that appear to bind cholesterol and chemical toxins in the digestive tract and help remove them from the body. Saponins may also inhibit cancer cell replication and increase levels of immune cells. Sources: asparagus, legumes (particularly soybeans), oats, potatoes.

saturated fat This type of fat is found in animal foods such as meat, poultry, and full-fat dairy products, including butter and whole milk. Tropical cooking oils, such as palm and coconut, are also sources of saturated fat. High intakes of saturated fat from red meat, particulary processed meats, are linked to cardiovascular disease.

selenium This essential trace mineral acts as an antioxidant by promoting the activity of an enzyme that neutralizes dangerous free-radical molecules. Selenium also works along with VITAMIN E to reduce dangerous free-radical damage linked to chronic diseases such as cancer, heart disease, and some eye diseases. Selenium is required for optimal immunity and thyroid function as well. Sources: Brazil nuts, mushrooms, sunflower seeds, whole grains.

sesaminol compounds Found in sesame seeds, sesaminol compounds—sesaminol, sesamolinol, and pinoresinol—are converted into LIGNANS and appear to possess anti-imflammatory, cardioprotective, and anticancer properties.

shogaols Present in dried or cooked ginger, these phytonutrients may help fight cancer and heart disease, as well as improve pain and reduce swelling of inflamed joints.

sodium The major constituent of table salt, sodium is a mineral that is required in small amounts by the body in order to regulate water balance, blood pressure, and blood volume. Most plant foods naturally contain minute quantities of sodium, but most processed foods and fast foods contain excessive sodium. Too much sodium is linked to high blood pressure and increased risk of stroke, kidney disease, osteoporosis, stomach cancer, and water retention. While many experts recommend a maximum sodium intake of 2,400 mg each day, the American Heart Association recommends a limit of 1,500 mg each day for ideal heart health.

sorbitol A natural sugar that has mild laxative properties, sorbitol may help relieve constipation. Note that excess sorbitol can cause diarrhea. Source: fresh and dried fruit, prunes (dried plums).

soy protein Protein derived from soy is high in quality and provides all of the essential amino acids. Eating 25 g of soy protein each day as part of a healthy diet can significantly improve cholesterol levels in people with high cholesterol. Sources: soybeans, soy foods.

sulforaphane A notable SULFUR COMPOUND classified as a GLUCOSINOLATE, sulforaphane may reduce the risk of cardiovascular and neurodegenerative diseases, increase the activity of cancer-fighting enzymes in the body, reduce tumor growth, block carcinogens from initiating cancer, and fight hormone-related cancers such as prostate and breast. Sources: broccoli, cabbage, cauliflower, cooking greens, including kale.

sulfur compounds Sulfur-containing phytonutrients abundant in garlic and the onion family are collectively called sulfur compounds and include ALLYL SULFIDE and AJOENES. Certain sulfur compounds may stimulate cancer-fighting enzymes. Sources: chives, garlic, leeks, onions, scallions, shallots.

syringic acid A phytonutrient found in a wide range of fruits and vegetables, syringic acid may play a role in repairing liver cells damaged by alcohol consumption.

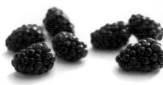

tangeretin A FLAVONOID present in tangerines, tangeretin may protect against neurodegenerative conditions such as Alzheimer's and Parkinson's diseases.

tannins Also called pro-anthocyanidins, tannins may detoxify carcinogens and scavenge harmful free radicals. Tannins in cranberries may protect against urinary tract infections and prevent the progress of age-related macular degereration. Note that tannins reduce IRON absorption. Sources: blackberries, blueberries, cranberries, grapes, lentils, tea, wine.

terpenes Terpenes are a class of phytonutrients that include PERILLYL ALCOHOL in cherries, LIMONENE in the zest of citrus fruit, SAPONINS in grains and vegetables, and eugenol in cloves and nutmeg. Terpene phytonutrients have antiviral, antifungal, and analgesic (pain-reducing) qualities and may help fight cancer, improve immunity, and help reduce inflammation.

thiamin Essential for normal development and growth, this B vitamin assists in energy metabolism and ensures proper functioning of the nervous and cardiovascular systems. Sources: corn, legumes, peas, nuts, rice, seeds.

thioproline A phytonutrient in fresh shiitake mushrooms, thioproline helps detoxify cancer-causing substances.

trans fatty acids These types of fats in foods are formed when vegetable oils are processed (hydrogenated) to improve their stability and convert them to solid fats. A food that has "hydrogenated vegetable oil" on its ingredient list contains trans fatty acids. Years of research have shown that high intakes

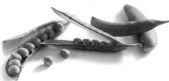

of trans fatty acids contribute to heart disease by elevating LDL ("bad") cholesterol and reducing HDL ("good") cholesterol and are linked to inflammation. Some margarines (especially stick margarines), solid shortenings, certain types of peanut butter, commercial frying fats (used in fast-food establishments), and baked goods are the major sources of trans fats.

tryptophan An essential AMINO ACID, tryptophan is converted by the body into the B vitamin NIACIN. Tryptophan stimulates production of serotonin, a neurotransmitter that supports mental health. COMPLEX CARBOHYDRATES enhance the absorption and use of tryptophan in the brain. Sources: bananas, peanuts, oats, prunes (dried plums), bread.

tyrosine A nonessential AMINO ACID, tyrosine is a precursor to numerous chemical messengers (neurotransmitters) in the brain and serves as a protein building block throughout the body. Sources: beans, lentils, nuts, oats, soy foods.

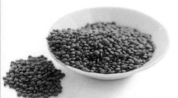

tyrosine kinase inhibitors These potent compounds in lentils and beans appear to team up with SOLUBLE FIBER to stabilize blood sugar levels.

vitamins, fat-soluble Fat-soluble vitamins—A, D, E, and K—dissolve in fat before they are absorbed in the bloodstream to carry out their functions. Because they are stored longterm in fatty tissues in the body, a buildup from supplement forms of these vitamins may result in toxic levels.

vitamins, water-soluble Water-soluble vitamins, C and the B vitamins, dissolve in water and are not stored in the body long term (with the exception of vitamin B_{12}, which is not readily excreted). Instead, they are eliminated in sweat and urine. Because they are not stored, we need to eat foods rich in these fragile vitamins each day.

vitamin A Known for its vision-enhancing properties, vitamin A is also vital for normal cell growth and maintaining immunity and healthy skin. This fat-soluble vitamin is synthesized in the intestines from BETA-CAROTENE and other CAROTENOIDS. Because high levels of vitamin A in supplement form may be toxic, it is best to obtain vitamin A from food. Sources: dried apricots, broccoli, carrots, peppers, spinach, sweet potatoes.

vitamin B_6 Also known as pyridoxine, vitamin B_6 is vital for the regulation of mental processes. Vitamin B_6 also helps maintain glucose (blood sugar) levels, healthy nervous and immune systems, and hemoglobin production. Along with VITAMIN B_{12} and FOLATE, vitamin B_6 is thought to lower blood levels of HOMO-CYSTEINE (a risk factor for heart disease). Sources: avocado, bananas, peas, potatoes, prune juice.

vitamin B_{12} Also called cobalamin, the best plant-based sources of vitamin B_{12} are fortified foods such as cereals and dairy-free milks and nutritional yeast. Vitamin B_{12} is required to produce DNA, the genetic material in all cells. Adequate amounts of vitamin B_{12} may help to prevent anemia, chronic fatigue syndrome, depression, heart disease, and infertility, and it is vital for healthy nerve cells and red blood cells.

vitamin C This vitamin, also known as ascorbic acid, has considerable ANTIOXIDANT power. Vitamin C may strengthen the immune system, support connective tissues, prevent nasal congestion, and enhance healing of wounds. Sources: berries, broccoli, citrus fruits, kiwifruit, peppers, pineapple, melons, tomatoes.

vitamin D Important for the absorption of CALCIUM and PHOSPHORUS, vitamin D is a fat-soluble vitamin that is often referred to as the "sunshine vitamin," because the body creates it when the sun's ultraviolet rays strike the skin for about 10 to 15 minutes a day. Sources: fortified dairy-free milk and orange juice, mushrooms.

vitamin E One of the fat-soluble vitamins, vitamin E is a potent antioxidant. The most useful form of vitamin E for our bodies, and the form most commonly found in foods, is alpha-tocopherol. Vitamin E may provide antioxidant protection against many ailments, including cancer, vision disorders, eczema, memory loss, and osteoarthritis. Note that large doses of vitamin E may adversely affect people on blood thinners or aspirin therapy. Sources: avocados, nuts, olive oil, sunflower seeds, wheat germ.

vitamin K This fat-soluble vitamin is critical for blood clotting as well as bone formation. Among various forms of vitamin K, phylloquinone is the form available in foods (vitamin K is also made in the gastrointestinal tract). Note that people who are on blood-thinning drugs should not take vitamin K supplements and should avoid foods high in vitamin K. Sources: broccoli, cabbage, cauliflower, soybeans, green leafy vegetables.

water Indispensable for life and comprising about 60 percent of body weight, water regulates temperature, provides lubrication, and serves as a fluid medium for metabolic processes throughout the body. Routinely drinking about eight glasses of water each day is essential to good health, as water is constantly lost from the body and must be replaced through regular consumption.

zinc This essential trace mineral is instrumental in maintaining normal skin, hair, immunity, protein metabolism, and numerous enzyme systems. Sources: beans, nuts, seeds, tofu, wheat germ, whole grains.

when to take a supplement

While reaping the multiple benefits of whole foods is the optimal way to prevent and/or manage symptoms of illness, there are situations in which the use of supplements is appropriate. For example, most foods that contain VITAMIN E (a fat-soluble vitamin) tend to be high in fat. So in order to get enough vitamin E, it may be helpful to take a supplement. And taking a general multivitamin every day can be beneficial—though a multivitamin is not a substitute for eating nutritious foods.

There are also specific medical conditions that warrant the use of supplements. Women of childbearing age should take supplemental folic acid (the synthetic form of the B vitamin FOLATE) to prevent possible birth defects in an unborn child. In addition, people at risk for osteoporosis should take a CALCIUM supplement. This is particularly important for postmenopausal women, who are most at risk for this debilitating bone-thinning disease, though older men are certainly also at risk.

Vegans may be at risk for vitamin B_{12} deficiency unless they include enough nutritional yeast or fortified food products, such as plant-based dairy substitutes, in their diets. And regardless of diet type, in order for B_{12} to be absorbed into your body, your stomach must produce enough of a substance called intrinsic factor, which attaches to B_{12} and moves the vitamin from your gastrointestinal tract into your bloodstream. Generally, your stomach produces less and less intrinsic factor as you age, reducing your body's ability to absorb vitamin B_{12}. (The good news is: Your liver can store excess B_{12} for up to five years, so deficiencies are rare.)

Another example of a nutrient that is difficult to get enough of through any type of diet is vitamin D. Plant-based dairy substitutes are often fortified with vitamin D but that may not be enough if it is your only source. Your health care provider can run a blood test to see if you are deficient in vitamin D and, if so, recommend specific types and amounts of supplements.

If you avoid any food group, if you are a woman who is pregnant, lactating or of childbearing age, or if you are elderly, ill, or at risk of developing a chronic medical condition, speak with your health-care provider to see if your situation warrants the use of individual nutrient supplements or multivitamin and mineral tablets.

foods that boost health

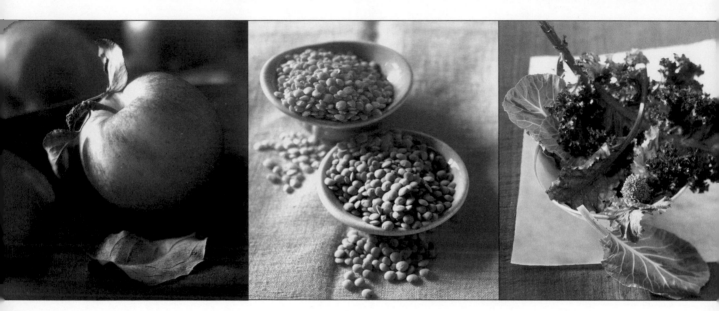

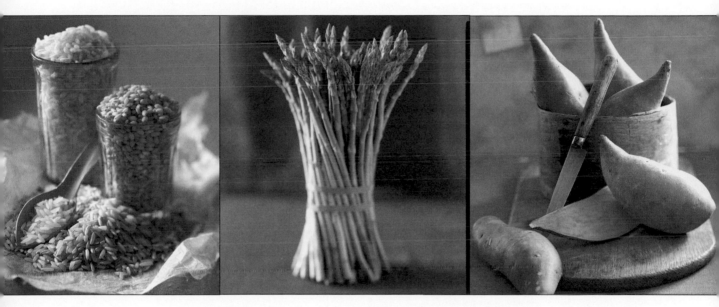

Plant Foods—and the

Nutrients in Them—That

Keep You Healthy

apples

Apples are packed with bushels of beneficial substances, such as pectin, vitamin C, and numerous phytonutrients that may help prevent heart disease and certain cancers, and also alleviate symptoms of allergies and asthma.

add more to your diet

► Top pancakes, waffles, or even fruit salad with applesauce instead of syrup.

► Stir diced apples into your breakfast oatmeal or other cereal.

► Applesauce makes a surprisingly creamy sorbet. Just freeze your favorite applesauce in an ice-cream maker.

► Substitute chopped dried apples for raisins in baked goods.

► Core apples and thinly slice them crosswise. Use these fresh, crunchy slices in sandwiches.

► Sprinkle diced apples on top of a homemade cheese pizza.

► Homemade applesauce is incredibly easy and quick to make: Cook chunks of apple with just a little bit of water or juice over low heat and in about 15 minutes you'll have applesauce. Certain apples will collapse to a puree by themselves; other types are sturdier and will have to be mashed a bit with a potato masher or fork.

what's in it

anthocyanins Natural food pigments, anthocyanins have antioxidant activity that may defend against carcinogens. They may also lower LDL ("bad") cholesterol and prevent blood clots.

glutathione This antioxidant may have anticancer actions and improve the immune system's ability to fight off infections.

pectin A type of soluble fiber that helps to lower artery-damaging LDL cholesterol, pectin in applesauce is also helpful in managing diarrhea. (A single unpeeled apple provides nearly 4 g of dietary fiber, almost half of which is heart-healthy pectin.)

phenolic acids Apples contain caffeic, chlorogenic, ellagic, and ferulic acids, as well as other types of phenolic compounds that may help to fight cancer.

quercetin A flavonoid linked to a reduced risk for cancer development, quercetin may also help to prevent cataracts and reduce symptoms associated with respiratory ailments.

rutin Rutin is a flavonoid that teams up with vitamin C to maintain blood vessel health.

maximizing the benefits

For **vitamin C** and **glutathione,** eat apples uncooked, as these nutrients are diminished by heat. For **pectin,** it's best to cook the apples, as the pectin is released when the apples' cell walls soften as they cook. For **insoluble fiber** and **anthocyanins,** which are found in the apple skin, use unpeeled apples (choose organic apples if you are concerned about pesticides).

health bites

You may breathe easier if you eat a lot of apples. A recent study linked apple consumption with a reduced risk for lung cancer. Researchers isolated quercetin, a powerful flavonoid, as the possible source of the anticancer effect—although the phenolic acids and vitamin C found in apples may also protect the lungs.

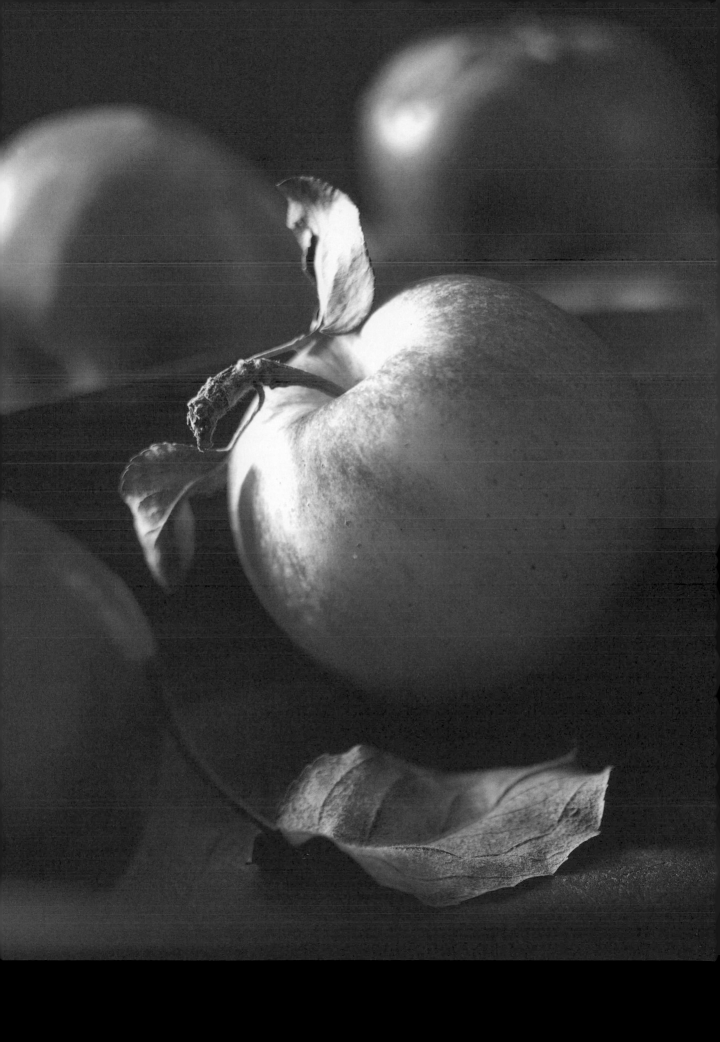

apricots

Apricots' deep golden color indicates the presence of carotenoids, specifically beta-carotene, an important antioxidant. Both fresh and dried apricots are packed with protective nutrients and phytonutrients.

what's in it

beta-carotene A carotenoid whose antioxidant power is linked with cancer prevention, beta-carotene is believed to combat free-radical damage, and is also thought to reinforce the immune system.

ellagic acid A compound that may reduce damage caused by carcinogens such as environmental toxins, ellagic acid is also being studied for its potential to inhibit the growth of cancer cells.

iron Dried apricots are a good source of iron (¼ cup provides 1.5 mg of this mineral). Adequate amounts of iron are important for everyone, particularly for pregnant women and children. Iron-deficient anemia can lead to fatigue and vulnerability to infections due to reduced immune response.

lycopene Apricots contain small amounts of this powerful antioxidant, which is believed to reduce LDL ("bad") cholesterol and protect the prostate against cancer.

pectin Pectin is a soluble fiber that lowers LDL cholesterol levels, which are linked to dangerous hardening of the arteries.

potassium This important mineral helps to prevent high blood pressure and is required for healthy nerves and muscles.

maximizing the benefits

Although eating fresh apricots is a way to get the most **vitamin C** (which is depleted by heat and exposure to air when apricots are dried), other substances—such as **beta-carotene, lycopene,** and **pectin**—are actually made more available to the body when the apricots (fresh or dried) are gently cooked.

health bites

If you are sensitive to the sulfites (sulfur dioxide) that are used to prevent dried apricots from turning brown, look for sulfite-free apricots in health-food stores and the health-food section of some supermarkets.

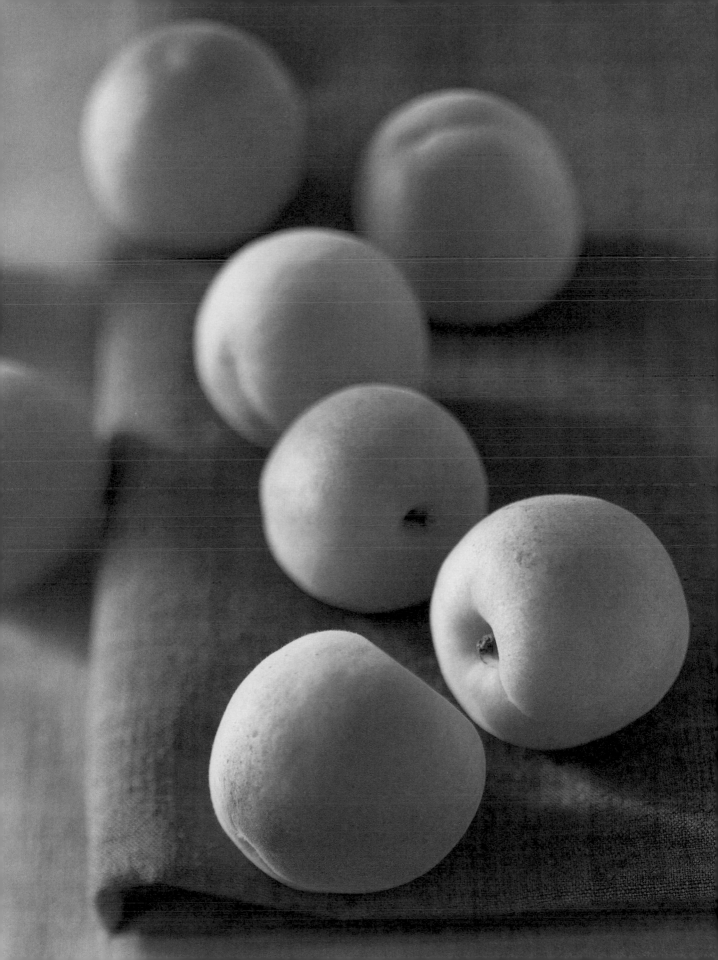

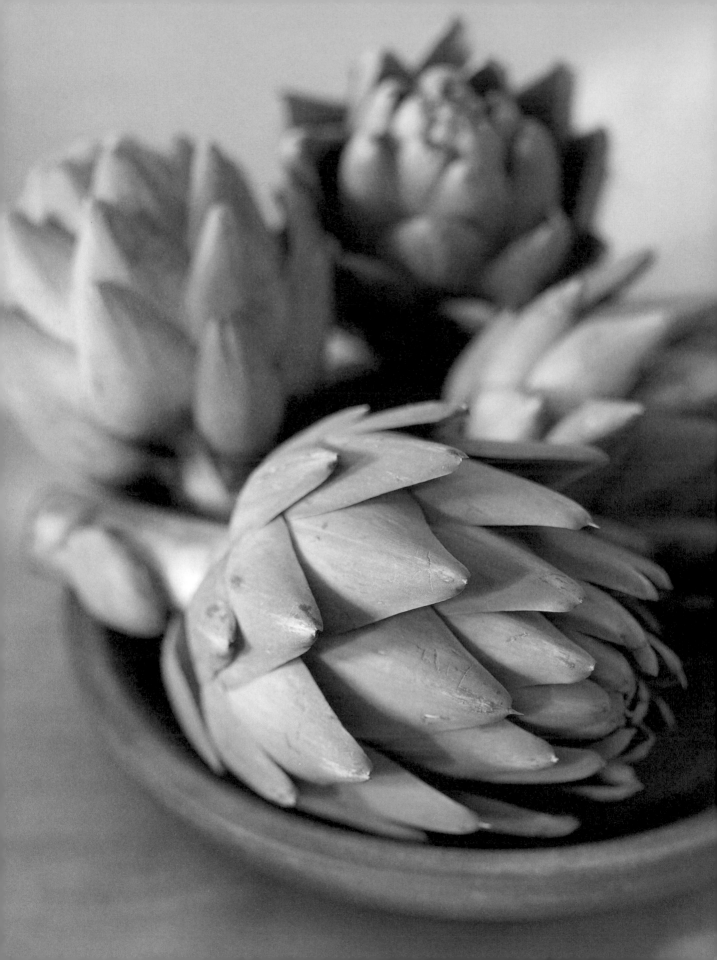

artichokes

This venerable vegetable contains several restorative nutrients. Used since ancient times as a digestive aid and for poor liver function, research reveals that artichokes may also confer cholesterol-lowering benefits.

what's in it

cynarin Cynarin is an organic acid found in artichokes that stimulates the sweetness receptors in the tastebuds of some people, causing the foods eaten afterward to taste sweeter. This phytonutrient may also offer antioxidant protection against carcinogenic and environmental toxins such as pollution and smoke. Cynarin also may have a beneficial effect on the liver by helping to promote bile flow (which assists in the removal of toxic substances from the body) and by preventing fat accumulation in the liver.

folate In addition to preventing certain birth defects, this B vitamin (also known as folic acid) may help lower heart disease risk by reducing levels of homocysteine, an amino acid that has been linked to atherosclerosis. Folate may also help to prevent cancer, since low levels of folate can be harmful to DNA.

luteolin With the potential to prevent LDL ("bad") cholesterol oxidation, this flavonoid may reduce the risk for heart disease. Studies suggest that luteolin also may block the release of histamines, which can trigger congestion and inflammation.

maximizing the benefits

Although frozen and canned "hearts" are the most available market form of artichokes, it's best to cook and eat fresh, whole artichokes as often as possible to take advantage of the phytonutrients found in the leaves. To preserve as much of the water-soluble **folate** as possible, steam or microwave rather than boil artichokes.

add more to your diet

▶ When steaming whole artichokes, add a mixture of herbs (such as rosemary, tarragon, and thyme) to the steaming water. This will add a subtle herb flavor to the artichokes themselves.

▶ Instead of dipping artichoke leaves in melted butter, try this: Make a puree of mashed roasted garlic, black pepper, silken tofu, and lemon juice.

▶ For a quick artichoke appetizer, puree jarred artichokes (rinsed and drained) with garlic and plant-based mayonnaise and yogurt. Serve as a dip with crudités.

▶ Fresh baby Italian artichokes, available seasonally, can be steamed or stewed and eaten whole with a drizzle of lemon juice and extra-virgin olive oil.

▶ Make an artichoke relish: Steam whole artichokes, then coarsely chop the tender part of the leaves and the heart. Toss with olive oil and vinegar and use on sandwiches or with salads.

health bites

Both the tender "heart" and the meaty leaves of the artichoke are edible, though it's the leaves that contain many of the vegetable's phytonutrients.

asparagus

Asparagus is delicious, low in fat, and low in sodium—a superb vegetable for those who are watching their weight. A nutrient-dense superfood, asparagus may help prevent heart disease, cancer, and certain birth defects.

add more to your diet

▶ When you're trimming the tough ends from asparagus stalks, save them and cook them in water until very tender. Use this B-vitamin-enriched water to boost the nutrition of an asparagus (or other) soup or pasta sauce.

▶ Fold cooked, cut-up asparagus into pasta dishes.

▶ Most people don't think of roasting asparagus, but it's delicious and a good way to preserve the B vitamins. Toss trimmed asparagus with a little olive oil and a sprinkling of garlic or fresh herbs such as thyme and roast in a 450°F oven for 10 to 20 minutes.

▶ Puree cooked asparagus with plant-based milk and herbs for a quick soup.

▶ Add cooked asparagus to pizzas, sandwiches, and wraps.

▶ For a twist on the classic guacamole, chop cooked asparagus very finely, add just a little avocado, and season as you would a traditional guacamole.

what's in it

fiber Insoluble fiber is important for promoting a healthy digestive tract, and soluble fiber helps to lower cholesterol.

folate Folate is vital during pregnancy as it prevents development of neural tube defects in the fetus. Folate is also cardioprotective, helping to reduce homocysteine, an amino acid linked to heart disease risk. Folate may also help prevent cancer (low folate levels may damage DNA and lead to cancerous changes in cells).

glutathione Functioning as an antioxidant, the enzyme glutathione may detoxify carcinogenic substances and protect cells from free-radical damage.

rutin This antioxidant flavonoid works hand-in-hand with the antioxidant vitamin C to maintain blood vessel health.

saponins These compounds may prevent heart disease by binding and preventing absorption of cholesterol in the digestive tract.

vitamin B$_6$ This immune-boosting vitamin, required for the production of disease-fighting antibodies, plays an important role in enabling the body to derive energy from food. Preliminary research suggests that vitamin B$_6$ also helps to relieve the discomfort of premenstrual tension as well as nausea in early pregnancy.

maximizing the benefits

To reap the full health benefits from this nutritional powerhouse, you should steam or microwave asparagus. Or, if you cook the stalks in water, use an asparagus cooker, which is designed to cook the asparagus with the tips facing up and not immersed in water: This is important because it's thought that most of the phytonutrients are in the tips.

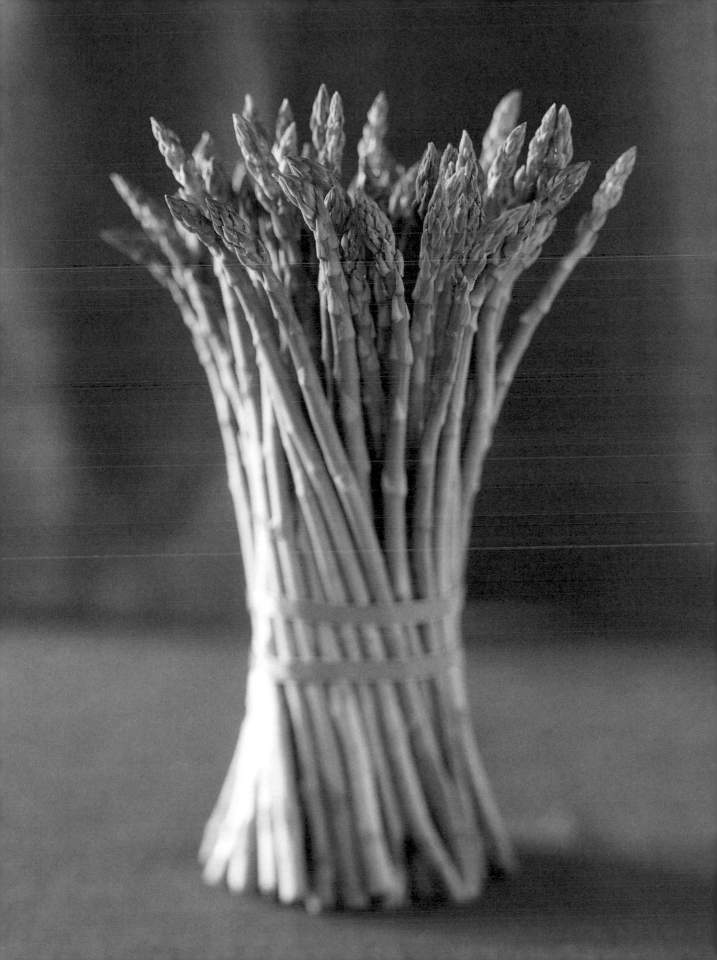

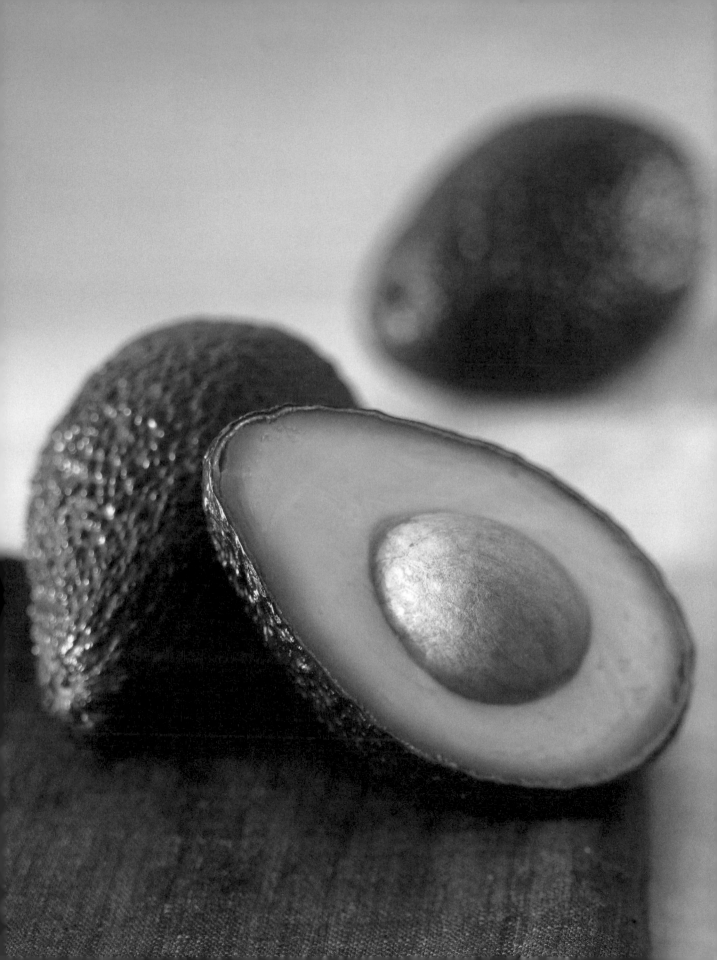

avocados

Creamy, luscious avocados are such a rich source of vitamins, minerals, healthful fats, and phytonutrients that many nutritionists and other health experts are urging Americans to eat more of them.

what's in it

beta-sitosterol This compound may block cholesterol absorption as well as reduce discomfort of BPH (benign prostatic hyperplasia). It is also under review for the potential to prevent breast cancer.

fiber The fiber content of avocados is high, which is good news since soluble fiber removes excess cholesterol from your body, and insoluble fiber helps to prevent constipation by keeping your digestive system running smoothly.

folate Avocados are good sources of folate. This important B vitamin is linked to the prevention of neural tube defects in fetuses as well as prevention of cancer and heart disease in adults.

glutathione Functioning as an antioxidant, this compound may neutralize free radicals that damage cells.

magnesium This mineral may help to reduce discomfort associated with premenstrual syndrome, migraines, anxiety, and other disorders.

oleic acid A type of monounsaturated fat in avocados, oleic acid has been linked to lower cholesterol levels when substituted for saturated fat in the diet.

maximizing the benefits

Avocado flesh turns brown rapidly when overripe or exposed to air, so it is a good idea to sprinkle it with lemon or lime juice while it's still bright green to prevent discoloration.

add more to your diet

▶ Make a salad dressing: Puree avocado with plain plant-based yogurt, lime juice or vinegar to taste, salt, and hot sauce, if you like.

▶ Make an avocado smoothie: In a blender, puree avocado, dairy-free milk, a touch of sweetener, and a couple of ice cubes.

▶ Mash avocado with lime juice and use as a spread on sandwiches.

▶ Try avocado toast: Rub toast with a clove of garlic and spread with mashed avocado.

▶ Mash avocado with a little salt (and perhaps some mustard) and use in place of mayonnaise in a bean, rice, or pasta salad.

health bites

If you avoid avocados because you think they're high in fat, think again. Avocados are indeed high in beneficial monounsaturated fat, which—when substituted for saturated fat in the diet—helps to lower LDL ("bad") cholesterol levels and the risk for heart disease.

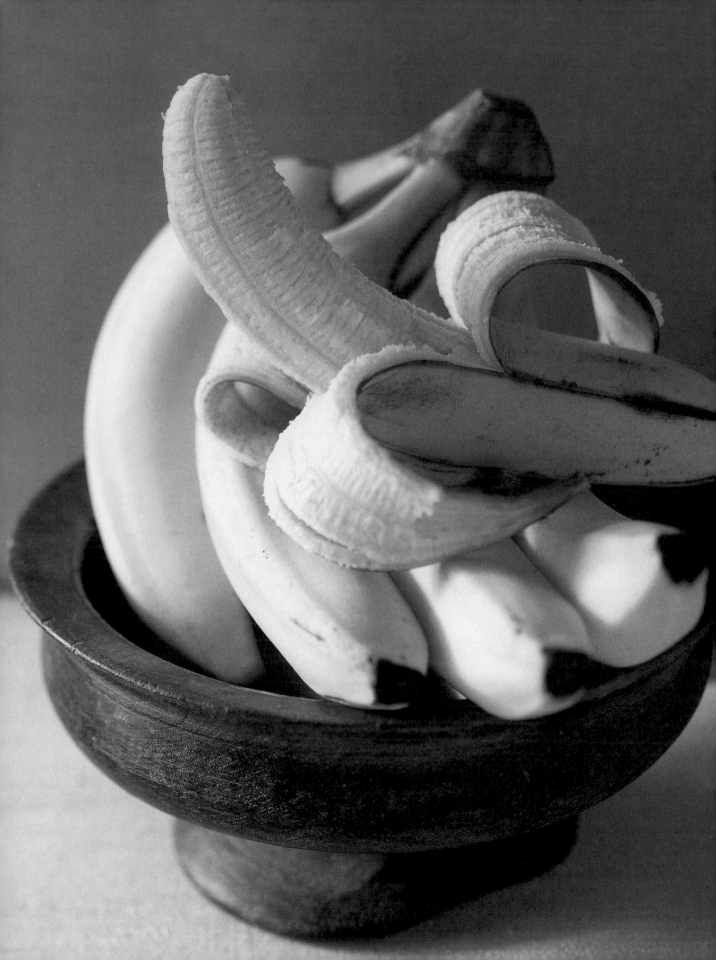

bananas

Next time you feel a bit anxious, try eating a banana. It contains vitamin B$_6$ as well as small amounts of tryptophan, both of which may promote a relaxed state of mind. This comforting fruit may also help ward off heart disease, stroke, and certain gastrointestinal woes.

what's in it

pectin In addition to being heart healthy, this type of soluble fiber is helpful in controlling diarrhea.

potassium A mineral with a wide range of benefits, potassium may play a role in lowering blood pressure and preventing stroke.

tryptophan An amino acid that stimulates the production of serotonin, a neurotransmitter that has a calming effect on the body, tryptophan may help to ward off depression, anxiety, and insomnia. Note that eating foods high in complex carbohydrates, such as pasta, rice, and beans, will help enhance the absorption of tryptophan.

vitamin B$_6$ This vitamin facilitates communication between muscles and nerves. It also helps to make red blood cells. It may also be useful in preventing the moodiness associated with premenstrual syndrome (PMS). Bananas are an excellent source of vitamin B$_6$.

maximizing the benefits

Cooking partially destroys **vitamin B$_6$,** so if you are interested in mood enhancement, it's best to eat bananas uncooked. If you are after extra pectin, cooked bananas make this soluble fiber more available.

add more to your diet

▶ Add cut-up bananas to curries for a little sweetness and to bring out the flavor of the curry spices.

▶ Bananas make a wonderful salsa: Toss diced bananas with scallions, red pepper, lime juice, and honey. Serve on tacos or in burritos.

▶ Freeze chunks of banana and puree in a blender along with a touch of nutmeg and lime juice to make an instant sorbet.

▶ Mash bananas with minced garlic and hot sauce and serve as a condiment alongside tofu or vegetable dishes.

▶ Banana raita, an Indian "side salad," is a sweet and cooling counterpoint to hot, spicy foods: Combine diced banana, plant-based yogurt, sliced scallions, and a touch of curry powder. Serve chilled.

health bites

Sugar molecules in bananas called fructooligosaccharides (FOS) are prebiotics that encourage the growth of beneficial bacteria in the intestine. These "friendly bacteria" may help to reduce toxins produced by unfriendly flora, improve nutrient absorption, and support communication between the gut and the brain.

beans

A nourishing and hearty source of plant protein, beans may help reduce LDL ("bad") cholesterol levels, stabilize blood sugar, and help control weight. They may also prevent certain types of birth defects and cancer.

add more to your diet

▶ You don't have to rely on canned beans (which are usually very high in sodium) for convenience. Just plan ahead a bit: Cook up a big batch of beans, then freeze in small batches.

▶ Puree cooked beans with herbs and spices and use as a topping for pizza in place of tomato sauce.

▶ Make a pasta sauce by pureeing cooked beans and garlic with broth and herbs, such as oregano or cumin.

▶ Instead of mayonnaise, make a sandwich spread of pureed beans, lemon juice, and some tomato paste.

▶ Puree cooked white beans and use them in place of pumpkin puree in a pumpkin pie.

▶ Use seasoned bean puree as a filling for stuffed mushrooms or eggplant.

what's in it

complex carbohydrates By making you feel full quickly, beans are a perfect food for people who are trying to control weight. Complex carbohydrates in beans also make them a great choice for people who want steady, slow-burning energy.

folate Essential for proper development of the fetus, folate also helps reduce the risk for heart disease by lowering homocysteine, an amino acid linked to the development of the condition.

insoluble fiber Beans are high in this beneficial fiber, which helps to prevent constipation by moving food through your system more quickly.

lignans Lignans may have cardioprotective and anticancer benefits, especially for prostate and breast cancer.

protease inhibitors Protease inhibitors have anitviral activity that blocks enzymes that lead to disease.

saponins These compounds may prevent cancer cells from multiplying, and they may also lower LDL cholesterol.

soluble fiber An important factor in lowering LDL cholesterol, soluble fiber may reduce heart disease risk. Fiber in beans also helps stabilize blood glucose levels, making this food a good choice for those with diabetes.

maximizing the benefits

The gas-causing culprits in beans are carbohydrates called oligosaccharides. Some theories suggest that presoaking dried beans, and then discarding the soaking water before cooking, will get rid of some of the oligosaccharides.

health bites

A serving of beans satisfies your appetite more than many other foods. The rich fiber content fills your stomach and causes a slower rise in blood sugar, staving off hunger for longer and providing a steady supply of energy.

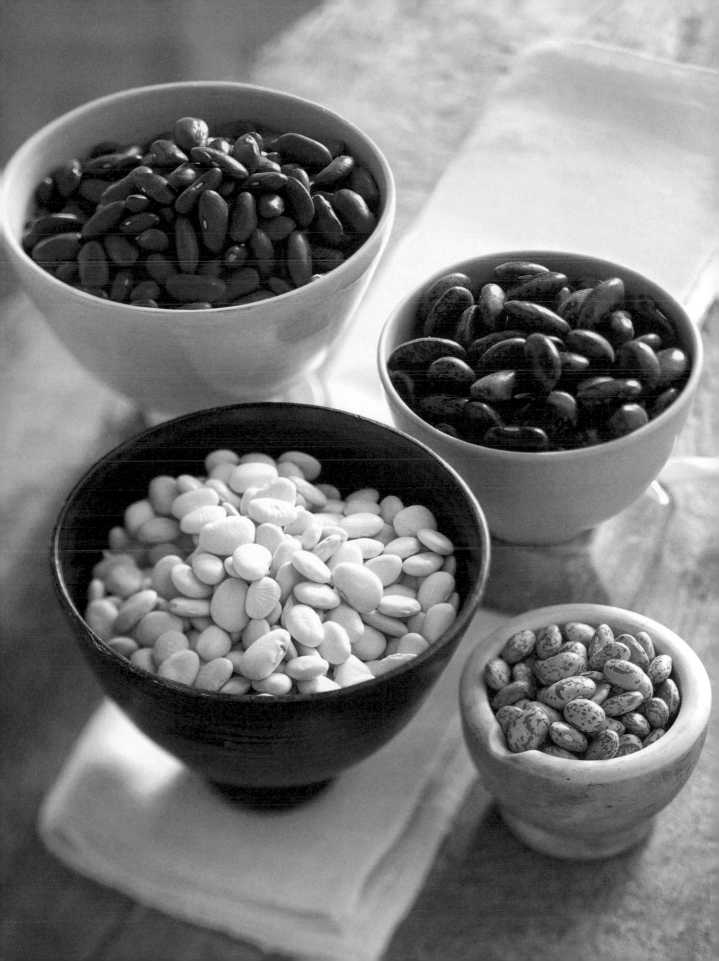

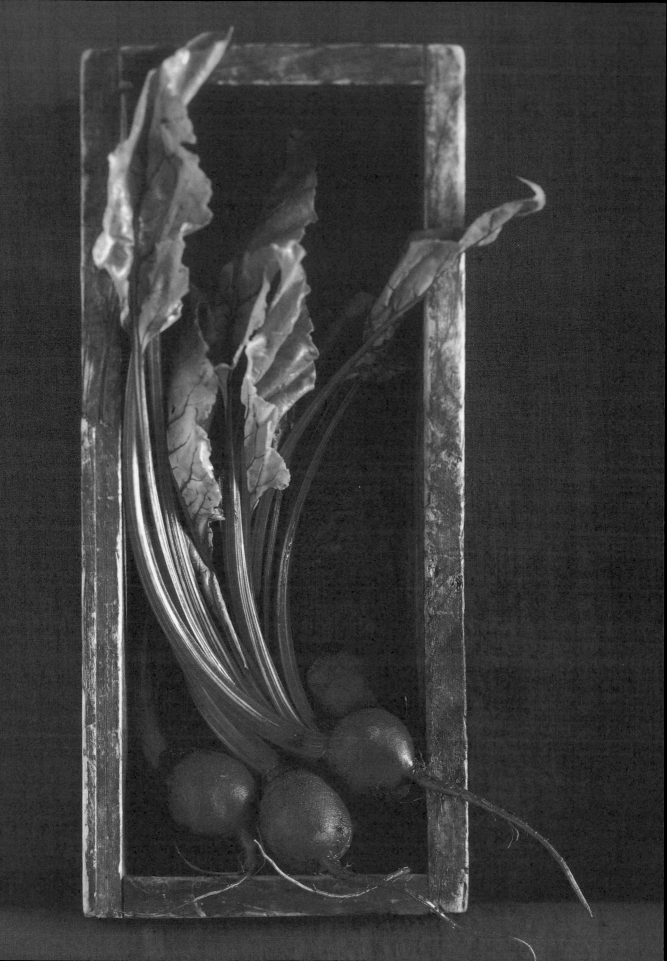

beets

Rich, sweet, and earthy in flavor, these ruby-red root vegetables are highly nutritious and provide fiber, folate, potassium, and such phytonutrients as anthocyanins and saponins.

what's in it

betacyanin A violet-red plant pigment, betacyanin is an antioxidant that protects against atherosclerosis, atherothrombosis, and ischemic heart disease.

betaine This substance can help lower blood levels of homocysteine, an amino acid associated with increased risk for heart disease, osteoporosis, and ocular issues.

fiber Soluble fiber in beets may be linked to the reduction of LDL ("bad") cholesterol levels.

folate Folate may help prevent birth defects and may also protect against heart disease and cancer.

oxalates If you are prone to kidney stones or gout, avoid beet greens; they are high in oxalates. Oxalates form tiny crystals that can contribute to the development of kidney stones.

saponins Available in small amounts in beets, saponins may bind cholesterol in the digestive tract, lowering the risk for heart disease.

maximizing the benefits

To preserve the **anthocyanin (betacyanin)** in beets, it's best to roast, bake, or microwave whole beets in their skins. If you cook peeled or cut-up beets in water, some of the vegetable's pigments (and thus the anthocyanins) and water-soluble B vitamin, **folate,** will leach into the cooking water.

add more to your diet

▶ Puree beets with plant-based yogurt or sour cream and vinegar to taste. Chill and serve as a refreshing summer soup.

▶ Add sliced, cooked (or pickled) beets to hummus sandwiches in place of sliced tomatoes.

▶ Shred peeled raw beets and use in place of carrots in carrot cake, carrot bread, or muffins.

▶ Make a slaw of shredded peeled raw beets, balsamic vinegar, mustard, and dill.

▶ Combine diced, cooked beets with olive oil and lemon juice and use as a sauce for steamed vegetables.

▶ For ways to use beet greens, see *Cooking Greens* on page 65.

health bites

Some people can't properly metabolize the pigments in beets and, as a result, their urine turns a bright red. Don't be alarmed if this should happen; it is a harmless metabolic reaction.

berries

Tiny powerhouses of nutrition, berries are bursting with healthy compounds, including folate, fiber, and phytonutrients, which may help improve memory in people with mild cognitive impairment and reduce the risk for developing heart disease and type 2 diabetes.

add more to your diet

▶ Do as the Italians do, and stir strawberries into savory rice dishes, such as pilaf or risotto. Stir in the chopped strawberries just before serving.

▶ Make your own cranberry sauce and use it in place of jam.

▶ Add berries to tossed green salads. Or make an all-berry salad and dress it with a lemon vinaigrette.

▶ Add fresh or frozen cranberries to soups and stews.

▶ Make a quick dessert "pizza": Spread sweetened plant-based yogurt or ricotta over a flour tortilla, spoon berries on top, and bake in a 400°F oven for 10 minutes, just until hot.

▶ Use berries as the basis of spicy salsas, chutneys, or relishes.

what's in it

anthocyanins These natural plant pigments in berries function as powerful antioxidants, which sweep out harmful free-radical molecules, preventing them from wreaking havoc on your body.

ellagic acid Ellagic acid is an antibacterial agent that may help prevent the growth of cancer cells. Blackberries, raspberries, and strawberries are particularly good sources.

kaempferol A flavonoid found in berries, kaempferol is believed to reduce the risk of chronic diseases, including cancer.

quercetin This well-studied flavonoid is thought to play numerous roles, including the ability to protect against heart disease, cancer, and possibly cataracts; it may also alleviate symptoms of allergies and asthma.

tannins Tannins (also known as proanthocyanidins) in cranberries and blackberries may prevent *E.coli* bacteria from attaching to the urinary tract and causing urinary tract infections. How they do this is currently under investigation.

vitamin C Among other functions, this important vitamin helps to strengthen the immune system and protect connective tissue that supports other tissues and organs in the body. Strawberries and cranberries are good sources.

maximizing the benefits

Cooking does not seem to destroy **ellagic acid** in berries. However, it will destroy some of their **folate** and **vitamin C.**

health bites

Blueberries may help prevent physical and cognitive issues related to aging. Though the specific substance in blueberries has not yet been identified, scientists speculate that the overall antioxidant power of the fruit and the abundance of anthocyanins protect brain cells from free-radical harm.

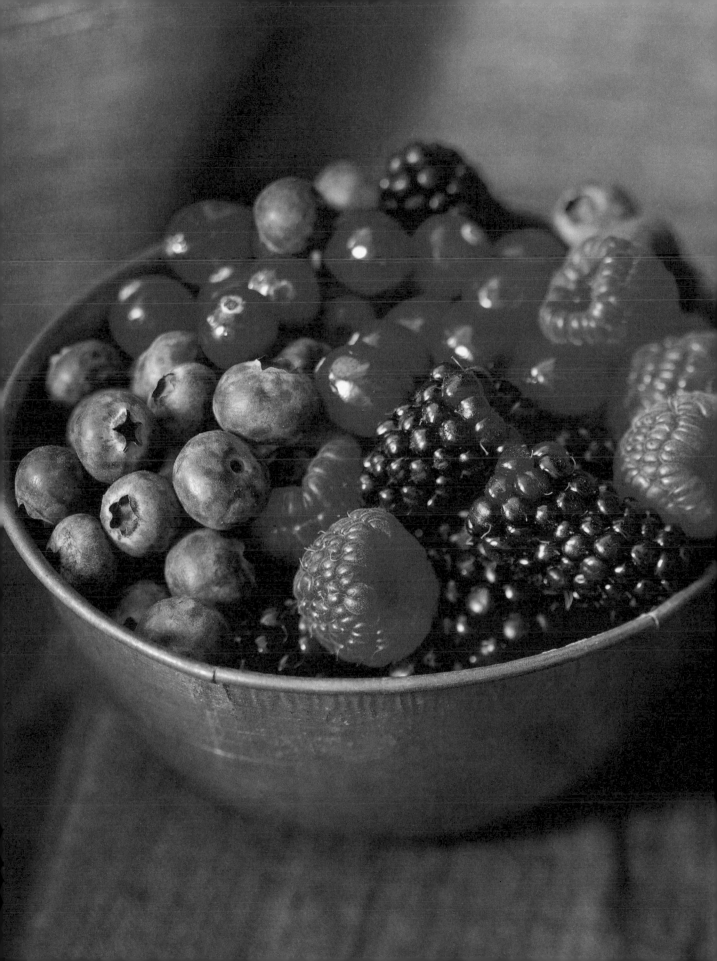

broccoli

One of the most studied of vegetables, broccoli's impressive status as a superfood is the result of its high level of phyto- nutrients and their potential to mobilize the body's natural disease-fighting resources.

add more to your diet

▶ Many recipes call for broccoli florets, but the stalks are delicious, too. With a paring knife, peel the stalks, then thinly slice crosswise.

▶ Puree cooked broccoli along with plant-based milk and seasonings, and serve as a soup. Top with nutritional yeast, if you like.

▶ Combine chopped, cooked broccoli and softened tofu and spread on flour tortillas or lavash bread. Top with sliced onion, lettuce, and tomato and roll up.

▶ Puree cooked broccoli along with olive oil, garlic, and crushed red pepper flakes and use as a sauce for pasta.

▶ Make a broccoli slaw: Shred raw broccoli, toss with shredded carrots, and season as you would a coleslaw.

what's in it

beta-carotene This powerful antioxidant may help to neutralize cell-damaging free-radical molecules.

calcium Broccoli is a good nonfat, non-dairy well-absorbed vegetable source of this bone-nourishing mineral.

dithiolethiones These anticancer agents may protect the gastrointestinal tract and help to stimulate the antioxidant glutathione, a cancer-protective compound.

folate This B vitamin may help to reduce the incidence of cancer and certain birth defects. It may also help to control levels of homocysteine, an amino acid linked to heart disease.

glucosinolates Once ingested, glucosinolates break down into various healthful compounds, including indoles, sulforaphane, and isothiocyanates, all of which may be potent cancer fighters.

indoles These compounds are thought to provide protection against hormone-related cancers, such as breast and prostate cancers.

insoluble fiber This type of fiber helps food move faster and with greater bulk through the digestive tract, promoting regularity.

isothiocyanates By stimulating the body's production of its own cancer-fighting enzymes, isothiocyanates may neutralize potential cancer-causing substances that enter the body, including carcinogens in smoke.

lutein This carotenoid may help prevent and improve age-related macular degeneration.

potassium Broccoli is a rich source of this mineral, which may help lower the risk for stroke and high blood pressure.

sulforaphane This powerful phytonutrient provides antioxidant, antimicrobial, anticancer, anti-inflammatory, antiaging, and neuroprotective benefits.

maximizing the benefits

Cooking broccoli with a lot of water can diminish broccoli's **glucosinolates, folate,** and **vitamin C.** Steam, microwave, or stir-fry it instead.

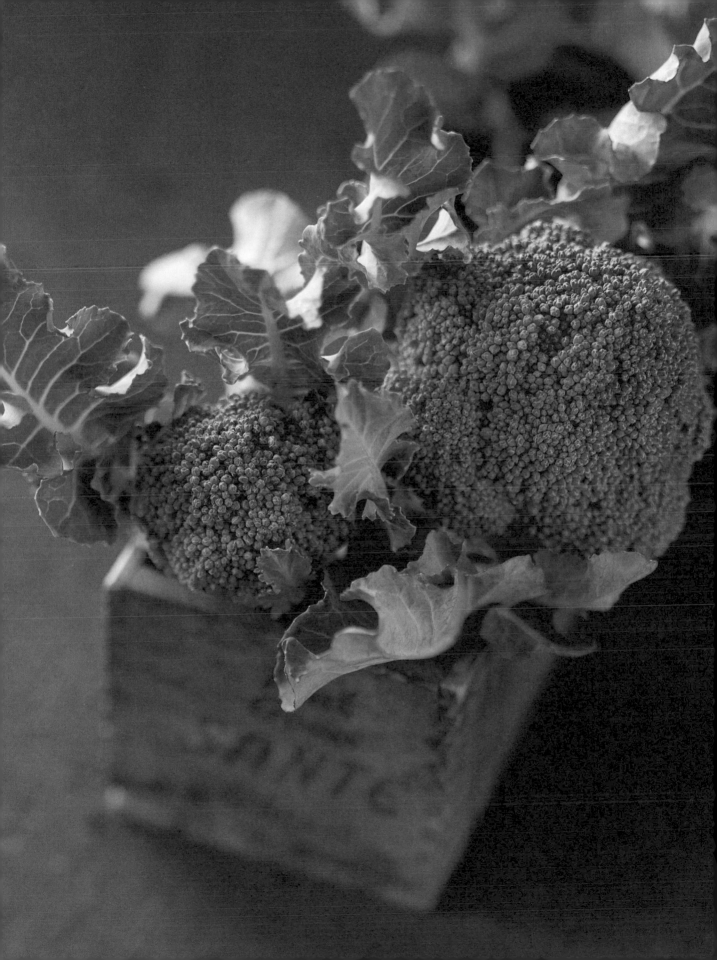

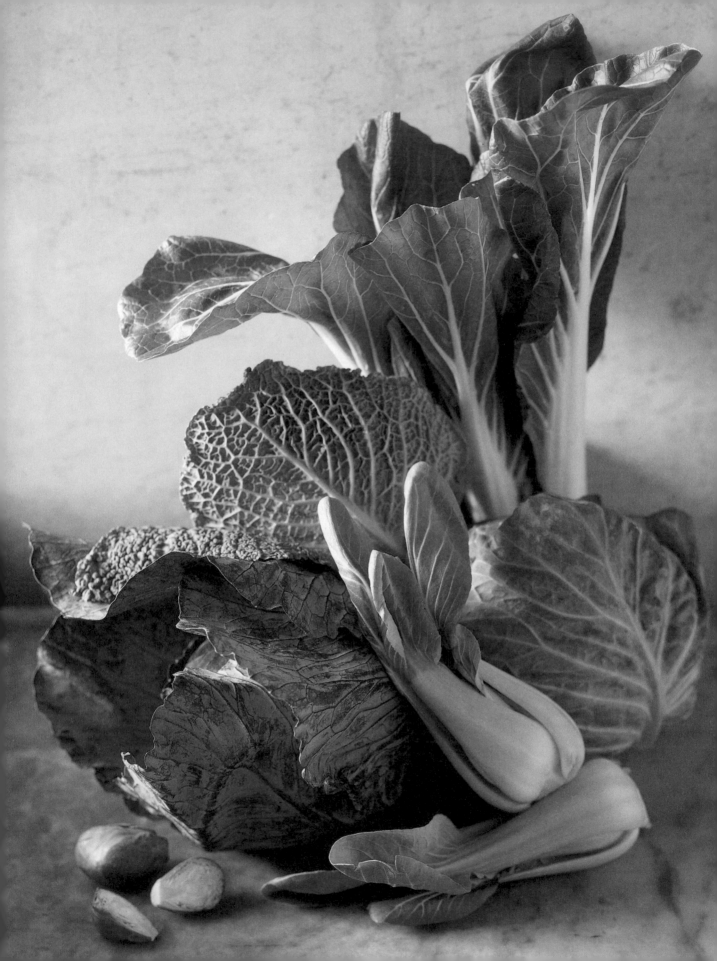

cabbage family

Cabbages are nutritional kings, as are their relatives, bok choy, kale, and brussels sprouts. Nutrient-rich and loaded with protective compounds, these members of the cabbage family may help to fight off cancer and heart disease.

what's in it

anthocyanins Found in red cabbage, these antioxidant pigments may protect cells from free-radical damage.

beta-carotene Bok choy is extremely rich in this important antioxidant and has more beta-carotene than other cabbages. Beta-carotene is linked to lower incidence of heart disease and certain kinds of cancer.

dithiolethiones These compounds may help protect against carcinogenic agents by increasing the body's reserve of glutathione, which has antioxidant properties.

folate This important B vitamin is believed to reduce the incidence of cancer and birth defects, and lower heart disease risk.

goitrogens Raw cabbage contains these compounds, which may slow down the thyroid. Consult with your physician if you have thyroid problems and you eat a lot of raw cabbage.

indoles Thought to deactivate estrogen, which stimulates tumor growth, indoles may protect against breast and prostate cancer. Savoy cabbage is an especially good source of indoles.

insoluble fiber This fiber helps to alleviate constipation.

isothiocyanates These compounds may stimulate the enzymes that impede hormones that promote breast and prostate cancers.

sulforaphane This isothiocyanate stimulates production of glutathione, a compound with antioxidant properties.

vitamin C Brussels sprouts supply four times the vitamin C of their cabbage cousins. Vitamin C may help to improve immune function and fight off infections and viruses.

maximizing the benefits

For **vitamin C,** raw cabbage is best. But when cooking, it's best to steam, microwave, or stir-fry for maximum retention of all nutrients.

add more to your diet

▶ Use cabbage leaves as edible steamer wrappers: Sprinkle thick tofu fillets with herbs (chervil, tarragon, or dill), wrap in cabbage leaves, and steam over seasoned broth (use more of the same herbs in the broth).

▶ Shred brussels sprouts and stir-fry with garlic, chopped nuts, and bread crumbs. Toss with cooked pasta.

▶ Steam cabbage or bok choy leaves and wrap around matchsticks of carrot and bell pepper. Serve the packets with a spicy dipping sauce.

▶ Stir-fry cabbage and onions, add to coarsely mashed potatoes, and serve surrounded by steamed veggies.

▶ Add shredded cabbage and apples to potatoes when making potato pancakes.

▶ Make a slaw with shredded brussels sprouts, carrots, red peppers, and pears. Dress the slaw with a light vinaigrette.

carrots

Gold mines of nourishment, these healthful vegetables provide impressive amounts of beta-carotene and a good-size helping of fiber. Consuming carrots may help to protect against heart disease, certain types of cancer, skin disorders, eye conditions, constipation, and high cholesterol.

add more to your diet

▶ Use carrot juice in place of water in homemade bread or pizza dough.

▶ To make a sauce to serve over pasta, sauté carrots with garlic in olive oil until very tender. Puree with carrot juice and some lemon juice to taste.

▶ Stir shredded carrots into rice pudding after the pudding is cooked.

▶ Use carrots instead of shredded coconut in macaroons or other cookies.

▶ Substitute carrot juice for broths in soups, stews, and pasta sauces.

▶ Cook carrots along with potatoes when boiling potatoes for mashing.

what's in it

beta-carotene Much more than the precursor for vitamin A, beta-carotene functions as an antioxidant that helps maintain good vision and a strong immune system. The more vivid the color of the carrot, the higher the levels of carotene in it. Carrots are one of the richest sources of this important carotenoid.

calcium pectate A unique type of pectin fiber, calcium pectate is thought to lower cholesterol by attaching to bile acids, a process that helps to remove cholesterol from the body.

insoluble fiber This type of fiber helps to prevent constipation by adding bulk to digested foods. It also makes you feel full, which may be helpful for weight loss.

vitamin A When you eat carrots or other plant foods high in beta-carotene, your body converts what it needs of the beta-carotene into vitamin A, which is important for numerous functions, including proper eyesight, normal cell growth, and healthy mucous membranes. Vitamin A helps eyes adjust to the dark, and it also promotes healthy skin and hair.

maximizing the benefits

Cooking carrots, especially with a little bit of fat (preferably monounsaturated fat, such as olive oil), makes **beta-carotene** more available for absorption by the body.

health bites

Although research suggests that beta-carotene in supplement form won't help prevent heart disease or cancer (and may, in fact, increase risk to your health), other studies suggest that eating fruits and vegetable high in beta-carotene may be protective against many chronic health conditions.

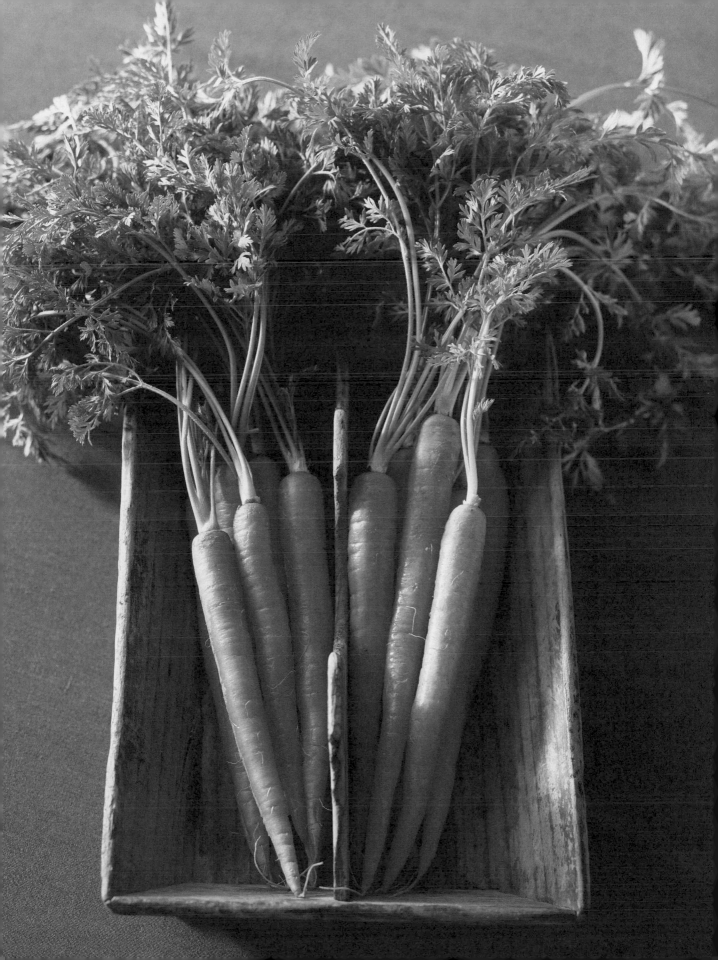

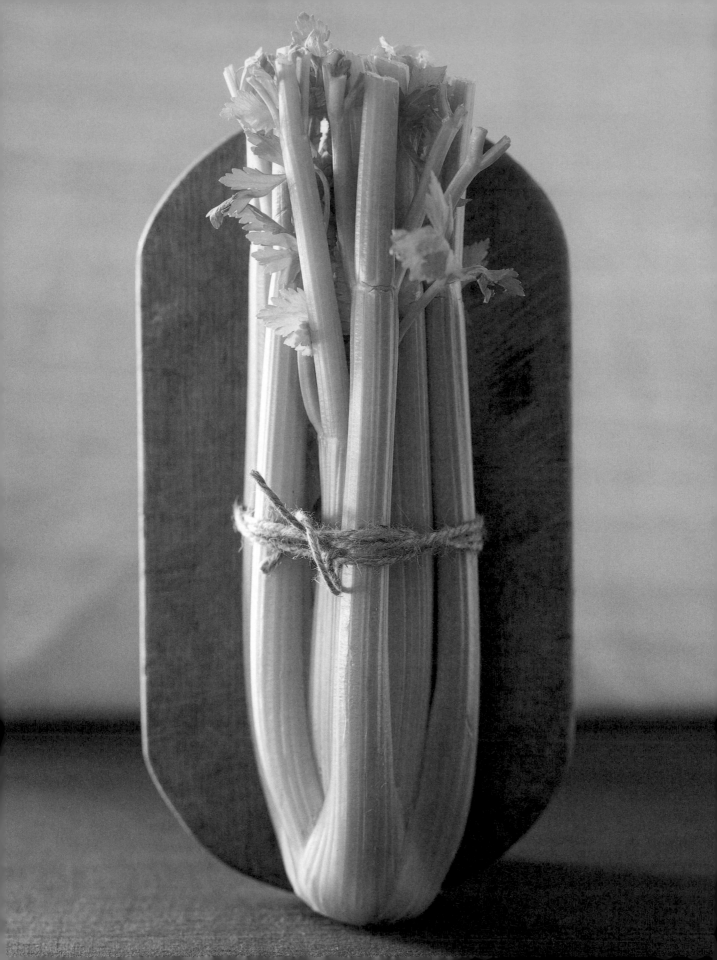

celery

Thought to contribute little in the way of nutrients, celery has finally achieved the status of a good-for-you food. Researchers are discovering many healthful compounds in celery, including those that may help lower blood pressure or reduce the risk for certain types of cancer.

what's in it

apigenin This flavonoid may offer protection against neurodegererative conditions such as Alzheimer's and Parkinson's diseases.

insoluble fiber Foods that are high in insoluble fiber tend to be low in calories, and they also promote feelings of satiety (fullness). An excellent choice for those who are trying to lose weight, insoluble fiber is filling because it absorbs water and adds bulk as it moves through the digestive tract, a process that also keeps your digestive system working properly.

phthalides (3-n-butyl phthalide) For a vegetable, celery is relatively high in sodium (35 mg per stalk)—a possible concern for people who suffer from hypertension but, at the same time, it also contains a unique compound that is believed to lower blood pressure. Some studies indicate that phthalides may reduce the body's levels of certain hormones that constrict blood vessels and raise blood pressure.

maximizing the benefits

If possible, include the celery leaves when cooking. They contain high concentrations of nutrients, such as **potassium** and **vitamin C.**

add more to your diet

▶ For a vegetable side dish, sauté matchsticks of celery in olive oil with chopped walnuts.

▶ Make a celery relish: Finely chop celery along with onion, garlic, and parsley. Add vinegar and mustard to taste and use as a topping for veggie patties, roasted vegetables, or salads.

▶ For a celery "tonic": In a blender, combine celery with tomato juice and horseradish, and puree.

▶ Make a triple-celery soup: Cook sliced celery, celery leaves, garlic, broth, a sprinkling of celery seeds, and herbs (such as marjoram or basil) and puree. Add plant-based milk for a creamy soup.

▶ Braise celery in seasoned broth until tender and serve as a side vegetable.

health bites

Celery seeds—whose pungency perks up the flavor of pickles or sauerkraut—contain potentially beneficial phytonutrients such as limonene, coumarins, phthalides, and apigenin. Modern science has found that celery seeds may have anti-inflammatory and other properties that may help alleviate pain and swelling associated with gout.

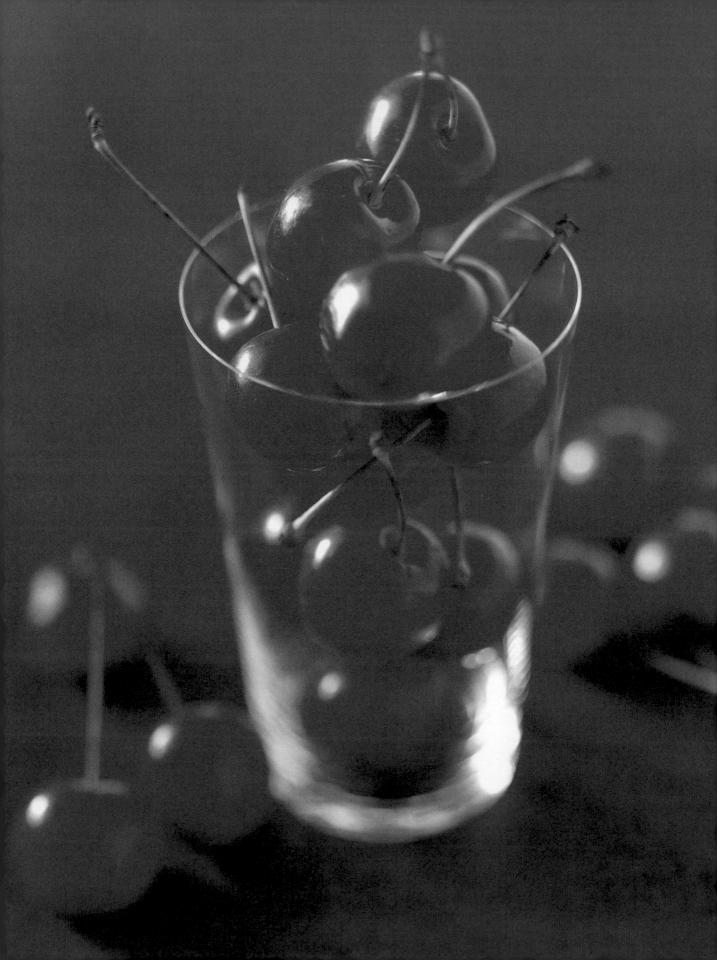

cherries

Sweet, juicy, and tantalizingly tart, cherries contain a number of healthful phytonutrients that may help decrease inflammation, lower blood pressure, improve arthritis pain, and promote better sleep.

what's in it

anthocyanins These plant pigments may reduce LDL ("bad") cholesterol oxidation and help prevent heart disease.

chlorogenic acid This phenolic compound may help thwart carcinogenic environmental toxins such as nitrosamines in cigarette smoke.

cyanidin A type of anthocyanin found in cherries, this compound may inhibit inflammatory enzymes.

perillyl alcohol Research suggests that perillyl alcohol reduces pancreatic, breast, liver, and lung tumors and may cause cell death in tumor cells without harming healthy cells.

quercetin A much-studied flavonoid, quercetin is known to protect body tissues from drug toxicity. Studies also link quercetin to a reduced risk for coronary artery disease and certain types of cancer. Cherries are believed to contain impressive amounts of quercetin.

rutin Rutin enhances the activity of vitamin C and helps in the production of collagen and maintenance of healthy veins and capillaries.

maximizing the benefits

Some studies involving natural, non-drug interventions have found that tart cherry juice (as well as acupressure, acupuncture, and mindfulness-based stress reduction) can help enhance sleep quality.

add more to your diet

▶ Chop cherries and combine with scallions, green bell pepper, and celery. Toss in a spicy dressing and use as a salsa to serve with sandwiches or salads.

▶ Add chopped cherries to your favorite brownie, cake, or cookie recipe.

▶ Add halved or chopped cherries to a savory stir-fry, stew, curry, or soup.

▶ Freeze cherry juice in ice-cube trays. Combine these cubes with more cherry juice, cherries, and plant-based yogurt in a blender, and puree to make a smoothie.

▶ Use cherry juice in place of red wine in savory sauces.

▶ Use dried cherries in place of raisins.

health bites

Although there is scant scientific evidence to support what many people believe, that cherries and cherry juice can relieve the pain of gout, some research suggests that a substance in cherries called cyanidin has anti-inflammatory properties that might help reduce the swelling and pain of this condition.

citrus fruits

Far from lightweights when it comes to nutritional power, citrus fruits have an abundance of vitamin C, potassium, pectin, and phytonutrients that may benefit numerous conditions, including allergies, asthma, cancer, cataracts, heart disease, stroke, and the common cold.

add more to your diet

▶ After juicing citrus fruits, pop the empty "shells" into the freezer and you'll have zest when a recipe calls for it.

▶ Combine orange or tangerine juice with seltzer for a healthy soda.

▶ Add grated orange or lemon zest to tea bread and cookie recipes.

▶ Substitute citrus juice for vinegar in your favorite salad dressing.

▶ Stir a healthy amount of lemon juice and honey into tea for a soothing drink.

▶ Add orange, tangerine, or grapefruit segments to a green salad.

▶ Sprinkle grapefruit halves with brown sugar and broil for a quick dessert.

▶ For a tropical fruit salad: Toss sliced bananas, strawberries, kiwifruit, and mango in orange juice.

▶ Segment oranges and add to green salads.

what's in it

beta-cryptoxanthin A carotenoid in oranges and tangerines, beta-cryptoxanthin may help prevent colon cancer.

folate This B vitamin is instrumental in the prevention of certain birth defects, and may also play a role in battling heart disease.

hesperidin This flavonoid is found in the zest (the thin, colored portion of the citrus peel) of oranges. Hesperidin may have anti-inflammatory and cholesterol-lowering effects.

limonene Found mainly in the zest of lemons, limes, and tangerines, limonene may help block cancer-causing chemicals.

naringin A flavonoid found in white grapefruit, this compound may protect the lungs against environmental toxins such as air pollution and cigarette smoke.

nobiletin This flavonoid, found in the flesh of oranges, may have anti-inflammatory actions.

tangeretin This flavonoid, found in tangerines, has been linked in experimental studies to a reduced growth of tumor cells in lung, breast, and prostate cancers.

maximizing the benefits

Don't spend too much time removing the pith (the spongy white layer between the zest and the pulp), because a good amount of the fiber and phytonutrients, particularly the flavonoids, is found in both the pulp and the pith. Freshly squeezed citrus juice also has more nutrients than frozen or bottled juices.

health bites

Compounds in grapefruit and grapefruit juice can interfere with the way some medications work, leading to dangerous side effects. If you are taking medication for cholesterol, high blood pressure, anxiety, Crohn's disease, heart conditions, or allergies, ask your physician if you should be avoiding grapefruit.

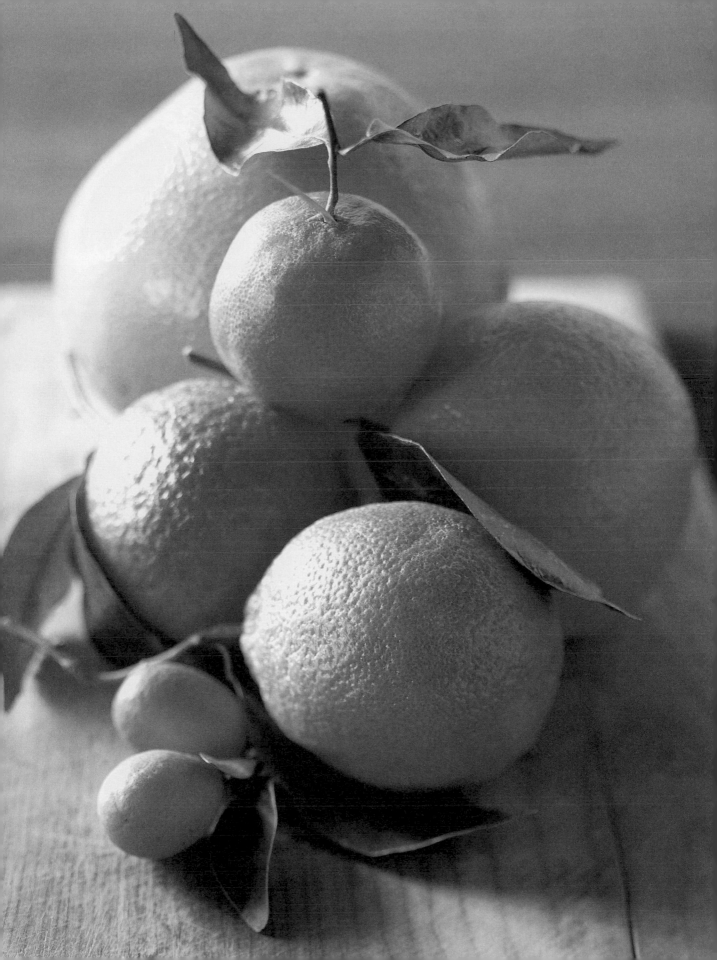

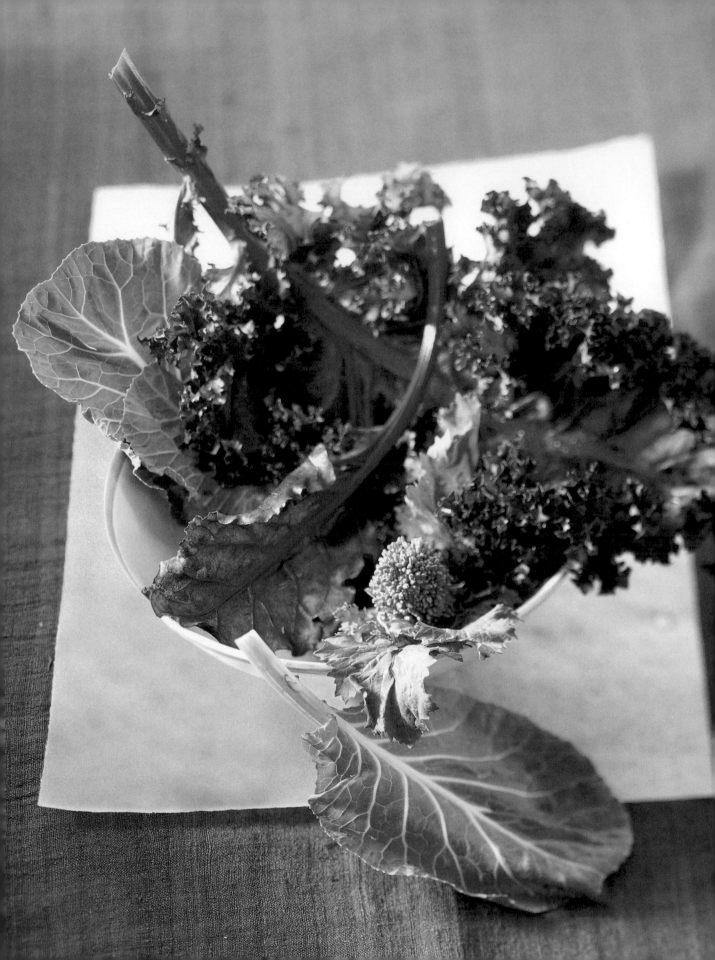

cooking greens

Cooking greens—kale and Swiss chard, and collard, beet, turnip, and mustard greens—are packed with vitamins, minerals, fiber, and an array of phytonutrients that may reduce heart disease risk, eye diseases, and certain cancers.

what's in it

beta-carotene Greens are rich sources of this antioxidant, which may help strengthen the body's defense system against harmful free-radical compounds. Kale has the most beta-carotene of all cooking greens.

calcium Although this mineral is found in greens, some greens, such as Swiss chard and beet greens, contain compounds called oxalates, which prevent calcium from being properly absorbed. If you are prone to kidney stones or gout, avoid foods high in oxalates.

chlorophyll This plant pigment may help to block the damaging changes that convert healthy cells to precancerous cells.

folate Cooking greens are a good source of this important B vitamin, which helps to ward off certain birth defects, cancer, and heart disease. Collards and turnip greens are the best for folate content.

indoles Indoles are thought to help protect against the risk for hormone-related cancers by blocking the action of estrogen.

isothiocyanates Partially responsible for the pungency of some leafy greens, these phytonutrients are thought to help protect against hormone-dependent cancers. These compounds are also believed to inhibit environmental carcinogens.

lutein and zeaxanthin These carotenoids are linked to the prevention of macular degeneration. Kale is an extremely rich source of these phytonutrients; collard greens are also a good source.

sulforaphane This phytonutrient may help prevent harmful carcinogens from initiating cancer.

vitamin K Found in huge amounts in cooking greens, this nutrient helps build bone, but can interfere with the effectiveness of blood-thinning medications.

maximizing the benefits

To enhance the bioavailability of **beta-carotene** in cooking greens, cook them with a small amount of olive oil. If you do cook greens in water, which can diminish **folate** levels, try to use the cooking water in the recipe or add it to a green smoothie.

add more to your diet

► Combine chopped sautéed kale with mashed firm tofu and nutritional yeast to use as a filling for lasagna or manicotti.

► Make a green bruschetta: Finely chop cooking greens and sauté with garlic in olive oil until melt-in-your-mouth tender. Use as a topping for thick slices of toasted Italian bread.

► Cook assorted greens in seasoned water with some olive oil and eat both the greens and their cooking liquid over slabs of cornbread.

► Chop and steam cooking greens, then fold into garlicky mashed potatoes.

► Stir finely chopped, cooked greens, such as Swiss chard, spinach, or kale, into grain dishes such as risotto, rice pilaf, quinoa sauté, or pasta or farro salad.

► Add chopped, cooked greens to your favorite lentil loaf mixture.

corn

A good source of complex carbohydrates, fiber, and thiamin, corn is a low-fat, high complex-carbohydrate food that provides abundant energy and may help to fight type 2 diabetes, heart disease, certain cancers, macular degeneration, and obesity.

add more to your diet

➤ Boost both the flavor and the health benefits of your next batch of cornbread by adding corn kernels to the batter.

➤ Season corn-on-the-cob with lime juice instead of butter.

➤ Combine corn kernels with chopped scallions, red bell pepper, hot pepper sauce, and lime juice, and use as a quick salsa for tacos or wraps.

➤ Serve an Italian-style polenta (made from cornmeal) as a side dish in place of rice or pasta.

➤ Add cornmeal to pancake batters, tea breads, and biscuits.

➤ For an interesting take on the Spanish soup gazpacho, substitute corn kernels for the cucumbers that most recipes call for, and stir in a generous amount of chopped cilantro.

what's in it

folate This B vitamin has been found to prevent neural tube birth defects in fetuses, and current research suggests that it also helps to reduce the risk for heart disease and cancer.

lutein and zeaxanthin Lutein and zeaxanthin are carotenoids that may help to prevent certain eye conditions such as age-related macular degeneration, one of the leading causes of blindness in older adults. Corn is especially high in lutein.

protease inhibitors These compounds may help to fight cancerous tumors by stopping the division of proteins that signal uncontrolled cell growth (tumorigenesis).

soluble fiber This type of fiber may help to lower cholesterol by binding with it and blocking its absorption. And if you are trying to lose weight, it is always helpful to consume high-fiber foods because they increase bulk and make you feel full sooner and for longer.

thiamin This B vitamin is required by the body for converting food to energy; a thiamin deficiency can result in fatigue. Thiamin is also essential for proper functioning of the nervous system.

maximizing the benefits

To preserve the water-soluble B vitamins in corn (**folate** and **thiamin**), it's best to steam rather than boil it. If this isn't practical, then be sure to cook for no longer than 10 minutes in boiling water to minimize nutrient loss.

health bites

One study showed that high blood levels of lutein and zeaxanthin are associated with better test scores on cognition, memory, and executive function in adults age 50 and older.

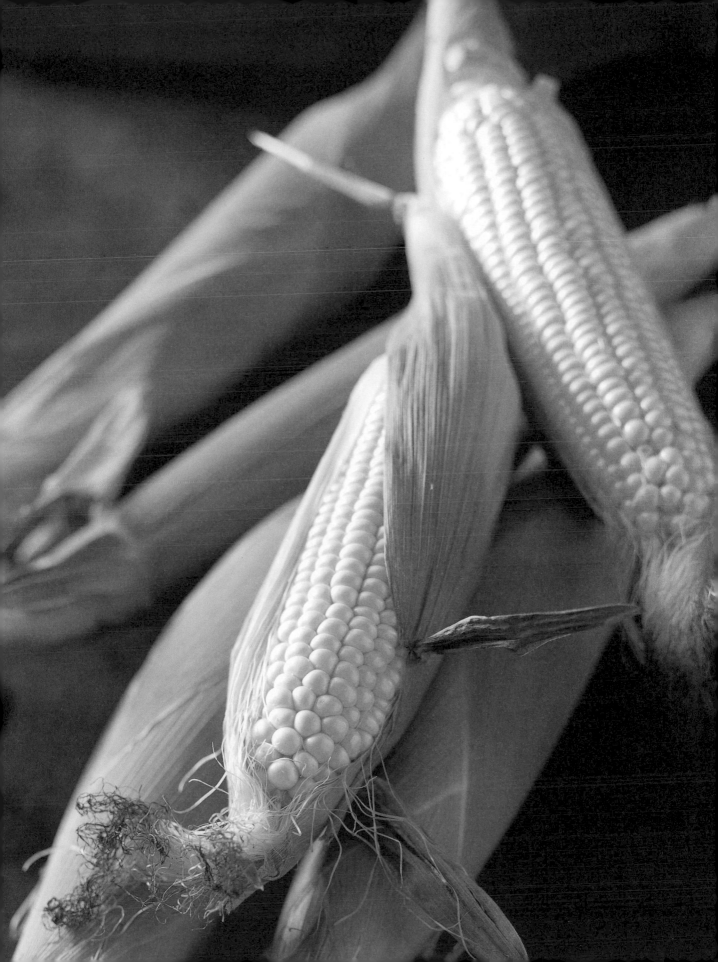

figs

The nutrients and phytonutrients in figs may help treat and prevent such ailments as cardiovascular disease, premenstrual syndrome, and hemorrhoids. Figs are especially rich in minerals, fiber, and phytonutrients.

add more to your diet

▶ Serve fresh figs with plant-based soft cheese and thin slices of prosciutto as an appetizer.

▶ Chop dried figs and add to granola.

▶ Poach dried figs in red wine sweetened with honey, and serve alongside vegetable dishes.

▶ Make a pasta salad with diced fresh figs, toasted pecans, and cooked pasta, and dress with a red wine vinaigrette.

▶ Cook dried figs in water until very tender. Puree with some of the cooking liquid and use as an all-fruit spread.

▶ Dice dried figs and add to cookie dough in place of raisins.

▶ Sauté sliced red onion in olive oil until just tender, add quartered figs, balsamic vinegar, and thyme leaves and cook until tender.

what's in it

fiber Figs are an excellent source of both insoluble and soluble fiber. Insoluble fiber may help to prevent constipation, diverticulosis, and hemorrhoids. The soluble pectin fiber in figs may help to lower blood cholesterol.

ficin An enzyme unique to figs, ficin has mild laxative properties that add to the fruit's ability to relieve constipation.

plant sterols These plant compounds may lower LDL ("bad") cholesterol and reduce the risk for heart disease.

polyphenols According to research, dried figs have up to 50 times more polyphenols than most other commonly consumed fruits and vegetables. Polyphenols neutralize damaging free radicals and help to prevent chronic disease.

potassium A diet rich in this powerful mineral may help to lower blood pressure and the risk for heart attacks and strokes.

vitamin B$_6$ This B vitamin may improve cardiovascular health and premenstrual syndrome (PMS). Fresh figs, in particular, are a good source.

maximizing the benefits

Fresh figs spoil quickly and should be consumed within a week of being picked. Dried figs, on the other hand, store well. And, because their water content is lower, dried figs are, ounce for ounce, more nutrient-dense than fresh. But remember, dried figs are more concentrated sources of sugar and calories.

health bites

Figs possess the highest overall mineral content of any of the most common fruits, providing significant quantities of bone-building, blood-nourishing, and cardioprotective minerals—calcium, iron, magnesium, manganese, and potassium.

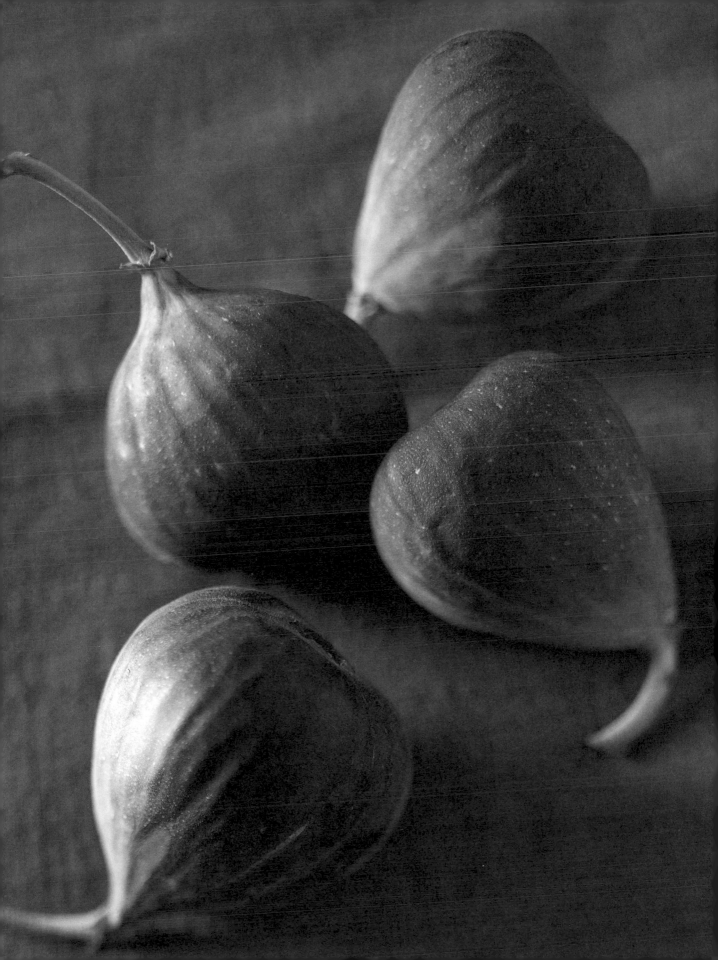

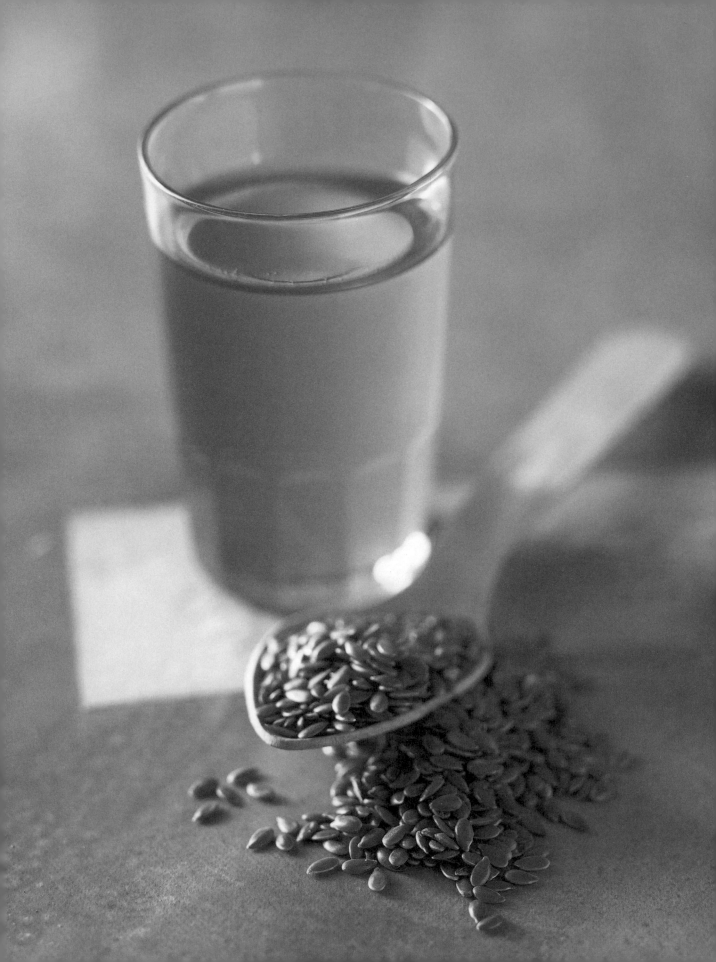

flaxseeds

The many merits of flaxseeds (and flaxseed oil) have propelled this ancient seed, which was cultivated as early as 4000 B.C., into the nutritional spotlight. Flaxseeds are being studied for the prevention or management of numerous conditions.

what's in it

alpha-linolenic acid (ALA) Because our bodies cannot manufacture this essential fatty acid, we must consume it in foods. Important for regulating blood pressure and for cell membrane health, ALA may have a wide range of beneficial health effects, including the ability to prevent heart disease by reducing the production of hormonelike substances that lead to blood clotting. ALA makes flaxseed oil healthful, though it should be noted that fiber and lignans are lost when the flaxseeds are processed into oil.

insoluble fiber This type of fiber keeps your digestive system running smoothly and helps to prevent constipation.

lignans Also referred to as phytoestrogens, lignans have mild estrogenic properties. Lignans may also play a protective role against autoimmune disorders such as systemic lupus erythematosus, rheumatoid arthritis, as well as fibrocystic breasts and some hormone-related cancers (breast, endometrial, and prostate).

soluble fiber The soluble fiber in flaxseeds forms a gel in the intestine, helping to trap and usher out harmful LDL ("bad") cholesterol particles.

maximizing the benefits

To get the most out of flaxseeds, they must be ground or they simply pass through the body, and you don't reap their health benefits. In addition, don't heat flaxseed oil—this will destroy its alpha-linolenic content as well as make the oil taste unpleasant.

add more to your diet

▶ Ground flaxseeds are easier to use and available in supermarkets but will become rancid faster than whole seeds. To prevent this, store them in the freezer. Or purchase whole seeds and grind them just before use in a mini-food processor or coffee grinder.-

▶ Use ground flaxseeds to replace one-fourth of the flour in pancake or waffle batter.

▶ Add ground flaxseeds to cookie, muffins, and quick breads.

▶ Make a pesto with fresh basil, garlic, ground flaxseeds (in place of nuts), flaxseed oil, and nutritional yeast. Toss with hot pasta.

▶ Grind flaxseeds and add to your cold cereal or stir into hot oatmeal.

▶ Make a plant-based egg substitute for baking and cooking by combining 1 tablespoon ground flaxseeds with 3 tablespoons water per egg and allow to stand for 5 minutes to thicken. Add to recipes in place of the eggs.

health bites

Adding flaxseeds to your diet may help to ward off heart disease and diabetes. Studies have also shown that flaxseed may help prevent and control complications associated with the progression of type 2 diabetes.

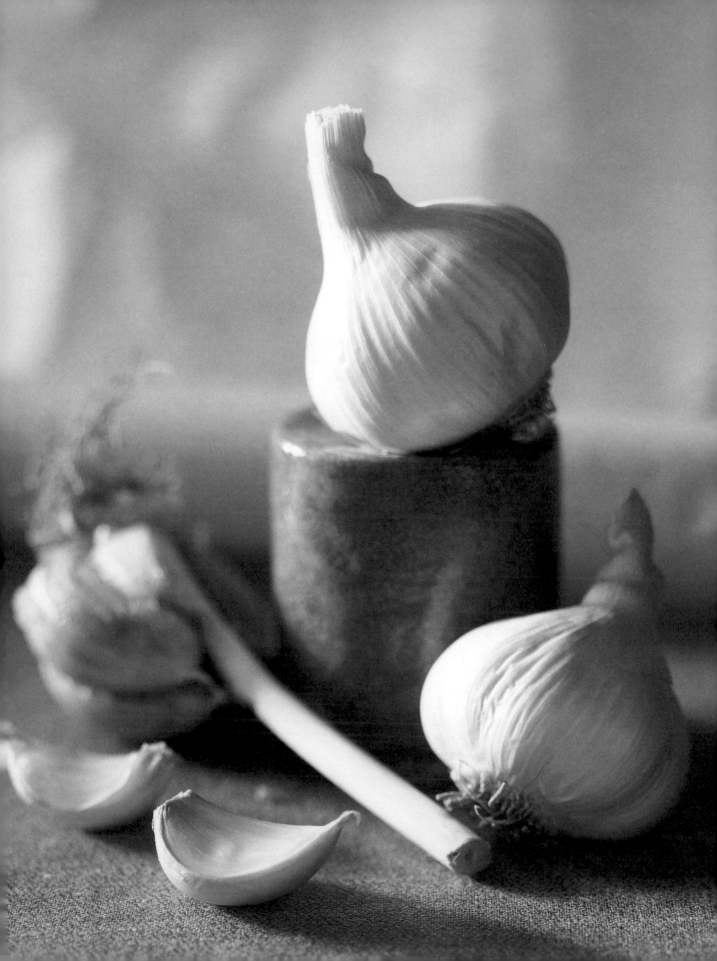

garlic

The medicinal application of garlic goes back as far as 1500 B.C., when the ancient Egyptians recommended it for a host of ailments, including heart disease, wounds, tumors, parasites, and headaches—some of the benefits modern science has also attributed to garlic.

what's in it

ajoenes Ajoenes may be responsible for garlic's antithrombotic (anticlotting) actions, and possibly may have antifungal activity.

allicin Allicin has antibacterial properties (it is also responsible for garlic's pungent smell) and is released when garlic is crushed or cut, producing numerous sulfur compounds.

allyl sulfides Believed to inhibit tumor growth, these sulfur compounds block the damaging effects of carcinogens and promote cancer cell apoptosis (cell death).

sulfur compounds These compounds, including ajoenes and allyl sulfides, may possess anticarcinogenic, anticlotting, antifungal, and antioxidant effects. Sulfur compounds also promote the activity of glutathione, a substance that may inhibit carcinogens.

maximizing the benefits

To activate garlic's full nutritional power, after chopping or crushing it, let the garlic stand for 10 minutes before cooking it. The brief standing period allows allicin and its potent derivatives to be activated.

add more to your diet

▶ Finely mince several cloves of garlic and stir into plant-based yogurt or sour cream. Serve as a dip for crudités.

▶ Roast whole, unpeeled cloves of garlic in olive oil. The garlic will get soft and creamy and can be spread on bread.

▶ Make a garlic-walnut sauce for pasta: Combine equal amounts of peeled garlic cloves and walnuts, a little olive oil, and fresh lemon juice, and puree until smooth. Toss with hot pasta.

▶ For appetizer nuts: Mince garlic, sauté in olive oil, and toss with toasted walnuts and almonds. Sprinkle with a bit of salt.

▶ In a blender, puree garlic, plant-based yogurt, and fresh cilantro for a savory drink.

▶ Chop garlic and stir into bread, biscuits, or potato pancakes. Or try it in corn muffins, and serve with savory soups and stews.

health bites

What's all the stink about? When garlic is digested, a portion of the sulfur compounds enters the bloodstream and is subsequently exhaled from the lungs or eliminated through the pores when we sweat. This is the price we pay to reap the benefits of the "stinking rose." And since the human nose can detect less than one part of these sulfur compounds in one billion parts of exhaled air, it's no wonder that garlic breath is so noticeable. Eating parsley might help to reduce these unpleasant odors, possibly because of its chlorophyll.

grapes

Nature's jewels, grapes contain phytonutrients that may help to reduce risk for heart disease, cancer, diabetes, and strokes. Studies also indicate that in addition to grapes, red wine, grape juice, and raisins are also rich in disease-fighting compounds.

add more to your diet

▶ Make roasted grapes by tossing grapes with a drizzle of olive oil and bake in a 400°F oven for 10 minutes, or until tender.

▶ Chop red grapes and combine with honey, fresh lemon juice, chopped red onion, and minced parsley, and use as a relish.

▶ Cook dried fruits such as apricots and raisins in purple grape juice until tender, then puree and use as an all-fruit spread.

▶ Prepare hot mulled grape juice or wine: Add cinnamon sticks, whole cloves, allspice berries, and whole black peppercorns to grape juice and cook over low heat until warm and fragrant.

▶ Finely chop grapes and toasted walnuts, stir into mashed tofu or plant-based soft cheese, and spread over flour tortillas. Add watercress and roll up for a sandwich wrap.

what's in it

anthocyanins Laboratory studies suggest that these pigments in red and purple grapes may suppress the growth of tumor cells.

ellagic acid This phenolic acid in grapes (and other berries) is thought to protect the lungs against environmental toxins.

flavonoids Grapes contain high levels of these heart-healthy antioxidant pigments, which may have the ability to prevent blood from clotting. Both red and purple grape juice are rich in flavonoids, which may help to prevent LDL ("bad") cholesterol from attaching to artery walls and creating blockages that can lead to heart attacks.

pectin This soluble fiber may help to lower LDL cholesterol.

quercetin A flavonoid linked to a reduced risk for cancer development, quercetin may also reduce clotting in blood vessels, and offer relief to people with respiratory ailments.

resveratrol This phytonutrient, found in the skin of grapes, has been linked to the ability to fight cancer, prevent strokes, lower cholesterol, and help manage diabetes and neurological disorders.

maximizing the benefits

To reap the full benefits of grapes, it is best to select red or purple varieties, which seem to contain the highest concentrations of healthful compounds.

health bites

Though the French eat a high-fat diet, they have a low incidence of heart disease, a phenomenon linked to resveratrol in red wine and described in 1992 as the "French Paradox." Since then, researchers have expanded their interest in resveratrol's protective effect on the cardiovascular system to benefit such conditions as obesity, non-alcoholic fatty liver, and neurological conditions.

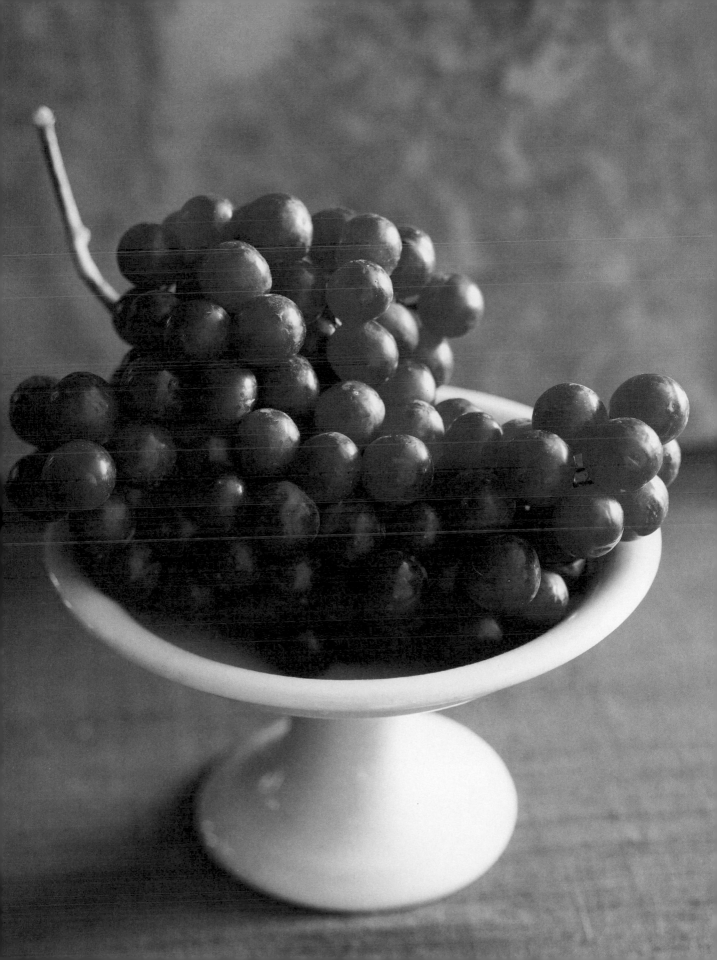

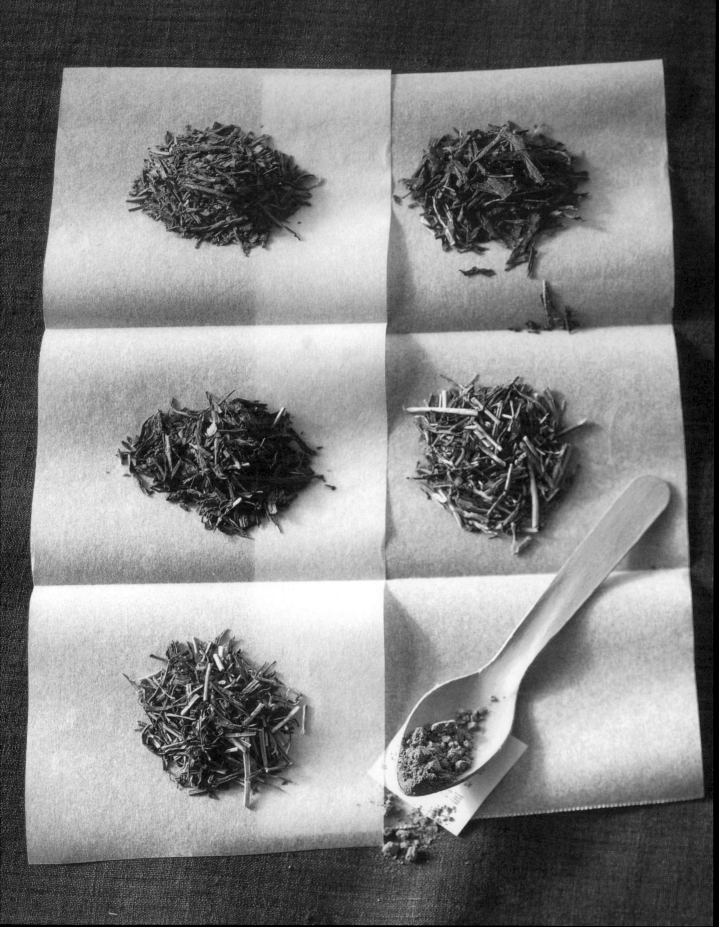

green tea

The healing powers of green tea have been valued in Asia for thousands of years. In the West, research suggests that drinking green tea may help to prevent cancer and cardiovascular disease, and support oral health.

what's in it

epigallocatechin gallate (EGCG) One of a class of flavonoids called catechins, EGCG is believed to be the most potent compound in green tea. With the purported capacity to fight cancer at all stages, EGCG may have (1) antioxidant power to seek out and destroy harmful free radicals, (2) the ability to inhibit an enzyme needed for the growth of cancer cells, and (3) a capacity to induce apoptosis (cell death) in cancer cells without damaging healthy cells. Researchers are also currently examining EGCG's potential role in reducing LDL ("bad") cholesterol.

maximizing the benefits

The level of protective catechins from freshly brewed green tea bags is higher than that of green tea extracts and ready-to-drink green tea beverages.

add more to your diet

▶ Brew green tea, sweeten with honey, chill, and serve over ice.

▶ Stir 1 teaspoon matcha into vinaigrette before dressing salads.

▶ Steep green tea leaves in warm dairy-free milk for 30 minutes, or until full-flavored. Use the milk in sweet puddings, cake recipes, soups, or pancake and waffle batter. Or use it in green smoothies or oatmeal.

▶ Make cubes of iced green tea and use to cool lemonade.

▶ Brew a pot of green tea and use it as the base for a vegetable soup or broth. Or, add to marinades.

health bites

Matcha (powdered green tea leaves) is a concentrated source of antioxidants that can be used to make tea and is also easily added to smoothies, baked goods, and other foods. Studies show that matcha tea provides at least three times the amount of EGCG in regular green tea.

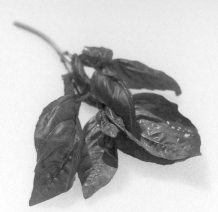

herbs

dill weed

A relative of fennel, wispy green dill weed is available both fresh and dried.

what's in it
Dill contains carvone, coumarins, flavonoids, limonene, and phthalides. Studies suggest that carvone and limonene have the potential to inhibit tumors, and flavonoids may neutralize harmful free radicals. Coumarins and phthalides show promise in stimulating cancer-fighting enzymes in the body.

add more to your diet
Use in: salads and salad dressings; creamy mustard sauces; muffins and savory turnovers. Matches well with potatoes and green beans.

basil

Fresh or dried basil is teeming with powerful antioxidants, responsible for basil's unique flavor.

what's in it
Flavonoid and terpene phytonutrients in basil are studied for their potential benefit in reducing total and harmful LDL cholesterol, as well as suppressing tumor growth.

add more to your diet
Use in: homemade pasta, pizza, and bread doughs; savory soups and stews; tomato sauces and pesto sauce; pilafs, risottos, and other grain dishes; and mashed potatoes. Use as whole leaves in salads and wraps.

horseradish

This pungent root is a member of the mighty cruciferous family, which includes broccoli, cabbage, and watercress.

what's in it
Horseradish's bite comes from a powerful substance called allyl isothiocyanate, which may alleviate congestion and respiratory inflammation, and possibly protect against foodborne pathogens. Kaempferol, also in horseradish, is believed to detoxify cancerous agents.

add more to your diet
Use in: salad dressings; creamy sauces, vegetable dips, and spreads; stirred into grain dishes or mashed potatoes; and potato salads.

cilantro

Cilantro's bold, distinctive taste is popular in Chinese, Indian, and Mexican cuisines. Fresh cilantro is far more flavorful than dried cilantro.

what's in it
Coumarin, phthalide, polyactylene, and terpene phytonutrients in cilantro are thought to stimulate anticancer enzymes in the body.

add more to your diet
Use in: salsas, relishes, condiments, and chutneys; pesto and other pasta sauces; rice, grain, bean, corn, and tomato salads; peach, pineapple, mango, plum, and papaya desserts; savory pancakes and carrot muffins.

mint

Fresh or dried peppermint and spearmint add a refreshing zest to any dish.

what's in it
Mint has traditionally been used to relieve abdominal pains, bad breath, and sore throats. Powerful terpene phytonutrients present in the mint family—carvone, limonene, menthol, and perillyl alcohol—may inhibit tumor growth.

add more to your diet
Use in: teas and drinks; plant-based yogurt or cheese sauces and spreads; sautéed vegetables; vinaigrettes; pasta sauces; fruit salads; and poached fruit.

oregano/marjoram

Quintessential Italian herbs, oregano and marjoram are similar in aroma and taste, as well as disease-fighting antioxidant power.

what's in it

Research suggests that quercetin and galangin, two antioxidant flavonoids in oregano, may inhibit the initial development of cancer in cells. Terpene compounds in both marjoram and oregano show promise in elevating levels of cancer-protective enzymes in the body.

add more to your diet

Use in: herb rubs and marinades; chili, pasta sauces, and soups. Matches well with mushrooms, potatoes, and summer squash.

parsley

A relative of the carrot, parsley is one of the most versatile and widely available fresh herbs. Choose flat-leaf (not curly) parsley for the best flavor, and avoid dried parsley altogether.

what's in it

Flavonoid, coumarin, and terpene phytonutrients in parsley are powerful antioxidants that are thought to stimulate the immune system and block cancer-causing substances. Parsley's high chlorophyll content may explain its use as a breath freshener.

add more to your diet

Use in: stuffings, grain, and rice dishes; soups and stews; salads; and pasta dishes.

rosemary

The distinctive taste of rosemary is faintly piney. It's available fresh and dried.

what's in it

Rosemary is rich in such anticancer compounds as carnosol, rosmanol, and a variety of flavonoids. Carnosol may be particularly effective as an antitumor agent. Additional anticancer substances in rosemary also show promise in blocking tumor growth.

add more to your diet

Use in: pizza and bread doughs; roasted vegetables especially winter squash and potatoes; and soups and stews.

sage

The bold, faintly earthy flavor of sage is a customary holiday seasoning. Sage is available as fresh whole leaves, or dried or "rubbed" leaves.

what's in it

Powerful anticancer terpene substances in sage may also lower heart disease risk. Studies suggest that cineole and perillyl alcohol (terpene compounds) may suppress tumor growth. A flavonoid, luteolin, shows promise in preventing the spread of cancer cells.

add more to your diet

Use in: roasted or mashed potatoes; homemade pizza, pasta, and bread doughs; grilled vegetables, sauces, and marinades.

tarragon

The bold, satisfying flavor of this fine French herb is often used to flavor vinegar and béarnaise sauce.

what's in it

Tarragon contains cancer-protective terpene phytonutrients that may interfere with tumor growth and help to stimulate cancer-protective enzymes in the body.

add more to your diet

Use in: beans and grain dishes; homemade vinegars, mustards, and relishes; poached and stewed fruit; sandwich and plant-based spreads. It matches well with carrots, artichoke, eggplant, and peas.

thyme

Fresh or dried thyme leaves are popular in French, Cajun, and Creole cuisines.

what's in it

Terpene compounds—cineole, limonene, and pinene—may suppress tumor growth and increase the body's production of protective anticancer enzymes. The flavonoid luteolin, common to peppermint, sage, and thyme, has shown promise in blocking cancerous changes in cells.

add more to your diet

Use in: soups, stews, and chowders. Matches well with roasted and steamed vegetables.

kiwifruit

This fuzzy, egg-shaped fruit, in addition to providing spectacular amounts of vitamin C, is richly endowed with phytonutrients that help to boost your immune system and may stave off age-related eye and other medical conditions.

add more to your diet

▶ For a healthful and delicious drink, combine peeled kiwifruit and lime juice in a blender and puree. Add seltzer and ice.

▶ Make a savory kiwifruit side dish: Combine kiwi wedges with cucumber, red bell pepper, and a little olive oil.

▶ Slice kiwifruit and serve in a salad with cucumbers, tomatoes, and romaine lettuce. Toss with balsamic vinaigrette.

▶ Boost a store-bought tomato salsa with chopped kiwifruit. Serve as a dip or as a spicy condiment for tacos, chips, or burritos.

what's in it

actinidin This enzyme is believed to aid digestion by helping to activate natural digestive reactions.

chlorogenic acid This compound is an antioxidant with the potential to prevent development of cancerous tumors.

chlorophyll Though not much is known about chlorophyll's health benefits, it is currently under review for its potential to block the absorption of cancer-causing substances in the body.

fiber Pectin is a type of soluble fiber that protects against heart disease and diabetes, while insoluble fiber keeps the digestive tract running smoothly and prevents constipation.

lutein This important carotenoid may possibly reduce the risk for colon cancer, cataracts, and age-related macular degeneration.

potassium Kiwifruit is an excellent source of potassium, a mineral that helps the heart work more efficiently, and plays a key role in controlling blood pressure.

vitamin C Kiwifruit is an exceptional source of this important vitamin, which functions as a powerful antioxidant. Vitamin C is believed to reduce the symptons and severity of the common cold and protect against heart disease. It also helps to build and repair the immune system and may protect against certain types of cancer. The antioxidant power of vitamin C is also thought to help prevent cataracts.

maximizing the benefits

To preserve the **vitamin C** content in kiwifruit, it is best to eat the fruit uncooked.

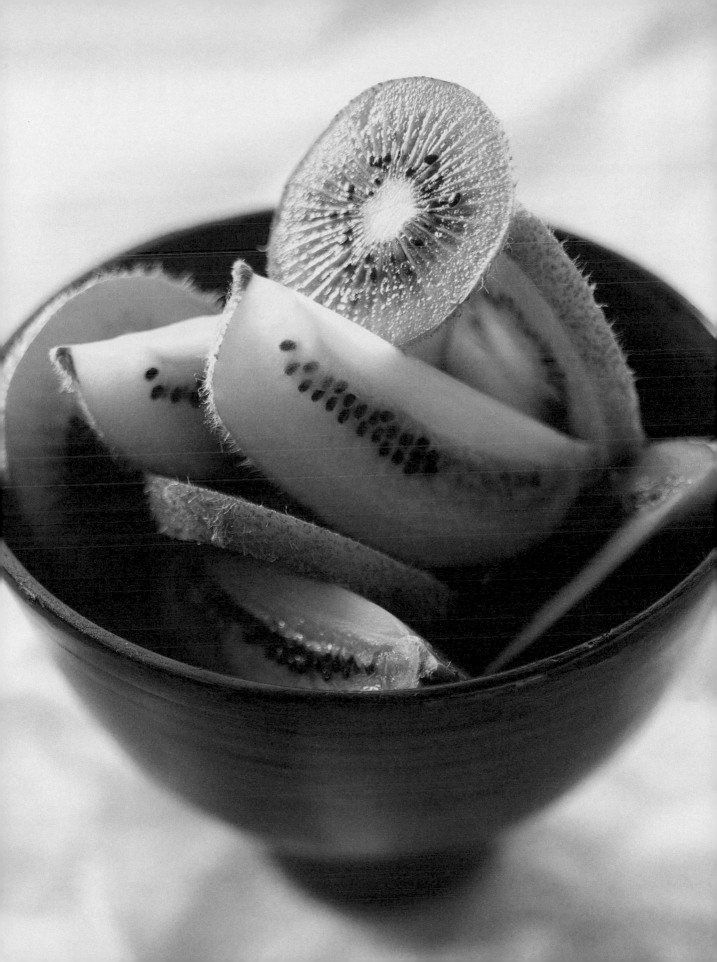

lentils

These low-fat, protein-rich legumes offer substantial phytonutrient power, folate, and an impressive amount of fiber, more than a quarter of which is the heart-healthy soluble type. They also have decent amounts of iron and calcium.

add more to your diet

▶ Cook lentils, puree along with garlic, tofu, and fresh lemon juice, and use as a dip or spread.

▶ Stir cooked lentils into pancake batter along with a touch of curry powder for an Indian-style main course.

▶ Mash cooked seasoned lentils; add sautéed onion and garlic, a flaxseed "egg" (see page 71), and enough bread crumbs to form into patties. Brown in a skillet until heated through or grill over low heat.

▶ Toss cooked lentils in a lemony dressing along with cherry tomatoes and diced red bell pepper.

▶ Make a lentil soup using carrot juice instead of water for the base.

▶ Add cooked lentils to pasta sauce.

▶ Stir cooked lentils into salads or Buddha-type bowls.

what's in it

fiber Lentils are rich in insoluble fiber, which may stave off hunger and alleviate constipation. The soluble pectin and gum fiber in lentils helps to lower cholesterol and stabilize blood sugar.

folate A half cup of cooked lentils provides almost half of the daily requirement for this B vitamin, which may be instrumental in preventing birth defects, cancer, and heart disease.

iron Most lentils are good sources of this mineral, which is vital for immunity, healthy pregnancy, and anemia prevention.

isoflavones These phytoestrogens may lower the risk for heart disease and manage some of the symptoms of perimenopause and menopause.

plant sterols Similar in structure to cholesterol, these compounds help reduce blood cholesterol levels by competing with dietary and body-synthesized cholesterol for absorption.

protease inhibitors Found in lentils (and other legumes), these plant chemicals may inhibit tumor growth by short-circuiting processes necessary for cancer cell survival.

saponins Plentiful in lentils, saponins may prevent cardiovascular disease by binding cholesterol before it is absorbed. Laboratory studies suggest that these phytonutrients may also inhibit cancer by increasing the number of natural killer immune cells, and by blocking cancerous changes in cells.

tyrosine kinase inhibitors These compounds may work with fiber to stabilize blood sugar levels. Preliminary studies suggest that tyrosine kinase inhibitors may lower levels of a chemical in the blood that contributes to premature cardiovascular disease in people with diabetes.

maximizing the benefits

Eat foods high in **vitamin C** along with lentils to enhance **iron** absorption. To protect the **B vitamin** content, do not cook lentils in too much water, and if there is any cooking liquid that needs to be drained off, try to use it in the recipe or save for soups or other dishes. **Soluble fiber** in lentils is made available as the lentils cook and the fiber dissolves (this also softens the lentils).

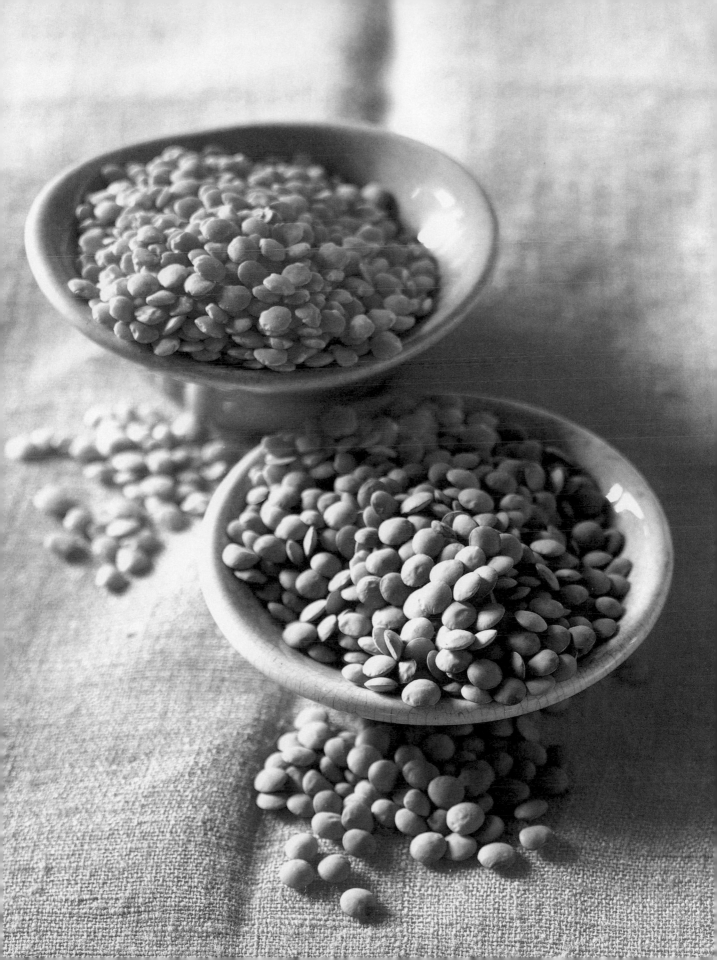

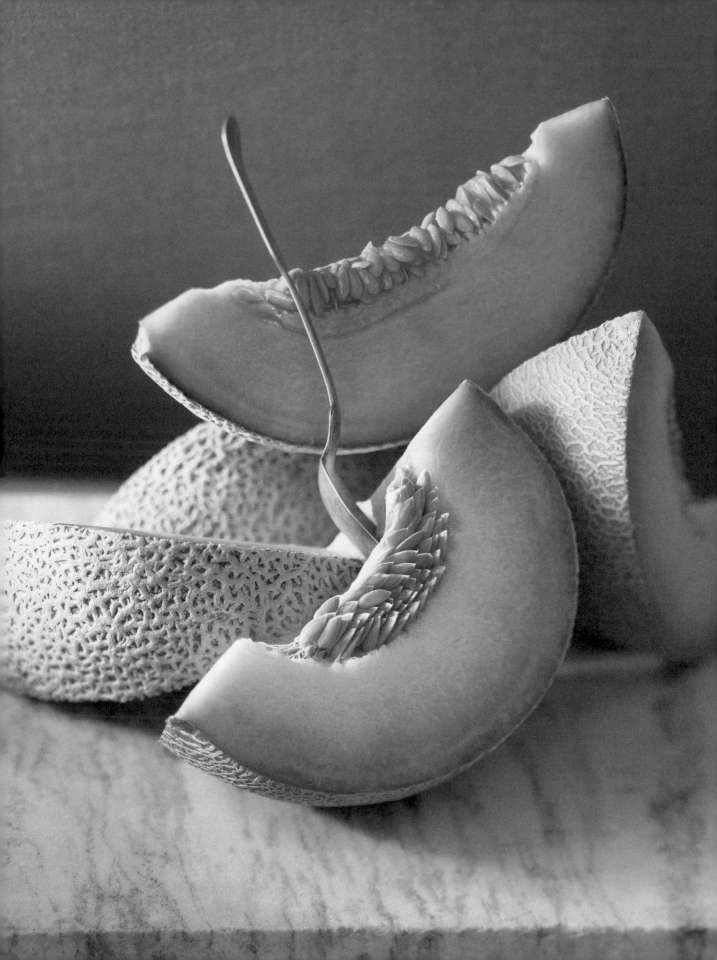

melons

The subtle scent of these fragrant fruits belies the muscularity of their nutritional powers. Melons—from cantaloupe to watermelon—may help prevent acne, cardiovascular disease, certain cancers, respiratory illness, and vision loss.

what's in it

beta-carotene Because of its orange hue, cantaloupe is the best melon source of this healthful orange-yellow pigment, which may protect against acne, certain forms of cancer, and vision loss.

lycopene Studies link a lycopene-rich diet with a low risk for heart disease and cancer, particularly prostate cancer. Watermelon is a particularly good source of this antioxidant pigment, which lends reddish color to watermelon flesh.

pectin The soluble pectin fiber in melons helps to lower cholesterol.

potassium Cantaloupe and honeydew are especially good melon sources of this vital mineral, which is linked to lower blood pressure and a reduced incidence of heart disease and stroke.

vitamin C Melon is a good source of this antioxidant vitamin, which may enhance the immune system and may be beneficial for respiratory infections. Cantaloupe and honeydew are particularly high in vitamin C.

zeaxanthin A vital component in the retina of the eye, this carotenoid helps to shield against damaging ultraviolet radiation, protecting against vision loss. Honeydew is the best melon source of zeaxanthin.

maximizing the benefits

To best preserve nutrient content, buy melons whole (some markets offer halves, quarters, or cubes). Certain nutrients, especially **vitamin C,** are diminished by exposure to the air.

add more to your diet

▶ Serve watermelon wedges with slices of smoked tofu.

▶ Puree honeydew with fresh lime juice, honey, and mint, and chill. Serve as a dessert soup.

▶ Make a salad with cut-up plum tomatoes, cantaloupe, and sliced red onion, and toss with a balsamic vinaigrette.

▶ Freeze chunks of assorted melon, then puree to make a sorbet.

▶ Make a fresh melon salsa with cantaloupe or honeydew, chopped fresh basil, lemon or lime juice, and pickled jalapeños. Serve with salads, tacos, and sandwiches.

▶ Add small chunks of cantaloupe to tomato sauces.

▶ Garnish hot tomato soup with a chilled, diced cantaloupe or honeydew.

health bites

An excellent choice for weight loss, these nutrient-dense (and water-dense) fruits average 50 calories per cup of cubes and provide ample fiber and just enough sweetness to satisfy the appetite.

mushrooms

The mushroom's ancient tradition as a healing food continues as modern science uncovers its disease-fighting compounds, which may help manage cancer, heart disease, high blood pressure, high cholesterol, and viral infections.

add more to your diet

▶ Mushrooms and potatoes taste especially good together, so add cooked mushrooms to potato salads or roast them along with roasted potatoes.

▶ Use mushrooms, especially shiitakes, to add a meaty texture to vegetarian stews and chilis.

▶ Make a relish: Sauté a mixture of finely chopped mushrooms, scallions, and garlic in olive oil; add vinegar and use as a topping for veggie burgers, tacos, and sandwiches.

▶ Grind dried mushrooms to a powder and use along with bread crumbs to make veggie balls, lentil loaf, and bean burgers.

▶ Top portobello mushroom caps with shredded plant-based mozzarella shreds and chopped tomato and serve as appetizer pizzas.

what's in it

B vitamins Though they lack vitamin B_{12}, mushrooms are high in riboflavin, niacin, and vitamin B_6, which may help to manage depression, heart disease, and migraines.

ergosterol This vitamin D precursor may promote bone health.

eritadenine Found in shiitakes, this compound may lower cholesterol by promoting cholesterol excretion.

lentinan Present in small amounts in shiitakes, this polysaccharide compound is under review for immune-enhancing properties.

lentinula edodes mycelium (LEM) These compounds in shiitake mushrooms may prevent cancer, heart disease, high cholesterol, high blood pressure, infection, and liver disease.

selenium This antioxidant mineral is thought to protect against cancer and macular degeneration.

thioproline Preliminary research suggests that this anticancer compound in shiitake mushrooms may block the formation of cancer-causing nitrogen compounds in the body.

maximizing the benefits

Since the **B vitamins** in mushrooms leach into water when heated, if you soak dried mushrooms to reconstitute them, try to use the soaking water in the recipe—it's packed with flavor. Since some people may react to the allergens and other substances in raw mushrooms, it's best to eat them cooked.

health bites

A review of the scientific literature found that cultivated mushrooms may improve glucose metabolism, destroy free radicals, stimulate digestion, and enhance nutrient absorbtion.

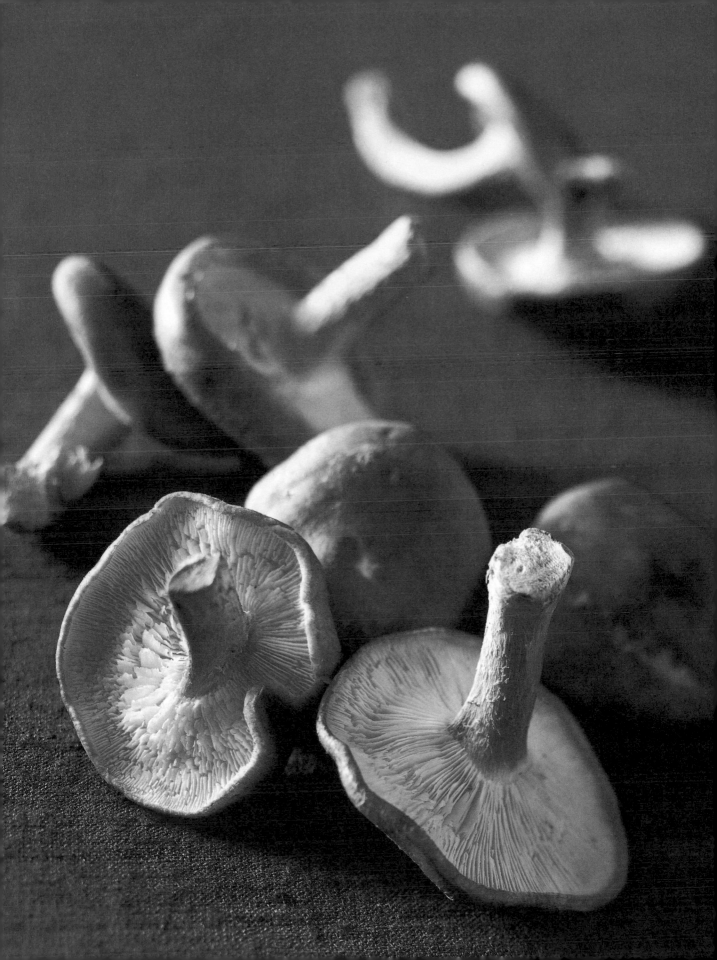

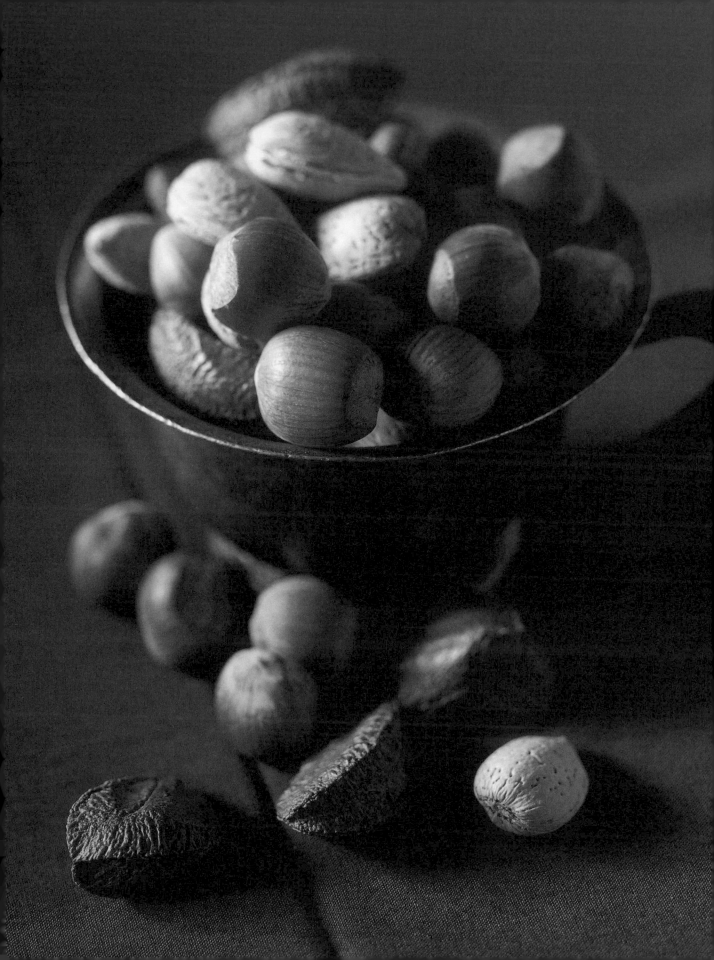

nuts

Energy-packed and protein-rich, nuts may also lower the risk for cancer and cardiovascular disease. In addition to the nutrients listed below, nuts are an excellent source of the cardioprotective amino acid, arginine, and also supply B vitamins.

what's in it

alpha-linolenic acid (ALA) Found in walnuts, this omega-3 fat may alleviate arthritis and lower risk for heart attack and stroke.

ellagic acid Walnuts are an especially good source of this antioxidant compound, which may inhibit the growth of cancer cells.

plant sterols Especially rich in pistachios, plant sterols help defend against certain forms of cancer and cardiovascular disease.

potassium High in pistachios, potassium may lower blood pressure and stroke risk.

resveratrol Found in peanuts, this phytonutrient may prevent cancer, high cholesterol, and stroke.

saponins These cancer-fighting phytonutrients may boost immunity and promote healthy levels of blood sugar and cholesterol.

selenium Brazil nuts are extraordinarily rich sources of this powerful antioxidant, which helps to prevent cancer, certain eye disorders, and heart disease.

vitamin E Nuts are one of the best food sources of this antioxidant vitamin, which may help prevent cardiovascular disease and cataracts. (Almonds and hazelnuts are particularly rich in vitamin E.)

maximizing the benefits

Refrigerate or freeze nuts to prevent their oils from going rancid. To enhance the flavor of nuts, toast them in the oven for 5 to 10 minutes, or until fragrant.

add more to your diet

▶ Sauté finely chopped nuts in olive oil along with bread crumbs and toss with freshly cooked pasta.

▶ Make your own nut butters: Place nuts in a food processor and process until pureed; add salt if you like.

▶ Toast and finely chop nuts, sweeten with maple syrup, and use as a topping for plant-based "ice cream" or fruit salad.

▶ Stir peanut butter into stews or curries to help enrich and add flavor.

▶ Use finely chopped nuts as a coating for tofu or tempeh cutlets.

health bites
Studies show that nuts protect against heart disease by improving blood levels of fat, reducing inflammation, and contributing unsaturated fats and plant sterols to the diet.

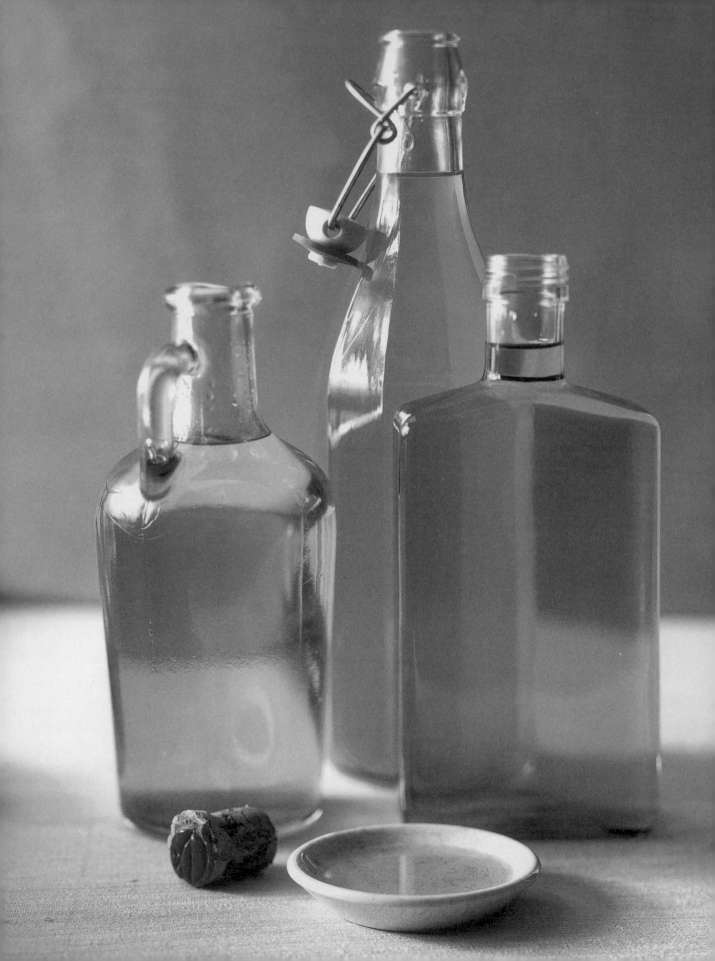

olive oil

Olive oil is rich in unique disease-fighting phytonutrients, vitamin E, and monounsaturated fat, which all help to clear cholesterol from arteries. Research also suggests that olive oil may help manage diabetes, rheumatoid arthritis, stroke, and breast and colon cancer.

what's in it

hydroxytyrosol and oleuropein These antioxidant phytonutrients may work together, according to laboratory studies, to help protect against breast cancer, high blood pressure, infection-causing bacteria, and heart disease.

lignans Present in extra-virgin olive oil, these potent antioxidants may protect against breast, colon, and prostate cancer by suppressing early cancer changes in cells.

monounsaturated fat When substituted for saturated fat, this cardioprotective fat helps to lower total and LDL ("bad") cholesterol and may increase HDl ("good") cholesterol levels. Research suggests that a diet deriving most of its fat calories from monounsaturates may reduce the risk for chronic disease, including arthritis, certain cancers, and cardiovascular disease. At 73% monounsaturated fat, olive oil has the highest percentage among common cooking oils: By contrast, coconut oil has 6% and corn or soy oil 24%.

vitamin E Olive oil is one of the best dietary sources of this elusive vitamin, which shields against damaging free radicals.

maximizing the benefits

To preserve flavor as well as disease-fighting compounds, store olive oil in an airtight container in the refrigerator or other cool, dark place, and use as soon as possible. Refrigerated olive oil will solidify, so you will have to let it reach room temperature before it's pourable.

add more to your diet

▶ Substitute a light, mild-flavored olive oil for other oils or melted butter in baked goods and baked desserts.

▶ Serve a fruity olive oil instead of butter at the table for drizzling on bread.

▶ Don't forget whole olives, which also add healing oils and delicate flavors to food. Chop and add to pasta sauces, salad dressings, or stews; or fold into bread or pizza dough.

▶ Use olive oil for sautéing pancakes or cooking waffles.

health bites

Since the heat and chemicals used in processing olive oil can diminish nutrient content, it's best to choose those oils that are minimally processed, such as extra-virgin or cold-pressed.

onion family

All members of the onion family—onions, chives, leeks, scallions, and shallots—are noted for their powerful phytonutrients and fiber, which may protect against cancer, cardiovascular disease, constipation, and other conditions.

what's in it

diallyl sulfide Most abundant in onions but also found in other members of the onion family, this cancer-protective phytonutrient appears to increase levels of cancer-fighting enzymes, particularly in the stomach. In areas where large amounts of onions are consumed, the death rate from stomach cancer is significantly reduced, and diallyl sulfide intake is thought to be a factor.

fiber The onion family is a source of both insoluble and soluble fiber, which may confer protection against constipation, hemorrhoids, high cholesterol, and possibly weight gain.

fructooligosaccharides (FOS) Shallots are a significant source of FOS, the indigestible carbohydrates that encourage growth of beneficial bacteria in the colon.

kaempferol This anticancer substance, found in leeks, may help to block the development of cancer-causing compounds.

lutein and zeaxanthin Present in the green tops of leeks and scallions, these pigments work together to help prevent cell damage that may lead to vision loss and cancer.

quercetin Found in red onions, this flavonoid has shown promise in inhibiting growth of breast, blood, gastric, lung, and skin cancer cells and in helping prevent cardiovascular disease.

maximizing the benefits

High-heat cooking significantly reduces the benefits of **diallyl sulfide.** Fresh, raw onion has the most health benefits, and mincing (even chewing) the onion helps to release the phytonutrient power.

health bites

Studies show again and again that quercetin's antioxidant and anti-inflammatory properties help reduce the risk of neurodegenerative disorders, hypertension, allergic conditions, arrhythmia, cancer, and atherosclerosis, as well as cancer and heart disease.

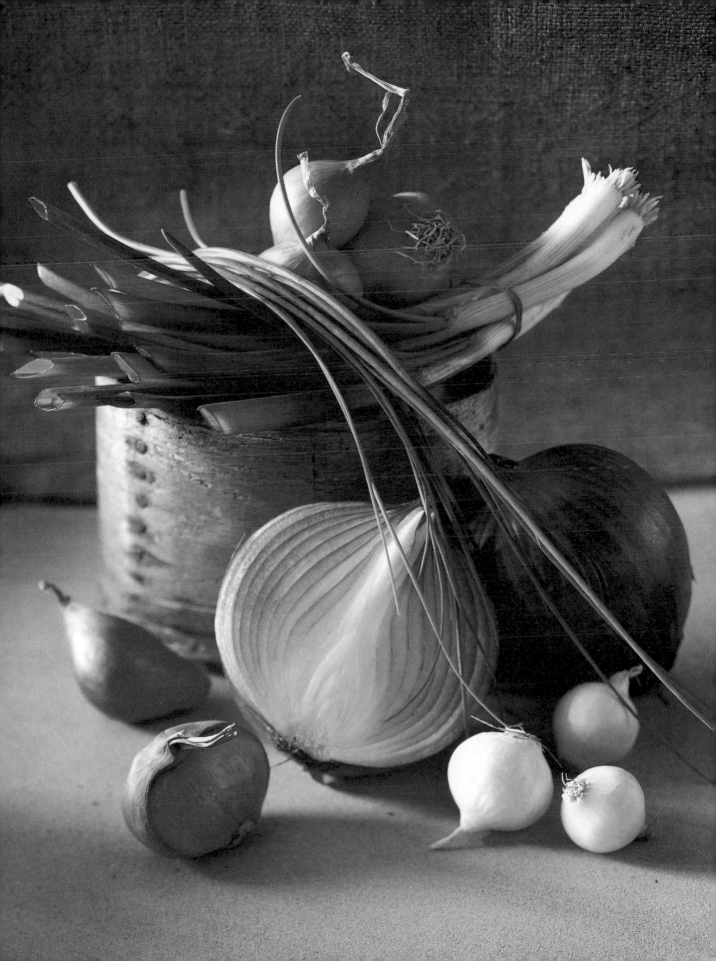

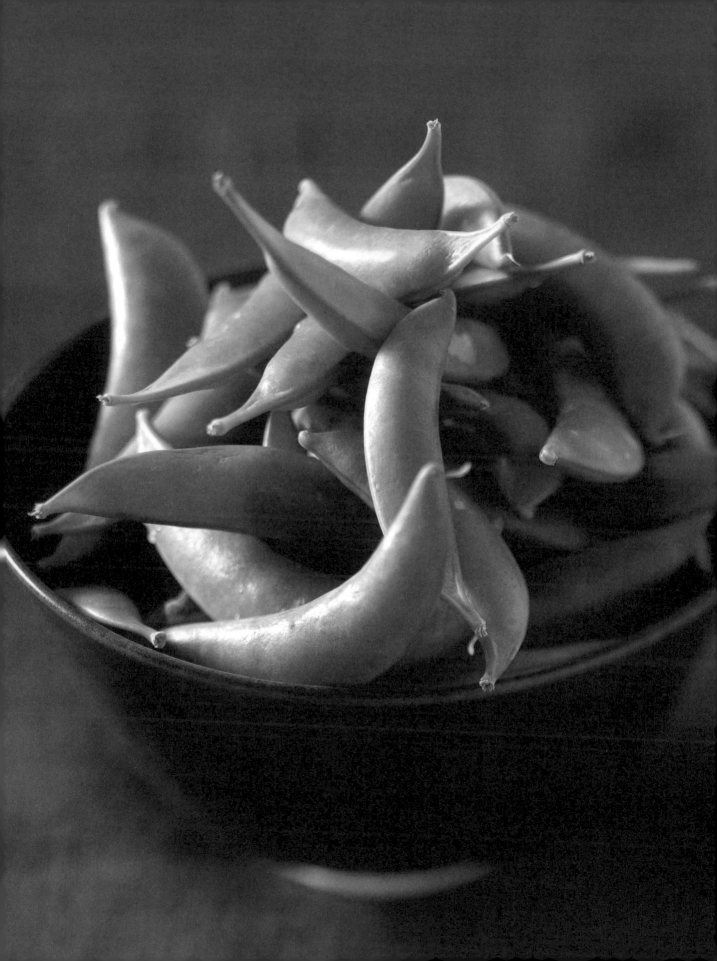

peas

Fresh, sweet garden peas are a good source of plant-based protein and nonheme (plant-derived) iron, making them an excellent food for vegetarians. Peas may help reduce the risk for developing certain cancers, depression, high cholesterol, and macular degeneration.

what's in it

chlorophyll Though the health benefits of chlorophyll are not fully understood, some studies suggest that it may deter certain chemicals from causing DNA damage to cells.

folate Important for all stages of life, this B vitamin is linked to reduced incidence of certain birth defects, cancer, heart disease, and possibly depression.

lutein This carotenoid may prevent colon cancer and eye diseases such as macular degeneration and cataracts.

lysine A building block for the manufacture of protein, this essential amino acid is vital for collagen synthesis and tissue repair. It may also help to slow down or block the effects of herpes-family viruses.

protease inhibitors These compounds may help to diminish the rate of division in cancer cells.

saponins Believed to lower LDL ("bad") cholesterol levels, saponins can bind cholesterol in your digestive tract and usher them out of your body.

tryptophan Found in small amounts in peas, this amino acid helps to maintain proper levels of serotonin, which regulates mood.

vitamin B_6 Preliminary studies show that this B vitamin may boost serotonin levels, which may prevent depression and anxiety.

vitamin C As an antioxidant, vitamin C may protect against cataracts by fighting the harmful effects of free radicals.

maximizing the benefits

Heat-sensitive vitamin C and water-soluble B vitamins (folate and B_6) are best preserved if you either quickly steam or microwave peas instead of boiling or cooking for long periods of time.

add more to your diet

- Steam peas, stir into hummus, and use as a filling for stuffed twice-baked potatoes.

- For a twist on the classic guacamole, add mashed cooked peas to avocado along with the usual seasonings.

- Cook peas in a small amount of water with thyme and scallions. Puree the peas with their cooking liquid, add plant-based milk, and serve as a soup.

- Buy edible-pod peas (such as sugar snaps) and eat as a snack.

- Stir cooked peas, chopped cilantro, and salsa into pancake batter for a Mexican-style main-dish pancake.

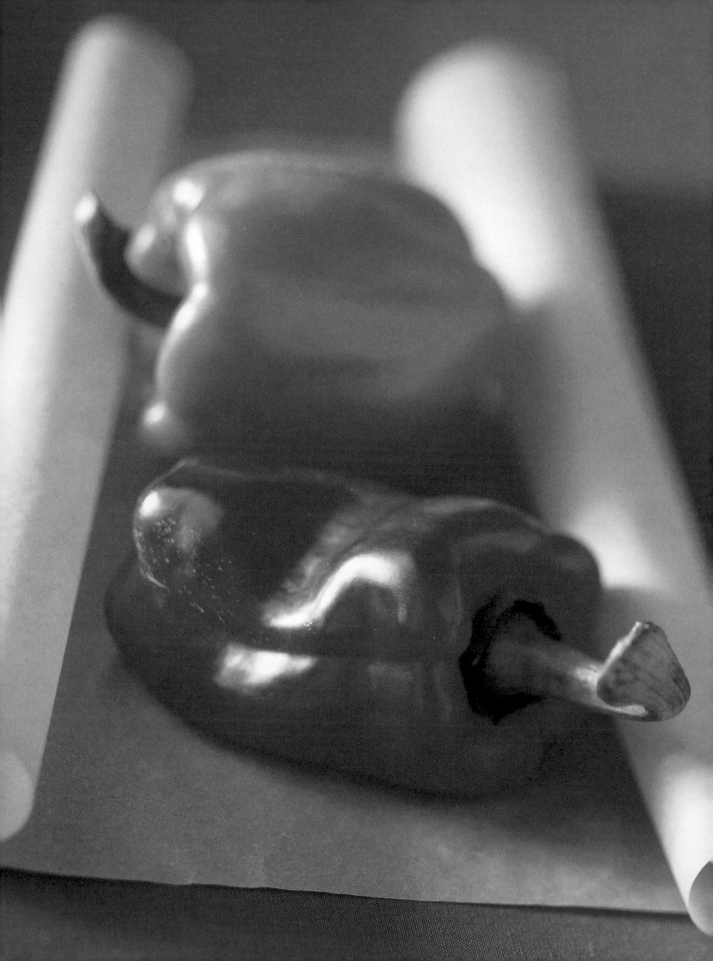

peppers

Sweet bell peppers and spicy chili peppers add color and zest to your favorite dish, while offering protection against heart disease, vision loss, and nasal congestion.

what's in it

beta-carotene This antioxidant pigment may help prevent eye diseases, certain cancers, and heart disease. Red peppers are particularly rich in beta-carotene.

capsaicin This pungent phytonutrient, which supplies the "heat" in chili peppers, may ease congestion by increasing secretions in the nose and airways. Studies suggest that capsaicin may also detoxify cancer-causing compounds and encourage cancer-cell death. The hotter the chili pepper, the greater the capsaicin content.

chlorophyll Preliminary research suggests that this plant compound may stop healthy cells from mutating into cancerous cells and may protect against environmental carcinogens.

lutein and zeaxanthin A diet rich in lutein and its antioxidant partner, zeaxanthin, may protect against certain forms of cancer, heart disease, macular degeneration, and cataracts. One cup of diced fresh red bell peppers offers tremendous quantities of lutein, while orange peppers are a top source of zeaxanthin.

vitamin C Peppers are a major source of this essential vitamin, which may enhance our defense against respiratory ailments. The combined antioxidant power of beta-carotene and vitamin C in peppers may help to prevent cataracts and macular degeneration. One cup of fresh bell peppers supplies even more vitamin C than 1 cup of fresh orange juice.

maximizing the benefits

For **vitamin C,** eat uncooked peppers, since this vitamin is easily destroyed by heat. To maximize the bioavailability of **beta-carotene** and also preserve other nutrients, cook peppers until they are crisp-tender, and eat with a little monounsaturated fat, such as olive oil, to aid absorption.

health bites

Red bell peppers are richer in vitamin C and supply more than ten times the beta-carotene of green peppers. But all peppers—green, purple, yellow, orange, and red—are rich in both nutrients.

add more to your diet

▶ Fill bell pepper wedges with bean puree and serve as an appetizer.

▶ Add roasted, peeled red bell peppers and spicy chipotle peppers to mashed potatoes for a side dish. Or thin the potato-pepper mixture with plant-based milk to make a soup.

▶ Add diced chili peppers to muffins or cornbreads.

▶ Puree homemade or bottled roasted red peppers with a little tomato paste, garlic, salt, and pepper, and serve as a vegetable dip. Or thin the mixture with a little olive oil and use as a pasta sauce.

▶ Make a hot and sweet pepper salsa: Mince red, green, and orange bell peppers along with chili peppers (jalapeño, chipotle); add minced red onion, vinegar, and cilantro. Serve the salsa, or toss it with freshly cooked pasta.

pineapple

Long used as a folk remedy to settle intestinal upsets and relieve constipation, this tropical fruit is also noted for its anti-inflammatory enzyme and healing nutrients, which help bolster immunity and bone and cardiovascular health.

add more to your diet

▶ Make a pineapple salsa: Chop pineapple, bell peppers, and red onion. Toss with ginger, honey, and lime juice. Serve with salads, tacos, or burritos.

▶ Use pineapple juice instead of vinegar in a salad dressing.

▶ Cook crushed pineapple in unsweetened pineapple juice until thick and use as a no-sugar-added all-fruit spread.

▶ Add thin slices of pineapple and spicy mustard to veggie burgers or sandwiches.

▶ Make a barbecue sauce substituting chopped pineapple and pineapple juice for half of the tomato in the recipe.

▶ Make a pineapple drink: Puree pineapple with dairy-free yogurt and a touch of honey.

what's in it

bromelain This antibacterial, anti-inflammatory enzyme is plentiful in pineapple and may help to control tissue swelling and inflammation associated with bronchitis, cough, osteoarthritis, rheumatoid arthritis, varicose veins, strains, and sprains. Preliminary research suggests that bromelain's anti-inflammatory property may reduce blood clot formation and break down existing clots, which may lower the risk for stroke and heart attack.

ferulic acid Pineapple is a good source of this phytonutrient, which helps prevent the formation of cancer-causing substances.

manganese One cup of pineapple provides more than the suggested Adequate Intake of manganese, the bone-building mineral.

plant sterols These plant compounds may help to lower cholesterol and reduce the risk for heart disease.

soluble fiber Pineapple is high in pectin fiber and gum fiber, which have cholesterol-lowering properties and promote healthy bowel function.

vitamin C Fresh pineapple is a good source of vitamin C, which may enhance immunity and wound healing, while also preventing heart disease and serious eye disorders.

maximizing the benefits

To preserve the **vitamin C** content, eat pineapple uncooked. However, the **soluble pectin fiber** in pineapple becomes available when the pineapple is cooked.

health bites

Preliminary research suggests that bromelain may reduce traveler's diarrhea by inhibiting *E. coli,* one of the bacteria responsible for the illness. Scientists believe bromelain may displace *E. coli* from receptors in the intestinal wall.

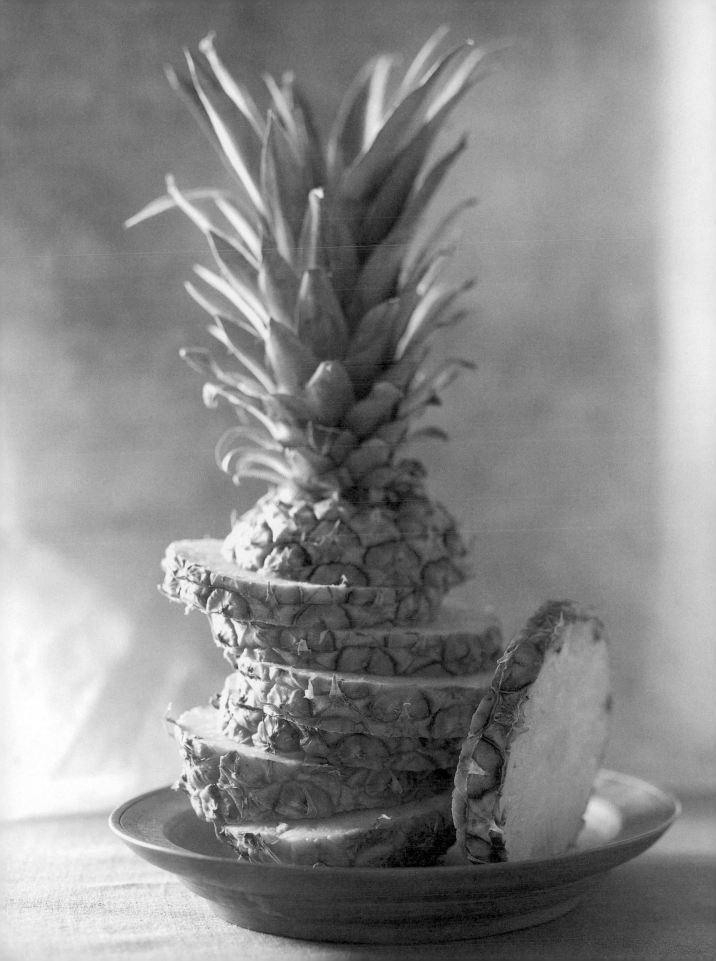

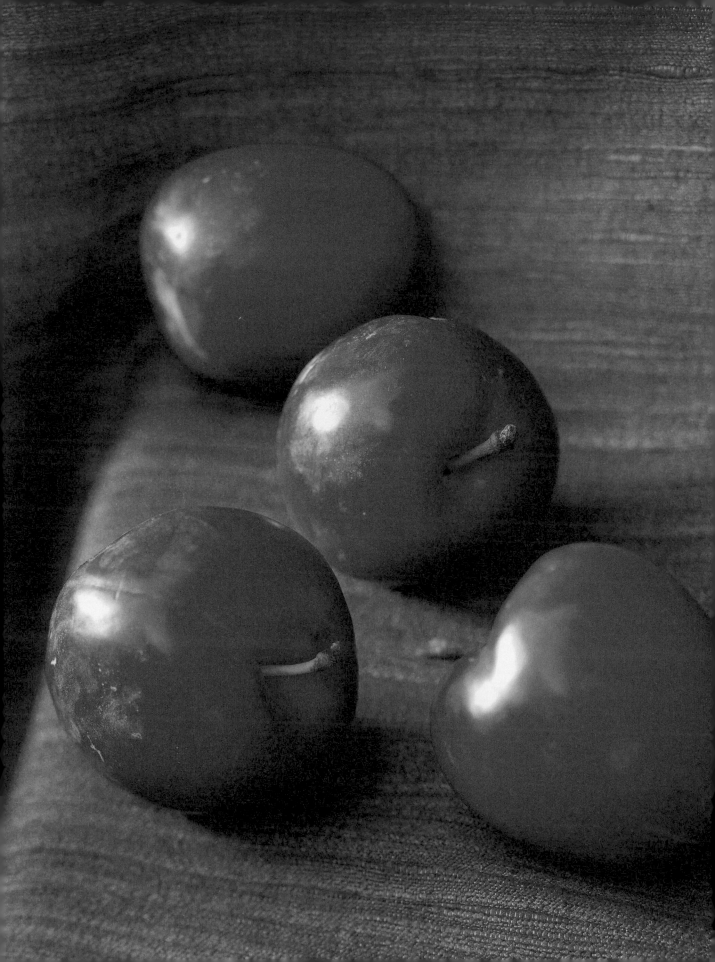

plums & prunes

Juicy, vividly colored plums and prunes (dried plums) are packed with disease-fighting antioxidants and natural sugars. Prunes and prune juice are a delicious, natural choice for relieving constipation (and boosting heart health).

what's in it

anthocyanins Reddish-blue pigments that lend intense color to plums, anthocyanins may protect against cancer and heart disease by mopping up harmful free radicals.

chlorogenic acid A phenolic phytonutrient, this potent antioxidant quenches damaging free radicals and is thought to help detoxify carcinogenic environmental agents, such as nitrosamines in cigarette smoke.

insoluble fiber The insoluble fiber in plums and prunes helps to bulk up the stool and ease elimination.

potassium A potassium-rich diet is associated with lower blood pressure and a reduced risk for kidney stones and stroke.

quercetin A potent free-radical fighter, quercetin may help to prevent estrogen-dependent cancer, including breast cancer, and may help to block oxidation of harmful LDL ("bad") cholesterol, a process that could lead to heart disease.

soluble fiber Plums and prunes are rich in soluble fiber, which helps to relieve constipation and lower cholesterol levels.

sorbitol A naturally occurring sugar, sorbitol may help to relieve constipation by absorbing water and bulking up the stool. Note that sorbitol can irritate the colon, especially in those with irritable bowel syndrome.

maximizing the benefits

If you stew prunes, be sure to drink the liquid or include it in the recipe to retain the **sorbitol,** which leaches into cooking water.

add more to your diet

▶ Make a fruit soup: In a blender, mix prune juice, plant-based oat milk, and a little fresh lemon juice. Chill and serve with diced fresh plums and minced fresh mint.

▶ Buy prune butter and use it as a fruit spread, as a filling for layer cakes, or as the basis for vinaigrette.

▶ Cook diced pitted prunes in vinegar and sugar along with onions and garlic and serve as a condiment alongside salads or sandwiches.

▶ Make a barbecue sauce: Cook diced pitted prunes in prune juice along with honey, vinegar, minced fresh ginger, and hot sauce.

▶ Add sliced fresh plums to savory soups and stews.

▶ Instead of cream cheese and jelly: Spread bread with plant-based cream cheese and top with thin slices of ripe plums.

health bites

Prune juice is an antioxidant-rich constipation remedy. Drinking prune juice at bedtime may promote a morning bowel movement (or one in the evening if you drink prune juice at breakfast).

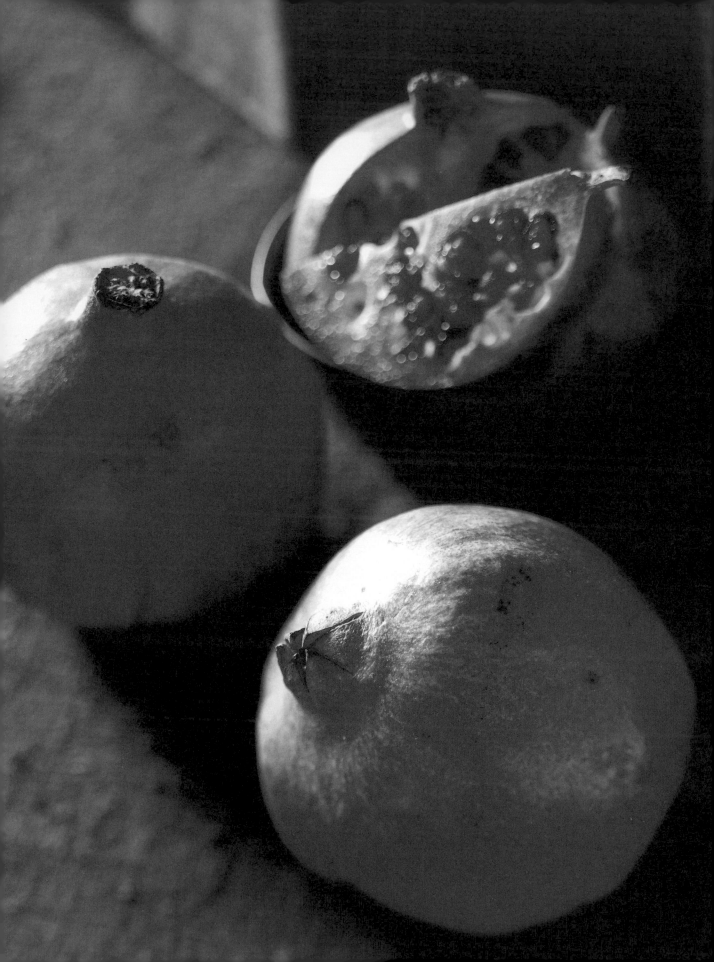

pomegranates

The word **pomegranate** is old French for "seeded apple," an apt name for this apple-sized fruit packed with jewel-like clusters of crimson seeds. The pomegranate is touted as an anti-aging fruit that may prevent hardening of the arteries.

what's in it

anthocyanins By protecting against free-radical cell damage, these pigments may help to prevent cancer and heart disease. Some evidence suggests that anthocyanins strengthen capillaries, which is beneficial for hemorrhoids and varicose veins. Research has shown that pomegranate juice has two to three times the antioxidant capacity of equal amounts of red wine or green tea, and anthocyanins make an important contribution to the pomegranate's antioxidant power.

catechins These phytonutrients may defend against cancer, heart disease, and infectious agents by protecting cells from dangerous free radicals.

ellagic acid Abundant in pomegranates, ellagic acid may work with other antioxidants to protect the body from environmental toxins, fight inflammation, and support brain health.

fiber Both soluble and insoluble fiber present in pomegranates help to relieve constipation, satisfy hunger, and lower cholesterol.

manganese Pomegranates are loaded with this mineral, which is essential for strong teeth and bones.

potassium Linked to lower blood pressure, potassium-rich foods may also reduce the risk for heart disease, kidney stones, and stroke.

maximizing the benefits

You can eat the pomegranate's seeds (its skin is inedible) as is, or crush them in a strainer to separate the juice from the kernels.

add more to your diet

▶ Keep a bottle of pomegranate molasses (found in Middle Eastern markets, gourmet stores, and online) on hand for a variety of uses. This condensed, syrupy form of pure pomegranate juice has a high concentration of antioxidants.

▶ Use pomegranate molasses in place of vinegar in a salad dressing.

▶ Brush red onion slices with pomegranate molasses and a touch of brown sugar and broil.

▶ Add pomegranate juice to orange juice for a refreshing drink.

▶ Stir pomegranate juice or pomegranate molasses into a barbecue sauce.

▶ Toss pomegranate seeds into fruit salad, green salads, or grain dishes like rice pilaf.

health bites

A recent study suggests that drinking pomegranate juice daily may improve cardiovascular health by reducing both systolic and diastolic blood pressure in patients with metabolic syndrome.

potatoes

This versatile American favorite, served in its high-fiber skin, is a nourishing, satisfying source of healing compounds. Spare yourself the added calories, fat, and sodium by enjoying potatoes in their naturally filling, unprocessed form.

add more to your diet

▶ Add potatoes to soups and stews and, once cooked, mash some of the potatoes to help thicken the dish.

▶ Make a quick, cold potato soup: Cook sliced, unpeeled potatoes until tender. Mash with dairy-free milk (enough to make the potatoes the consistency of a thick but spoonable soup) and salt. Stir in chopped fresh dill and scallions.

▶ When making mashed potatoes, cook potatoes in their skin and use some of the potato cooking water when mashing. Save the remaining water to use in soups and stews.

▶ Make a salad dressing using mashed potatoes as a substitute for some of the oil, then stir in chopped garlic and lemon juice or vinegar.

▶ For a colorful potato salad, use purple, red, blue, yellow, and white potatoes, and leave the skins on.

▶ Add small cubes of cooked potato to lentil loaf and bean burger mixtures.

what's in it

anthocyanins Found in purple, blue, and red potato skin, these antioxidant pigments may be cancer- and cardioprotective.

caffeic and ferulic acids Present in the potato skin, these phytonutrients may team up to help destroy harmful carcinogens, fight inflammation, and protect the brain.

chlorogenic acid This phytonutrient may help prevent cancer by blocking the formation of cancer-causing nitrogen compounds.

complex carbohydrates These energy-producing nutrients help manage depression, heartburn, and memory function.

potassium Potassium-rich foods such as potatoes are linked to enhanced cardiovascular health and a lower risk for kidney stones.

protease inhibitors These compounds show promise in suppressing cancer at both the primary and secondary stages.

saponins These may remove toxins before they're absorbed.

vitamin B$_6$ This cardioprotective B vitamin may lessen symptoms of depression, insomnia, and premenstrual syndrome (PMS).

vitamin C Because such vast quantities of potatoes are eaten, they are a leading source of vitamin C in the American diet. This important antioxidant vitamin may protect against free radicals and enhance immune function.

maximizing the benefits

For the most nutrients, eat potatoes with their skin, and bake, microwave, or steam. If peeling, remove the thinnest layer possible. If boiling, leave the skin on and try to reuse the cooking water, where many of the **B vitamins** wind up.

health bites

A study of healthy elderly people with poor memory found that eating 1 cup of mashed potatoes significantly improved their short- and long-term memory. Scientists hypothesize that potatoes may enhance the production of memory-enhancing brain chemicals.

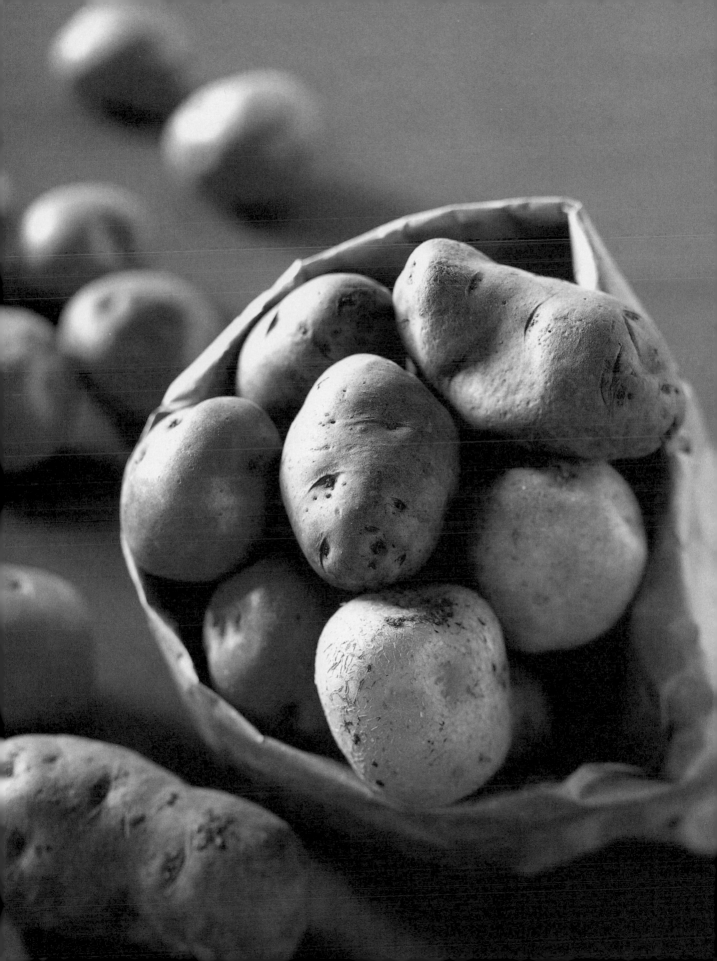

rice

A staple ingredient in cuisines worldwide, rice is an important source of complex carbohydrates, fiber, and essential nutrients. Free of gluten, rice is a natural choice for people with celiac disease or wheat gluten allergies.

add more to your diet

▶ Have rice for breakfast: Combine rice and vegetable broth and cook very slowly until the rice breaks down and the mixture becomes a porridge.

▶ Add cooked rice to pancake batter, along with herbs, to make a savory rice pancake to serve alongside main dishes.

▶ Add cooked rice to a cornbread batter to add an interesting texture.

▶ Make a rice pie crust: Combine cooked rice, a flaxseed "egg" (see page 71), and some herbs, grated vegetables, and bake as you would a savory pie crust.

▶ Make puddings with rice milk.

what's in it

complex carbohydrates Energy-providing complex carbohydrates help to absorb excess fluids, contributing to white rice's reputation as a remedy for diarrhea and heartburn.

folate Enriched white rice is an excellent source of this B vitamin, which helps to lower the risk for birth defects and heart disease.

magnesium Brown rice provides high levels of this mineral, which may improve PMS and reduce the risk of kidney stones.

oryzanol Research is exploring this compound's potential to reduce oxidative stress related to aging and the development of age-related diseases. Oryzanol—a mixture of different forms of ferulic acid and terpene phytonutrients—is found in the bran layer of brown rice.

selenium This antioxidant mineral is associated with prevention of allergies, asthma, cataracts, infertility, and prostate problems.

vitamin B$_6$ This vitamin may help to thwart allergies, anxiety, asthma, depression, and heart disease. Brown rice provides substantial quantities of this B vitamin.

maximizing the benefits

Unless package directions say otherwise, when cooking rice, do not rinse it before (or after), because that washes away essential nutrients. Also avoid cooking with excess water to retain **B vitamins.**

health bites

Choose brown rice because it has more vitamins and minerals than plain milled white rice—stripped of many of its nutrients—and is also high in oryzanol and insoluble fiber. However, many rices—brown and white—are "enriched" by adding back many of the nutrients lost in processing.

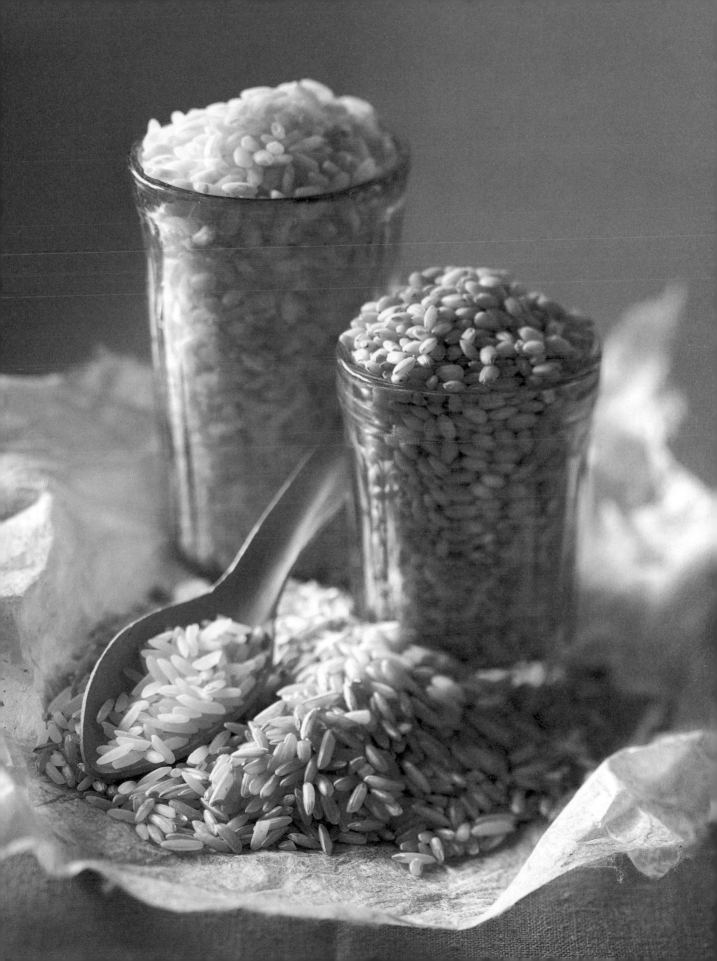

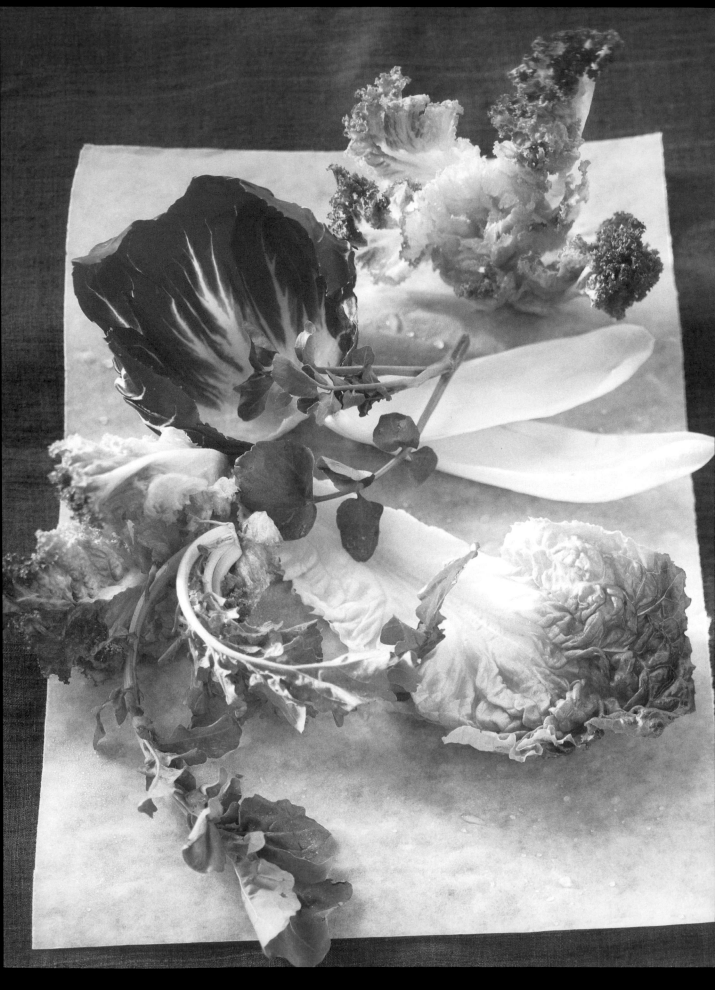

salad greens

Toss your salad with a variety of greens to elevate your fiber intake and antioxidant levels. Arugula, chicory, dandelion greens, escarole, radicchio, and watercress offer myriad nutrients and health benefits.

what's in it

beta-carotene Watercress, escarole, and especially chicory and dandelion greens are sources of this healing pigment, which helps lower the risk of death from stroke, heart disease, and cancer.

folate One cup of raw chicory provides almost half the daily requirement for folate, which helps to protect against cardiovascular disease and birth defects. Arugula also supplies ample folate.

fructooligosaccharides (FOS) and inulin These prebiotic, indigestible carbohydrates may promote the growth of beneficial bacteria in the digestive tract and improve gastrointestinal health. FOS and inulin from chicory are known for their potential to protect against constipation, diarrhea, irritable bowel syndrome, and high blood fats.

insoluble fiber This type of fiber may satisfy your appetite and relieve constipation by improving intestinal function.

potassium Salad greens, particularly chicory, provide appreciable amounts of this cardioprotective mineral.

vitamin C Chicory, dandelion greens, and watercress are very good sources of this antioxidant, which benefits immunity, blood vessels, skin, cartilage, and cardiovascular health.

vitamin E Chicory and dandelion greens contain appreciable amounts of vitamin E compounds, which may protect against cancer and vision loss.

maximizing the benefits

Vegetable oils enhance the absorption of **beta-carotene,** so vinaigrettes are beneficial partners to beta-carotene-rich greens.

add more to your diet

▶ Sauté watercress or arugula in olive oil with garlic and red pepper flakes and serve as a hot vegetable side dish.

▶ Toss chicory with smoked tofu and whole-wheat croutons in a warm red wine vinaigrette.

▶ Make a sauce for pasta: Sauté dandelion greens in olive oil with golden raisins and pine nuts, and toss with pasta.

▶ For a cool summer soup, combine tomato juice, watercress, vinegar, and a couple of ice cubes in a blender and puree until smooth.

▶ Serve hot foods, such as sautéed vegetables, tofu, or tempeh on a bed of cool, dressed salad greens.

▶ Add bitter salad greens such as arugula, watercress, or radicchio to sweet fruit salads.

health bites

The antioxidants in dark green leafy vegetables are well known for their abillity to inhibit the growth of many different types of cancer cells.

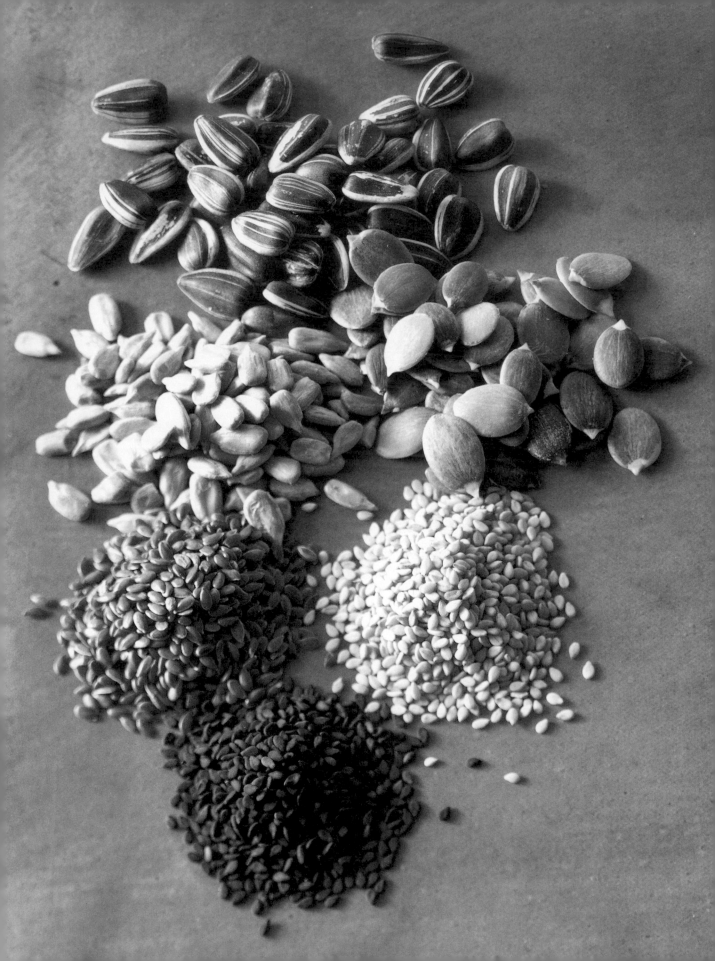

seeds

Rich in heart-healthy fat, pumpkin, sesame, and sunflower seeds possess an enormous amount of phytonutrients that may protect against cancer, cardiovascular disease, cataracts, chronic fatigue syndrome, and macular degeneration.

what's in it

essential fatty acids Seeds are rich in these nourishing fat compounds, which may improve fibrocystic breasts, cardiovascular health, immunity, and skin health.

magnesium This mineral may prevent chronic fatigue syndrome, heart disease, and kidney stones.

plant sterols Pumpkin seeds are particularly high in these compounds, which may lower both total and LDL ("bad") cholesterol, and may prevent the development of BPH (benign prostatic hyperplasia).

selenium This antioxidant mineral works with vitamin E to fight the free-radical cell damage that can lead to cancer, heart disease, and vision problems.

sesaminol compounds Sesame seeds contain sesaminol, sesamolinol, and pinoresinols—all precursors to lignans (phytoestrogens under review for anticancer and cardioprotective potential).

syringic acid Present in sesame seeds, this phytonutrient is under review for its potential to work with other plant antioxidants in the seeds to help combat UV sun damage in skin cells.

thiamin Sunflower seeds are a good source of this essential B vitamin; thiamin supports healthy brain function, including memory.

vitamin E Seeds are one of the best dietary sources of this antioxidant vitamin, which may have the potential to improve age-related bone dysfunction and enhance muscle repair and strength.

zinc Pumpkin and sesame seeds provide generous amounts of this vital mineral, which enhances immune function, protects DNA, and supports male reproductive health.

maximizing the benefits

To preserve their **essential fats** and nutrients (and to prevent them from going rancid), refrigerate or freeze seeds in airtight containers.

add more to your diet

▶ Puree toasted pumpkin seeds with lime juice, garlic, cilantro, and some pumpkin seed oil. Use as a sauce for steamed vegetables or pasta.

▶ Substitute sunflower or pumpkin seeds for walnuts in a chocolate chip cookie dough.

▶ Substitute pumpkin seed oil for half of the olive oil in a salad dressing.

▶ Coat thin tofu cutlets in a mixture of crushed sunflower and pumpkin seeds, and pan-fry.

▶ For a super-quick pasta sauce: Stir dark sesame oil into plain plant-based yogurt and toss with hot pasta. Garnish with sliced scallions and toasted sesame seeds.

▶ Add sesame seeds or chopped pumpkin or sunflower seeds to pie crusts.

▶ Whisk together soy sauce and dark sesame oil or pumpkin seed oil and drizzle over stir-fried vegetables and tofu.

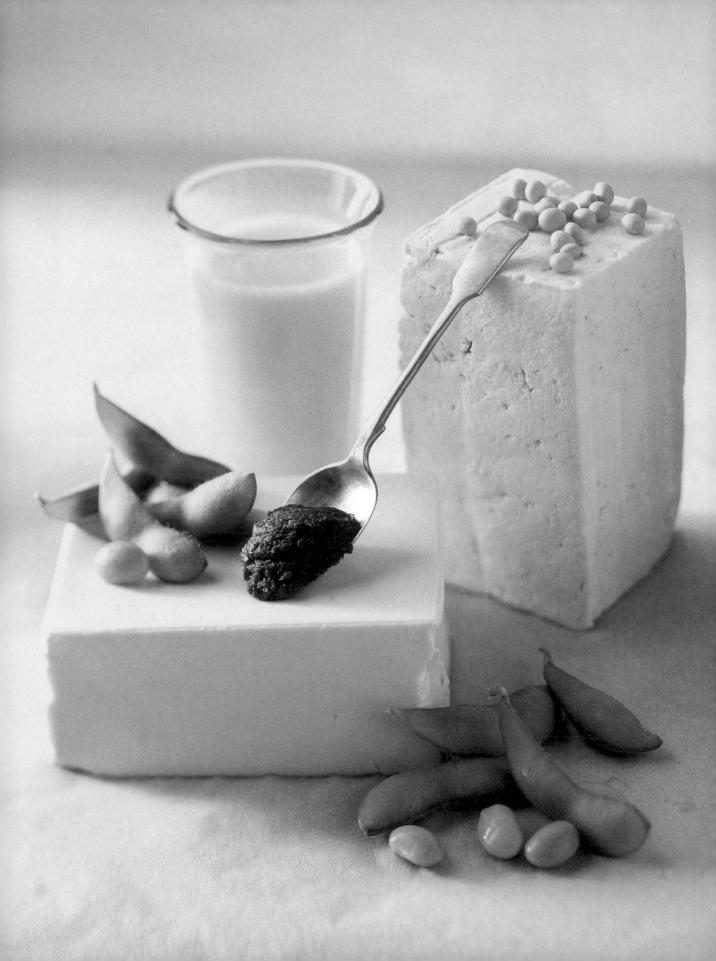

soy foods

The richest dietary sources of phytoestrogens, soy foods that include tofu, edamame, dried soybeans, soy milk, miso, and tempeh possess high-quality plant protein, lots of soluble fiber, and a wealth of phytonutrients.

what's in it

beta-sitosterol A type of phytosterol (plant sterol), beta-sitosterol is under review for its potential to lower cholesterol and to relieve symptoms associated with prostate enlargement.

genistein and daidzein These two powerful isoflavone phytoestrogens may protect against osteoporosis by inhibiting calcium loss from bones and increasing bone mineral density and content. Genistein and daidzein may also help to prevent heart disease, prostate cancer, and some forms of breast cancer. Soy foods are the richest sources of the isoflavones genistein and daidzein.

lignans Experimental research suggests that these phytoestrogens with antioxidant properties may prevent harmful changes in cells, particularly those leading to breast, colon, and prostate cancer.

phytic acid This phytonutrient may protect against kidney stones and neutralize cancer-causing free radicals in the intestines.

protease inhibitors Research indicates that a protease inhibitor unique to soy foods, Bowman-Birk inhibitor (BBI), may slow enzyme production in cancer cells and reduce tumors.

saponins These plant compounds have anticancer and cardioprotective properties and may help to raise levels of cancer-fighting immune cells, prevent bile acids from becoming cancerous agents in the colon, and lower cholesterol levels.

maximizing the benefits

To preserve **phytoestrogen** content, minimize cooking time for tofu and miso by adding them late in the cooking process.

add more to your diet

▶ Use tofu to replace the cheese in lasagna or macaroni and cheese.

▶ Substitute soy milk for cow's milk in puddings, custards, or smoothies.

▶ Steam edamame (fresh soybeans) in their pods, then shell them. Add the beans to grain or vegetable salads.

▶ Make a miso-carrot salad dressing: Whisk a couple of tablespoons of shiro miso into carrot juice along with a couple of teaspoons of sesame oil, some ground ginger, and some wasabi paste.

▶ Use soybeans in classic bean recipes such as chili or baked beans, but precook them before starting the recipe, because they can take several hours to soften.

▶ Puree soft silken tofu with basil, garlic, almonds, and a little nutritional yeast, and use as a pasta sauce.

▶ Cut up firm silken tofu, drizzle honey over it, and serve in a fruit salad with melon and grapes.

▶ Add slices of smoked tofu or tempeh in wraps or sandwiches, or diced tempeh or smoked tofu in salads and pasta dishes.

health bites

The cholesterol-lowering effect of soy is well established. Studies also indicate that whole soy products—cooked soybeans and soy nuts—may help manage blood sugar.

spices

cinnamon

Derived from the inner bark of a tree, cinnamon is a sweet, warm, aromatic spice, most commonly used in baking.

what's in it

Cinnamon may have antibacterial and antimicrobial properties, and it may also reduce discomfort from heartburn by decreasing stomach acid. Cinnamaldehyde in cinnamon may prevent blood clots and ward off bacteria such as *H. pylori*, which has been linked to ulcers.

add more to your diet

Use in: soups, stews, and chilis; pancake and waffle batters; hot cocoa mixes.

caraway

Caraway is part of the carrot family and is available as a whole seed. It is the seed used to flavor rye bread and other Middle European dishes, such as sauerkraut and goulash.

what's in it

Limonene in caraway may help prevent cancer. Caraway also has small amounts of perillyl alcohol, which may have the potential to reduce tumor size.

add more to your diet

Use in: savory soups and stews; salad dressings and relishes; savory muffins and bread doughs. It matches well with cabbage, carrots, beets, cauliflower, and sweet and white potatoes.

cloves

A strong and highly fragrant spice, cloves are the dried flower bud of a clove tree. They are available whole or ground.

what's in it

Cloves may fight off bacteria, such as *E. coli*, that can cause food poisoning. Eugenol, an oil in cloves, can slow down blood clotting. Cloves are also used as a natural breath freshener, though they may numb the mouth and gums.

add more to your diet

Use in: spice rubs and barbecue sauces, tomato sauces and salsas, sweet fruit-poaching liquids. It is commonly used in gingerbread, mulled cider, and other cool weather favorites.

cayenne

This is a fiery spice derived from the dried pods of a particular variety of chili pepper.

what's in it

Cayenne may help to reduce discomfort from allergies, colds, and flu. Capsaicin is the compound that gives cayenne pepper its bite, and it is thought to reduce congestion by opening up the nasal passages.

add more to your diet

Use in: tomato sauces and salsas; chilis, stews, and soups; chocolate sauces, cookies, and cakes; salad dressings and fruit salad; spice rubs, marinades, and barbecue sauces.

coriander seed

Coriander seed comes from the cilantro plant and has a mild, citrus-like flavor. Coriander is used in curry powder and as a pickling spice.

what's in it

Coriander seed is thought to be helpful in relieving stomach cramps and may have the ability to kill bacteria and fungus. It contains limonene, which is a flavonoid thought to help fight cancer.

add more to your diet

Use in: sauces; savory soups and stews; spice rubs and marinades. It's an important flavor in curries and roasted vegetables.

cumin

Cumin is used in Indian and Mexican cooking and is available as the whole seed or ground.

what's in it

Examined for its potential to ward off bacteria and foodborne microbes, such as *E. coli*, cumin also has potential antioxidant and anticancer effects.

add more to your diet

Use in: savory soups, stews, and chilis; spice rubs and marinades; salsas, chutneys, and relishes; bread doughs and savory pancake batters; pasta and rice salads. It matches well with corn, cabbage, carrots, onions, lentils, beans, and potatoes.

ginger

Ginger is sold as the fresh root, powdered, pickled, and sugar-preserved. All forms of ginger have an aromatic spiciness.

what's in it

Substances in ginger—gingerol, shogaol, and zingiberene—have antioxidant capabilities, which may help to prevent heart disease and cancer. Ginger is thought to reduce motion sickness, nausea, and vomiting; and it has also been shown to possess anti-inflammatory properties.

add more to your diet

Use in: hot apple and pineapple ciders; cakes, cookies, and muffins; fruit desserts; savory soups, curries, and stews.

mustard seed

Mustard seed and mustard powder have a pungent, slightly smoky flavor. Note that some brands of prepared mustard contain turmeric, which make it bright yellow.

what's in it

Mustard seeds contain allyl isothiocyanates, which studies suggest inhibit the growth of cancer cells. The volatile oils in mustard may clear congestion due to colds and flu.

add more to your diet

Use in: relishes and salsas; pickling and preserving; cabbage and carrot slaws; salads and salad dressings; curries and stews.

nutmeg

Nutmeg is the seed of a tropical fruit. Its sweet, aromatic, warm flavor tends to be strong, so it is advisable to use small amounts.

what's in it

Eugenol, a monoterpene in nutmeg, is thought to prevent heart disease by preventing blood cells from forming too many clots. Nutmeg may also have antibacterial properties that may help destroy the foodborne bacteria *E. coli*.

add more to your diet

Use in: cookies, cakes, and pies; puddings and custards; white sauces. It matches well with spinach, green beans, broccoli, carrots, and sweet potatoes.

saffron

One of the most expensive spices in the world, saffron has a flavor that is unique, delicate, and difficult to compare with any other spice. Use in minute amounts as it is fragrant and intense.

what's in it

Laboratory studies suggest that saffron may be an important memory-enhancing and disease-fighting spice, due possibly to the pigment crocetin, as well as carotenoids, compounds that are believed to fight heart disease and cancer.

add more to your diet

Use in: soups, chowders, and stews; fresh pasta, pizza, and bread doughs; white sauces.

turmeric

The spice that gives curry powder its deep yellow color, turmeric has a delicate flavor.

what's in it

The curcumin in turmeric is thought to have a wide range of beneficial effects, and its antioxidant properties may fend off heart disease and cancer. Curcumin can relieve joint pain in arthritis and holds promise in reducing cataract development, and other eye disorders.

add more to your diet

Use in: curries, savory soups, and stews; spice rubs and marinades; pickled vegetables and condiments; sauces.

spinach

Endowed with a tremendous wealth of disease-fighting carotenoids, phytonutrients, and vitamins, spinach helps protect against cancer, high cholesterol, and vision loss.

what's in it

beta-carotene A half cup of cooked spinach provides close to a full day's supply of this antioxidant. Beta-carotene may help to protect against cancer and macular degeneration.

folate The folate in spinach helps protect against anemia, birth defects, and possibly heart attacks.

lutein and zeaxanthin Spinach is a rich source of these two carotenoids, which work together to help prevent macular degeneration and possibly cataracts and colon cancer.

oxalates Oxalates inhibit absorption of calcium and iron from spinach. Spinach and other foods high in oxalates are not recommended for people with gout and certain types of kidney stones.

plant sterols Researchers believe these plant substances help reduce high cholesterol.

vitamin C This antioxidant vitamin may help to prevent macular degeneration, osteoarthritis, and stroke.

maximizing the benefits

Serve spinach either raw or cooked, but avoid overcooking. To preserve loss of water-soluble **B vitamins,** steam or stir-fry spinach. Cooking helps to convert **protein, lutein,** and **beta-carotene** in spinach into more well-absorbed forms. To enhance **carotenoid** absorption, eat spinach along with heart-healthy fat.

health bites

Phylloquinone is the most common form of vitamin K found in green vegetables and is particularly high in dark greens, such as spinach. Vitamin K is necessary for proper blood clotting and possibly may play a role in preserving bone health. However, if you are on blood-thinning medications, consult with your physician before consuming vegetables high in vitamin K. High amounts may interfere with the anticlotting action of the medication.

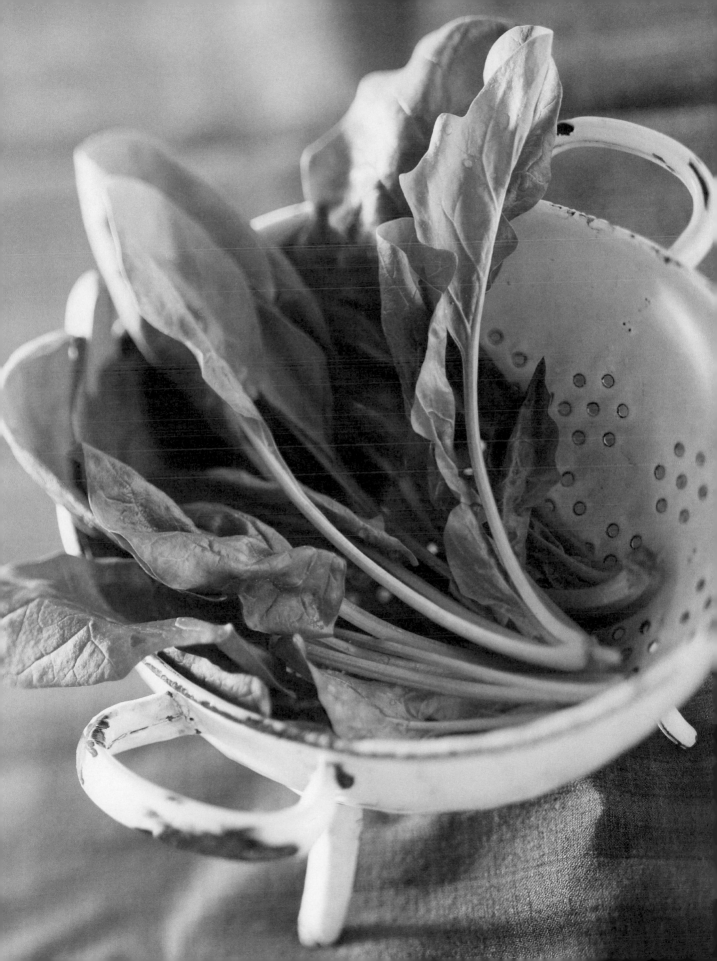

super grains

Ancient high-protein foods with healing properties, so-called super grains—amaranth, buckwheat, teff, and quinoa—are filling and rich in fiber, B vitamins, and phytonutrients.

add more to your diet

► Add teff flour to pancakes and biscuits, using 2 parts wheat flour to 1 part teff flour.

► Cook buckwheat, quinoa, or amaranth and make a salad with smoked tofu, green peppers, tomatoes, and cucumber. Toss with a lemon dressing.

► Grind amaranth in a mini food processor and use the amaranth flour to replace up to one-fourth of the wheat flour in a muffin recipe.

► Make a pilaf with quinoa, onions, dried cherries, and toasted pecans. Serve as a side dish instead of rice.

► Stir cooked buckwheat groats or quinoa into savory tea bread batters.

what's in it

complex carbohydrates Amylopectin and amylose, carbohydrates in buckwheat, may help to control blood sugar levels.

lignans These phytoestrogens may help to lower LDL ("bad") cholesterol and risk for breast, colon, ovarian, and prostate cancer.

lysine Quinoa is a good source of this essential amino acid, which may help to prevent and manage viruses of the herpes family.

magnesium Amaranth and quinoa are good sources of heart-healthy magnesium, which may also help to prevent allergies, asthma, kidney stones, and premenstrual syndrome (PMS).

phytic acids These phytonutrients may help to protect against free-radical cell damage in the intestines.

plant sterols These may help significantly reduce cholesterol.

protease inhibitors These antiviral compounds may also inhibit the formation of cancer cells.

rutin Present in buckwheat, rutin may help minimize cancer risk by detoxifying cancer-causing substances and preventing cancer agents from taking hold in the body. Rutin is also under review for its ability to help control diabetes, lower blood pressure, strengthen blood vessels, and reduce levels of harmful cholesterol.

saponins Quinoa is an especially good source of these substances, which may help to prevent cancer and heart disease.

vitamin E Working with other antioxidant phytonutrients in super grains, vitamin E may help to prevent cancer, cataracts, heart disease, and macular degeneration. Quinoa is a particularly good super grain source of vitamin E.

maximizing the benefits

To preserve nutrients, cook grains without excess water and until just tender; overcooking diminishes phytonutrients.

health bites

Laboratory studies suggest that buckwheat protein decreases cholesterol absorption into the body and increases cholesterol excretion from the body.

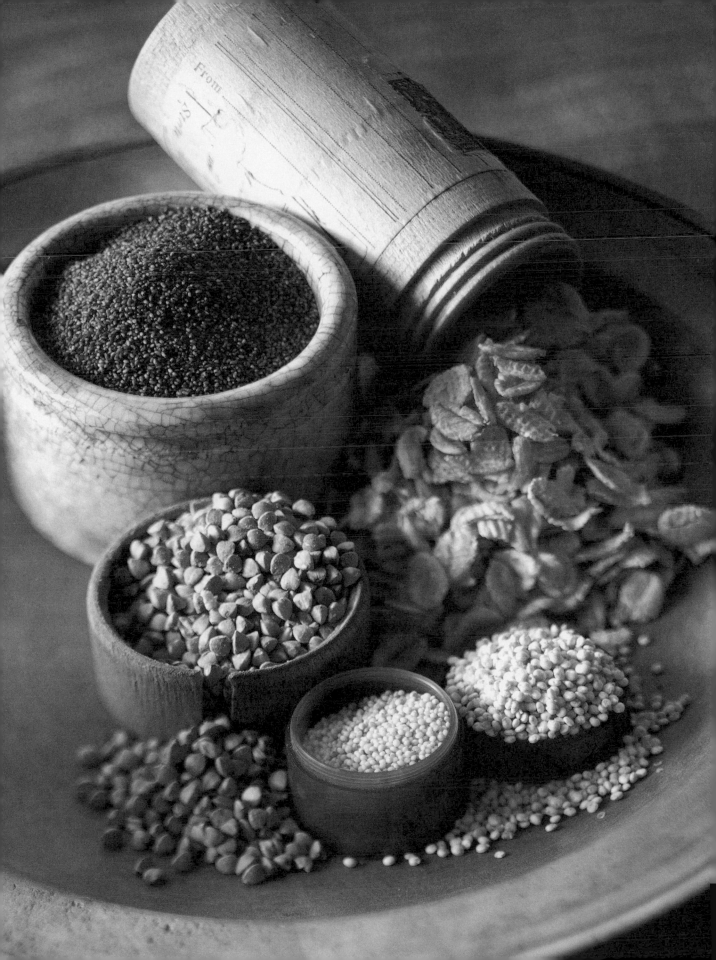

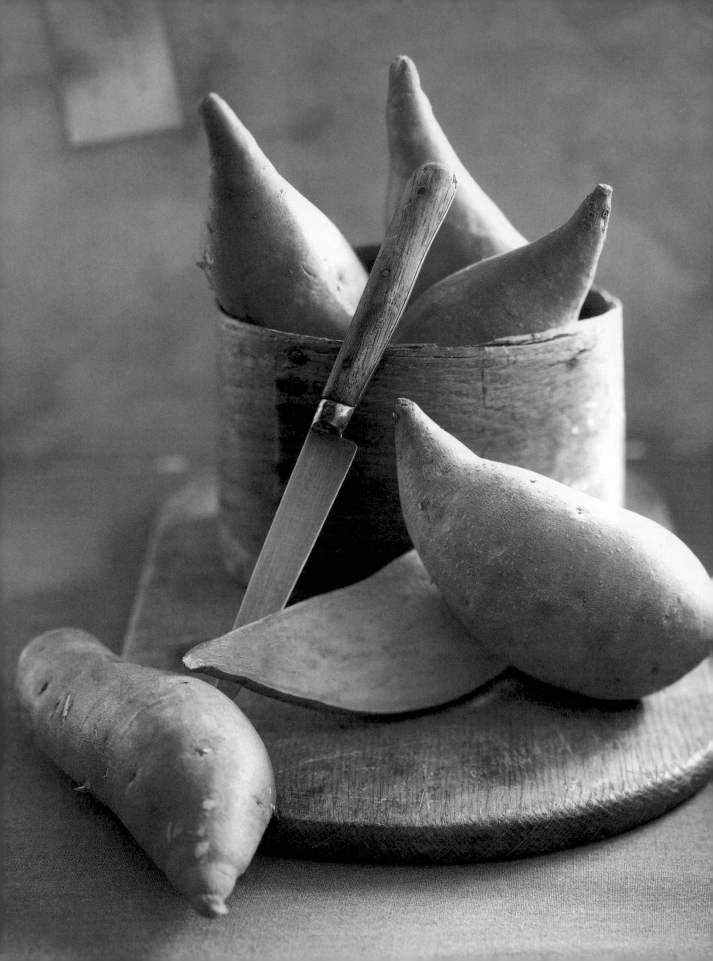

sweet potatoes

Vibrantly colored with carotenoids and filled with fiber, sweet potatoes are one of the most nutrient-dense vegetables. These roots may help prevent cancer, degenerative eye disease, depression, and heart disease.

what's in it

beta-carotene Sweet potatoes are an exceptionally rich source of this plant pigment. Beta-carotene may help to prevent certain cancers (stomach, pancreas, mouth, and gums) and age-related macular degeneration.

caffeic acid This phenolic compound shows promise in fighting cancer and virus-related disease.

chlorogenic acid Preliminary studies suggest this anticancer phytonutrient may help detoxify harmful carcinogens and viruses.

insoluble fiber When eaten with its skin, a sweet potato is an excellent source of insoluble fiber, which may help to prevent constipation, diverticulosis, hemorrhoids, and weight gain.

lutein and zeaxanthin These two carotenoid pigments lend bright orange color to sweet potatoes and may help to protect against atherosclerosis, certain types of cancer, and eye diseases.

pectin About half of the fiber in sweet potatoes is soluble pectin fiber, which may help control cholesterol.

plant sterols These cholesterol-lowering compounds may reduce cancer risk by binding carcinogenic agents in the digestive tract and removing them from the body.

potassium This heart-healthy mineral, found in abundance in sweet potatoes, is associated with lower blood pressure and a lowered risk for heart disease, kidney stones, and stroke.

vitamin B$_6$ Sweet potatoes provide good amounts of B$_6$, which may help to prevent heart disease, stroke, depression, and insomnia.

vitamin C Plentiful in sweet potatoes, vitamin C may help to bolster immunity and wound healing, as well as prevent degenerative eye conditions.

maximizing the benefits

Eat sweet potatoes with their skin to get more **beta-carotene** and **fiber.** Baking or broiling enhances beta-carotene and sweetens the potato as its starches turn to sugar.

add more to your diet

▶ Mash sweet potatoes with maple syrup for an unusual dessert.

▶ Make sweet potato chips: Thinly slice sweet potatoes, drizzle with olive oil, and bake in a 400°F oven until crisp.

▶ For a twist on mashed potatoes, use half sweet potatoes and half all-purpose potatoes.

▶ Add slices of cooked sweet potatoes to savory sandwiches.

▶ Mash cooked sweet potatoes with nutritional yeast and spinach and use in place of the cheese in lasagna recipes.

▶ Substitute mashed sweet potatoes for pumpkin in pies.

▶ Shred raw sweet potatoes and use in place of shredded carrots in cakes, muffins, and tea breads.

▶ Make a sweet potato salad: Cook sweet potatoes and while the potatoes are still warm, peel and cut into chunks. Toss in a dressing of lime juice, olive oil, minced scallions, curry powder, and salt.

tomatoes

Heartily indulge in phytonutrient-rich tomatoes (as well as tomato products), because the nutrients in this vegetable seem to work in concert to protect against cancer, clogged arteries, and skin conditions.

add more to your diet

▶ Cook fresh tomatoes with sugar, cinnamon, and orange zest for a sweet and savory jam.

▶ Combine tomato juice and carrot juice and chill. Serve as a refreshing summer soup garnished with chopped tomatoes and a dollop of dairy-free yogurt.

▶ To give a nutritional boost to savory soups, replace half of the water with tomato or tomato-vegetable juice.

▶ Make a quick sauce for pasta salad: Combine tomato paste, tomato juice, olive oil, balsamic vinegar, and chopped fresh basil, mint, or parsley.

▶ Brush bread with olive oil and garlic, top with tomato paste, and broil. Top with chopped fresh tomatoes.

what's in it

beta-carotene This bioactive pigment may help to prevent acne, certain forms of cancer (stomach, pancreas), and vision loss.

caffeic and ferulic acid These anticancer substances may help enhance the production of the body's cancer-fighting enzymes.

chlorogenic acid Found in greatest amounts in freshly picked tomatoes, this compound may be cancer-protective by inhibiting environmental toxins such as nitrosamines in cigarette smoke.

lutein and zeaxanthin These carotenoids present in tomatoes may team up to help prevent vision loss and possibly cancer.

lycopene Abundant in red tomatoes, this antioxidant pigment may prevent cell damage that leads to heart attacks and cancer. One study found that men who consumed lycopene-rich diets cut their heart attack risk in half, and several studies indicate lycopene may protect against prostate cancer. Tomato juice and tomato paste are particularly concentrated sources of lycopene.

vitamin C Present mainly in the jellylike substance around tomato seeds, vitamin C may protect against heart disease, respiratory infections, skin cancer, and vision loss.

maximizing the benefits

Lycopene is best absorbed from concentrated forms of tomatoes, such as tomato paste, juice, ketchup, sauce, and soup. The more concentrated the tomato source, the more concentrated the lycopene. Heat and oil enhance absorption of lycopene and **beta-carotene,** though some **vitamin C** is lost.

health bites

Lycopene-rich foods such as tomatoes, tomato paste, and watermelon may reduce the risk of developing prostate cancer but don't protect against the progression of advanced prostate cancer.

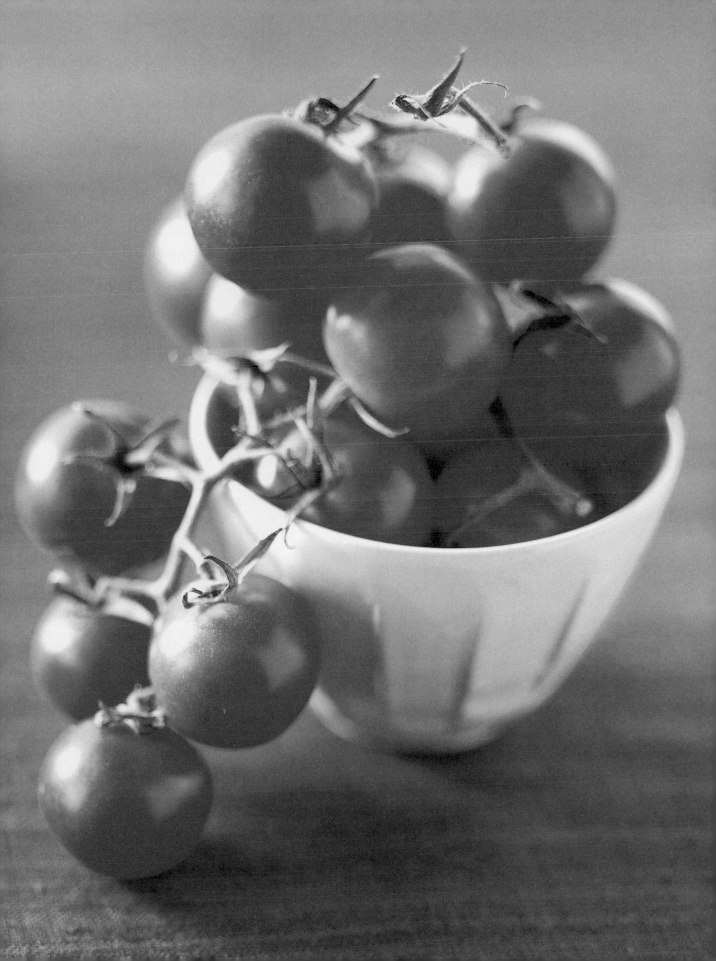

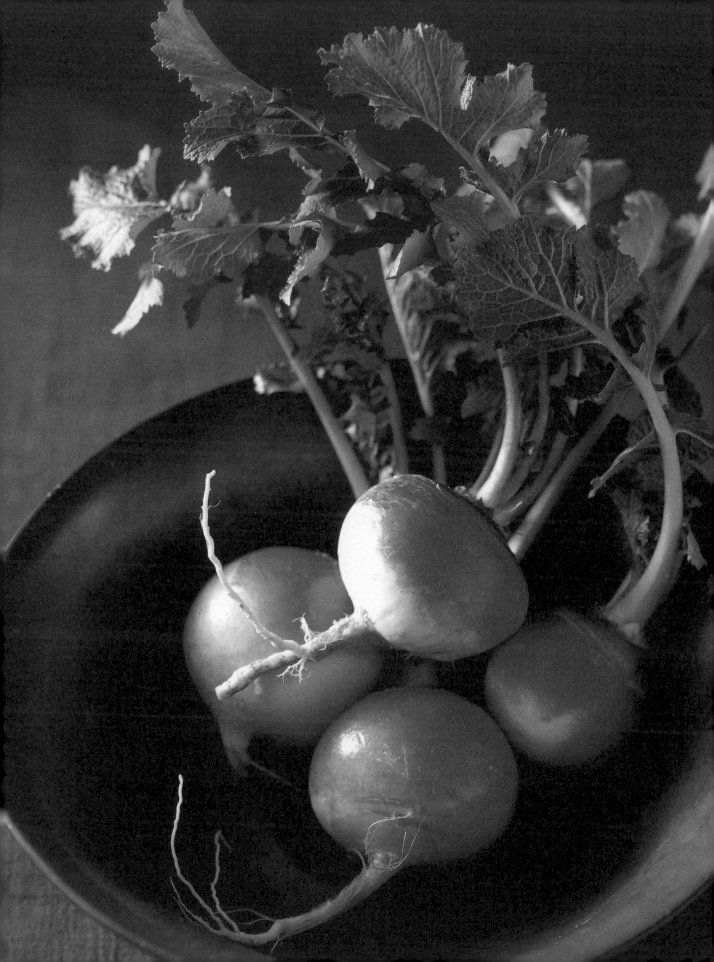

turnips

Earthy roots, with a sweet, smoky flavor, turnips (including the yellow rutabaga) are full of vitamin C and some essential amino acids. Complex carbohydrates and fiber add to the healing power of this cruciferous cousin to cabbage.

what's in it

complex carbohydrates An excellent fuel source for the body, complex carbohydrates tend to release a slow, steady supply of energy. They may also enhance memory, absorb stomach acid associated with heartburn, and improve tryptophan absorption.

goitrogens Found in raw turnips and other cruciferous vegetables, these compounds may suppress thyroid function.

insoluble fiber Insoluble fiber helps to alleviate constipation, and possibly varicose veins and hemorrhoids.

lysine This essential amino acid may help to prevent and manage cold sores and viruses of the herpes family.

soluble fiber This type of fiber helps to soak up cholesterol, lowering blood levels of artery-damaging LDL ("bad") cholesterol.

tryptophan A precursor to the B vitamin niacin, this essential amino acid may help to ease anxiety, depression, and insomnia.

vitamin C Acting as a powerful antioxidant, vitamin C helps to control damaging free radicals and may enhance immunity.

maximizing the benefits

Cooking appears to deactivate **goitrogens** and some **vitamin C** may be lost; on the other hand, cooking increases the availability of **soluble fiber.**

add more to your diet

▶ Combine sliced rutabaga, carrots, and potatoes and cook as for mashed potatoes.

▶ Shred rutabaga or white turnips, add to shredded potatoes along with chopped fresh dill, and make turnip-potato pancakes.

▶ Sauté cubed white turnips in olive oil with garlic and shredded turnip greens.

▶ Shred turnips and toss with shredded red and green apples, and a mixture of apple cider, apple cider vinegar, and Dijon mustard. Serve as a slaw.

▶ Roasted rutabagas have an earthy, nutty flavor: Peel rutabagas and cut into chunks. Toss with olive oil, wrap in foil, and bake at 400°F for 20 to 30 minutes, or until tender.

health bites

Goitrogens are present in raw cruciferous vegetables, including turnips, and may interfere with the synthesis of thyroid hormone. These compounds do not pose a risk for healthy people who eat moderate amounts of cruciferous vegetables. Individuals with hypothyroidism need to eat a varied, well-balanced diet that includes all kinds of vegetables, but also may want to cook cruciferous vegetables to deactivate goitrogens.

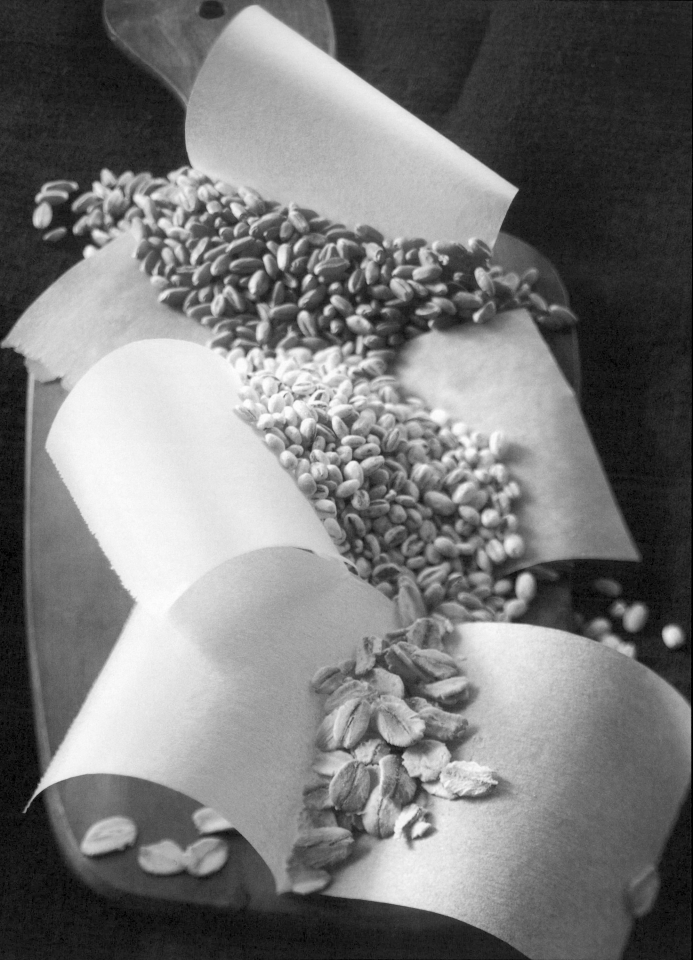

whole grains

The nutritious germ and bran layers of a whole grain are packed with phytonutrients and insoluble fiber. Whole grains—barley, buckwheat, bulgur, farro, oats, quinoa, rye, and wheat—are linked to a lower risk for cancer, cardiovascular disease, and diabetes.

what's in it

beta-glucan Most studies show that soluble beta-glucan fiber in oatmeal, oat bran, and barley may help to significantly reduce total cholesterol and LDL ("bad") cholesterol levels in the blood.

complex carbohydrates These substances may be why one study found that 1 cup of barley improved memory function in healthy elderly adults. Indigestible oligosaccharide carbohydrates may help prevent cancer, cardiovascular disease, and diabetes.

flavonoids These antioxidant compounds in the bran and germ may help to prevent cancer, diabetes, heart disease, and vision loss.

gluten A protein found in barley, oats, rye, and wheat, gluten triggers an immune response that causes discomfort and illness for people with gluten-sensitivity or celiac disease.

lignans Estrogenlike substances found in the bran and germ layers, lignans may lower cholesterol and help inhibit the damaging effects of estrogen, protecting against breast cancer particularly in postmenopausal women.

phytic acids These compounds may protect against free-radical cell damage and also slow starch digestion, thus helping to stabilize blood sugar levels.

plant sterols These substances may help reduce total and LDL ("bad") cholesterol by binding it in the digestive tract.

saponins Oats are an especially good source of these substances, which may bind cholesterol and interfere with cancer growth.

selenium Barley is an outstanding source of this antioxidant mineral, which partners with vitamin E to fight damaging free radicals.

vitamin E This antioxidant may help to prevent cancer, heart disease, skin disorders, and vision loss. Wheat germ is an exceptionally concentrated source.

maximizing the benefits

Cook these grains in a minimum of water and only until tender; overcooking will diminish the nutrient content.

add more to your diet

► Cook cracked wheat or soften bulgur (precooked cracked wheat) in boiling water. Use in salads, pilafs, stuffings, soup, salads; or add to a lentil loaf.

► Cook whole wheatberries, farro, or rye berries until soft, and fold into homemade whole-wheat bread dough.

► Substitute barley for rice in a rice pudding recipe (the cooking times will be longer for barley).

► Toast oat groats (this brings out flavor), then grind them to make a flour. Use the toasted oat flour to make cookies and cakes.

► Although not technically a grain, quinoa boasts all the health benefits of a grain and can replace rice, barley, or bulgur in salads, soups, or stews.

► Add wheat germ to homemade pizza doughs and savory pie doughs.

winter squash

Pumpkin and its orange-fleshed relatives—acorn and butternut squash—are colorful and delicious vegetables that may help to prevent heart disease, macular degeneration, and weight gain.

what's in it

beta-carotene Pumpkin and butternut squash supply extraordinary amounts of this nourishing orange-yellow pigment, which may help to prevent cancer and macular degeneration.

fiber Squash contains appreciable amounts of soluble fiber, which helps to lower harmful LDL cholesterol. Insoluble fiber in squash helps to make you feel full, so you are satisfied with less food, and can also help relieve constipation.

lutein Pumpkin is a particularly significant source of this carotenoid, which may stave off macular degeneration and possibly help prevent cataracts and colon cancer.

magnesium Acorn and butternut squash are good sources of this vital mineral, which may be beneficial for allergies, asthma, cardiovascular health, high blood pressure, kidney stones, and premenstrual syndrome (PMS).

potassium A diet high in this mineral may help to lower the risk for high blood pressure, kidney stones, and stroke. Acorn and butternut squash supply generous amounts of potassium.

thiamin A serving of acorn squash (1 cup cooked) contributes beneficial amounts of this necessary brain-boosting B vitamin, which may help to improve memory and mood.

vitamin B$_6$ Acorn squash supplies an impressive quantity of this essential B vitamin, which is linked to a reduced risk for heart disease and possibly depression.

vitamin C This powerful antioxidant may prevent cataracts and chronic disease. Butternut is the best winter squash source of vitamin C.

maximizing the benefits

For **beta-carotene,** boiling, steaming, baking, and broiling are all fine; but some **B vitamins** will be lost if the squash is cooked in water for a long period of time.

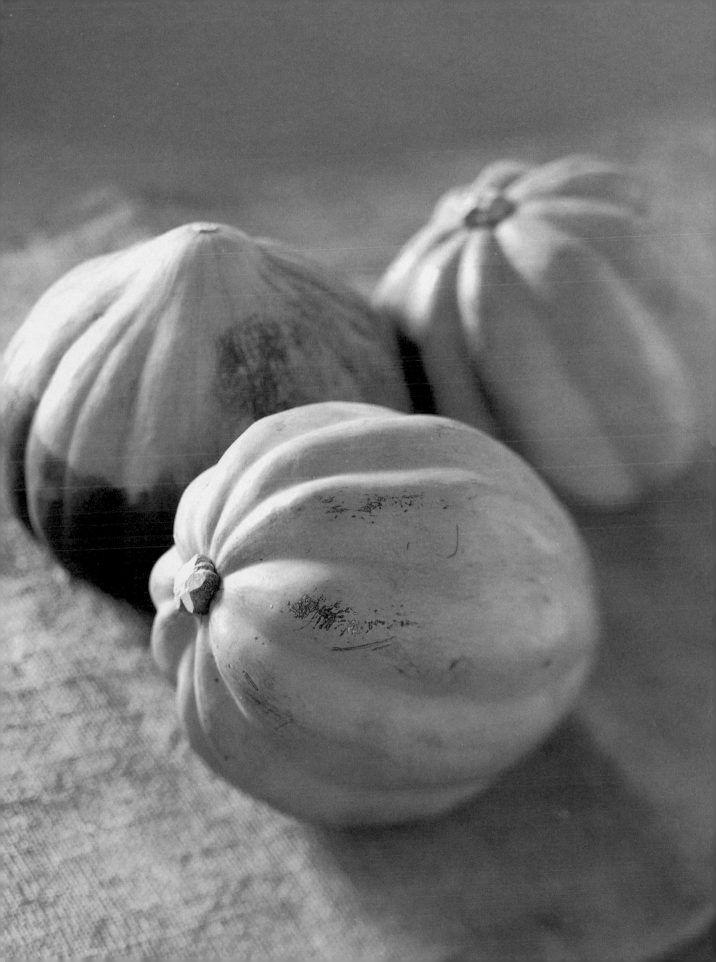

what ails you?

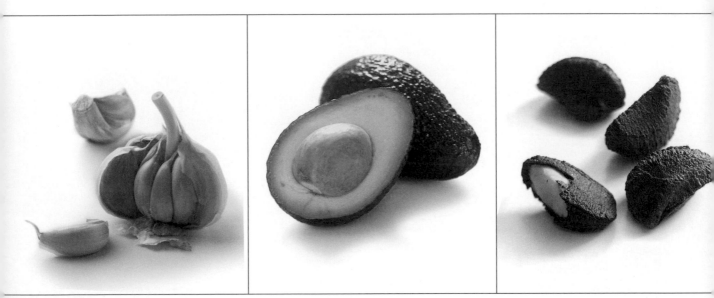

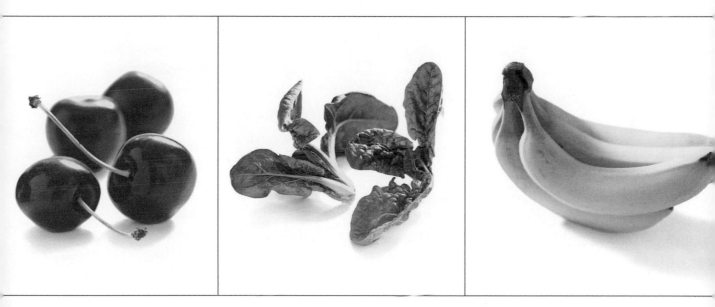

How to Reverse or
Prevent Common Ailments
and Diseases with a
Plant-Based Diet

acne

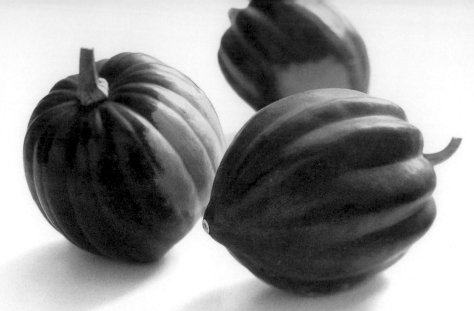

what it is

Acne, an inflammatory condition, occurs when an excess amount of sebum (an oily substance produced by glands that lubricates and moistens the skin) blocks the skin's pores at the base of hair follicles, causing small pus-filled eruptions to appear on the face, chest, shoulders, and back.

Pimples, blackheads, and whiteheads are the characteristics of this condition, which can be managed by simple self-care measures, over-the-counter topical medications, or under the supervision of a dermatologist. Though most forms of acne are mild, in its severe form (cystic acne), permanent pits and scars can occur, especially if skin lesions are picked at and squeezed.

One of the most common of all skin problems, acne generally afflicts adolescents, teenagers, and young adults, though some older people also suffer from acne. Although it is not a dangerous condition, acne can nonetheless cause distress and discomfort for young people in particular, who may, as a result, suffer from poor self-image, social isolation, depression, and anxiety.

what causes it

Acne is often triggered by hormonal activity, which can increase the production of sebum. Though the hormonal shifts of adolescence make teenagers the primary sufferers of acne, women who are pregnant, menstruating, or in menopause are also susceptible. Certain medications (such as steroids or oral contraceptives) that affect hormones, as well as stress, can all contribute to the overproduction of sebum and therefore to acne. For some people there may be a genetic component that contributes to the onset of the condition.

how food may help

One of the prevailing beliefs about acne is that certain foods—such as chocolate or pizza—can cause it or make it worse; but there is no solid evidence to support this. Although more research is needed on the role of diet in acne, certain nutrients are known to promote optimal skin health.

Many skin conditions seem to respond to **vitamin A,** which appears to have a beneficial effect on cell growth and maturation. The best dietary sources of vitamin A are found in foods rich in **beta-caro-tene,** which is converted by the body into vitamin A. Some studies indicate that beta-carotene protects the skin from free-radical stress, and, though research is conflicting, there is also some evidence that it reduces sebum production.

Since inflammation is one of the characteristics of acne, **essential fatty acids** may help alleviate the condition by hindering the body's production of certain inflammatory compounds. **Vitamin E** is also helpful in maintaining healthy skin by teaming up with **selenium** to promote an enzyme called glutathione perox-idase, which may help to reduce inflammation.

The immunity-building mineral **zinc** may help to improve acne, perhaps through its involvement in hormone metabolism as well as the role it plays in healing. And some evidence shows that **vitamin B$_6$** may help to stabilize hormonal fluctuations that can cause acne.

There also appears to be a strong connection between skin inflammation, acne, and gastrointestinal dysfunction. Growing evidence indicates that adding probiotics to the diet can help resolve acne.

recent research

Several studies have linked moderate to severe acne in adolescents and young adults to a high-glycemic or high-sugar diet. One study found significant increases in acne severity among those who drank more than 3½ ounces of carbonated soda, sweetened tea, and fruit-flavored drinks per day.

your food arsenal

foods	nutrient	health benefits
apricots asparagus sweet potatoes winter squash	beta-carotene	Beta-carotene may reduce sebum production by affecting sebaceous gland activity. Too much sebum is one of the causes of acne.
avocados bananas potatoes	vitamin B$_6$	By helping to regulate levels of hormones implicated in the development of acne lesions, vitamin B$_6$ may reduce outbreaks.
beans nuts tofu	zinc	Zinc has been linked to optimal skin health by enhancing immune function, reducing inflammation, and promoting tissue regeneration and healthy hormone levels.

allergies &
asthma

what it is

Though both allergies and asthma are characterized by an immune response to substances that are triggers only in certain people, the two conditions are not the same. Allergies usually result in watery and itchy eyes, runny nose, excessive sneezing, congestion, difficulty breathing, and sometimes hives. Asthma is a chronic inflammatory respiratory disorder. An asthma "attack" takes place when the bronchial tubes that conduct air to the lungs become constricted, causing difficulty in breathing, shortness of breath, wheezing, and coughing. Inflammation is present in the lungs (bronchial tubes) of people with asthma, even those with mild cases, and this plays a key role in all forms of the disease. Inflammation is also present in some people who suffer from allergies.

what causes it

Allergies or asthma may be linked to a genetically inherited tendency. Preliminary research also suggests that asthma may be *caused* by allergies (it is important to note, however, that while many asthma sufferers also have allergies, not all people with allergies have asthma). The release of a chemical called histamine can cause many of the physical manifestations of both allergies and asthma. Histamine has been linked to inflammation, congestion, and excessive mucus secretion and muscle contraction in the airways, as well as itching accompanied by hives.

Numerous irritants such as dust and dust mites, mold, cockroaches, pollen, and pet dander can set off both allergies and asthma. Other asthma triggers include tobacco smoke, cold air, humidity, exercise, food or drug allergies, as well as respiratory infections such as colds, flu, and bronchitis. (For dietary advice for *Colds & Flu*, see *page 152;* for *Bronchitis*, see *page 140*.)

how food may help

It is prudent to eat a low-fat diet rich in fruits and vegetables, which are linked to respiratory health.

Magnesium may help the lungs to relax and may also reduce inflammation. There is also some research that indicates magnesium may help to usher you into a calm sleep, which is important, since insomnia (usually caused by coughing) tends to occur frequently in people with allergies and asthma.

Believed to be a potent lung protector, the flavonoid **quercetin** is thought to also have the capacity to reduce the release of histamine. Another flavonoid, **luteolin,** may also have this effect. Quercetin also appears to have anti-inflammatory properties.

The antioxidant mineral **selenium** teams up with **vitamin E** to protect cells against free-radical damage, and this protective effect is thought to benefit membranes in airways. Selenium may ensure adequate levels of glutathione peroxidase, which is believed to be a potent free-radical-fighting enzyme.

A diet rich in **omega-3 fatty acids** may help to reduce inflammation, and immune-boosting foods rich in **zinc** may help maintain a strong immune system. **Vitamin C** functions as an antioxidant and helps to shield the lungs from environmental pollutants, which can often exacerbate asthma.

recent research

One study showed that eating at least 5 apples a week may strengthen your lungs. The study discovered that men who ate nearly an apple a day had slightly stronger lung function than those who excluded apples from their diets.

Although the researchers were unable to provide a scientific explanation for the protective attributes of apples, a reasonable theory may be that apples are loaded with healthy compounds, including antioxidants and flavonoids, which are thought to fight disease by protecting the body from free-radical damage.

As apples are rich in myriad healthy compounds, it may be the combination of these nutrients that creates the effect. Current research proposes that quercetin, in particular, stands out as a very potent flavonoid that helps to maintain lung health and fight allergic respiratory diseases.

your food arsenal

foods	nutrient	health benefits
amaranth avocados quinoa sunflower seeds	magnesium	Scientists speculate that magnesium may help relax muscles in the lungs.
apples berries cherries red onions	quercetin	Preliminary studies indicate that the anti-allergenic activity of quercetin may be due to its ability to reduce the release of histamine.
Brazil nuts sunflower seeds	selenium	Though the jury is still out regarding selenium's role in asthma, low blood levels of this mineral have been reported in asthmatics.
broccoli citrus fruit peppers strawberries	vitamin C	Vitamin C may help to reduce the harmful effects of environmental oxidants that can worsen allergy and asthma symptoms.

anemia

what it is

Anemia is a fairly common condition that results when the body doesn't have enough iron to produce the hemoglobin (the blood's oxygen-carrying protein) needed to make red blood cells. Proper production of red blood cells helps to supply and transport oxygen to the body's tissues and organs. If your cells don't have a normal supply of oxygen, you feel tired and weak, symptoms associated with iron deficiency anemia (the most prevalent type of anemia), which is a reversible condition. In addition to iron deficiency anemia, there are folate deficiency anemia, pernicious anemia, and more rare types of anemia such as aplastic anemia, hemolytic anemia, thalassemia, and sickle cell anemia.

what causes it

Iron deficiency anemia can result from either an iron-poor diet, intestinal problems that interfere with proper iron absorption, or blood loss (from an acute incident, such as a hemorrhage; from benign causes, such as hemorrhoids or menstruation; or from gastrointestinal bleeding). Young children and pre-menopausal women are at highest risk for developing iron deficiency anemia. Vegetarians may also be at higher risk. Pregnancy can also increase the risk for anemia because the iron requirements of the fetus can potentially deplete the mother's stores of the mineral.

how food may help

To produce red blood cells, the body requires, among other nutrients, iron, folate, and vitamin B_{12}. For iron deficiency anemia, you can help build up your iron stores by eating foods rich in "nonheme" (plant-sourced) **iron** but your doctor may also prescribe supplements. It is important for vegetarians to eat ample amounts of nonheme iron along with foods rich in vitamin C, which improves nonheme iron absorption. To enhance your iron stores, cook in iron pots and pans.

Vitamin C also improves **folate** absorption, which is important in managing folate deficiency anemia. Folate is required for the body's metabolism of amino acids, as well as for the formation of healthy red blood cells. Foods rich in this important B vitamin should be consumed on a regular basis, because folate is water-soluble and the body cannot store a lot of it.

It may also be useful to eat foods rich in **beta-carotene,** since this carotenoid is converted in our bodies to **vitamin A,** which may help to mobilize stored iron from the liver. Foods rich in **vitamin B$_6$,** which assists in the formation of hemoglobin, are also beneficial. Vegans and vegetarians may be at risk for developing pernicious anemia, which results from a chronic lack of **vitamin B$_{12}$.** Make sure you consult a physician before you embark on a nutritional plan to correct your anemia.

foods to avoid

Note that some foods contain substances that may reduce your body's ability to absorb iron: tannic acid in tea; calcium phosphate in dairy products; oxalates in spinach, rhubarb, Swiss chard, and chocolate; and phytates in bran, peas, seeds, and soybeans. All of these may hinder the entry of iron into your digestive system. A high-fiber diet in general may act as an iron inhibitor.

your food arsenal

foods	nutrient	health benefits
asparagus black-eyed peas chicory lentils pinto beans	folate	Folate, along with other nutrients, is important for the manufacture of red blood cells. Adequate intake of this vital B vitamin can also help to prevent development of a type of anemia called folate deficiency anemia. Alcohol addiction and poor diet increase the risk for developing this type of anemia.
amaranth quinoa tofu	iron	Iron is required for the formation of hemoglobin, which carries oxygen in red blood cells to organs and tissues. Fatigue and weakness associated with iron deficiency anemia are due to insufficient red blood cells and the resulting inadequate distribution of oxygen to the cells.
nutritional yeast	vitamin B$_{12}$	Required for the production of red blood cells, this vitamin may help to prevent the onset of a type of anemia that is often found in strict vegans or people whose general diet is poor and lacking in variety.
broccoli citrus fruit peppers strawberries	vitamin C	Folate and iron are best absorbed from plant sources when accompanied by a source of vitamin C.

anxiety & stress

what it is

Anxiety and stress, though slightly different emotional states, are both natural reactions to danger or to an uncomfortable situation. A basic human survival instinct left over from our primordial roots, stress is an automatic protective mechanism that may actually help to alert us to danger.

Stress is a normal part of everyone's life. However, reactions to stress can culminate in anxiety, which, depending upon its severity, can interfere with health. Symptoms of anxiety include a heightened sense of self-awareness and an exaggerated awareness of surroundings, muscle tension, nervousness, insomnia, heart palpitations, intense worry, and feelings of dread and doom. Prolonged feelings of anxiety may signal a more serious anxiety disorder, which can lead to depression. For most people, though, anxiety and stress are all too common hallmarks of living in a fast-paced world that often seems out of our control.

what causes it

Certain factors (the list of potential triggers could be endless) can spur anxiety and stress, including real physical threats, job changes, hormonal changes, medications, financial problems, marital woes, illness, grief, and withdrawal from caffeine, alcohol, tobacco, sedatives, narcotics, or other addictive drugs.

how food may help

Because anxiety and stress can often overstimulate nerves and cause muscles to be tight and tense, it may be helpful to eat foods rich in **calcium** and **magnesium,** two minerals that work together to help regulate nerve conduction and muscle contraction.

Dietary support from **complex carbohydrates,** which are found in most "comfort foods," is another nutritional defense against stress and anxiety. The amino acid **tryptophan** is instrumental in the manufacture of serotonin, a mood-enhancing neurotransmitter that will help you to relax and feel more calm. Complex carbohydrates not only ensure proper absorption of tryptophan but they also may dampen the stress response by elevating levels of serotonin.

A number of B vitamins help to release energy from carbohydrates, maintain proper nervous system function, and control glucose levels—all of which are useful during stress and anxiety. Specifically, **vitamin B$_6$** assists in the manufacture of brain chemicals—such as serotonin, dopamine, and melatonin—that control mood.

Because stress can create temporary high blood pressure by triggering the release of certain hormones, it would be wise to consume foods that can combat high blood pressure (see *page 174*). As another side effect of anxiety and stress, the body can experience gastrointestinal woes such as diarrhea (see *page 160*).

Also important are immune-building foods rich in **vitamin C** and **zinc**, whose substances may help fight off viruses (the common cold and flu) brought on by the body's weakened state due to stress. Cold sores, too, are frequent companions of stress; see page 150 for some dietary advice that can help you evade and/or manage them.

recent research

A small study recently showed that a vegetarian diet may be linked with reduced anxiety and depression levels. The study participants were divided into two groups, 40 vegetarians and 40 nonvegetarians. Diet analysis of the two groups showed that the vegetarian group consumed more antioxidant-rich foods than did the nonvegetarian group.

Psychological tests were administered to both groups to determine differences in anxiety and depression between both groups. Interestingly, significantly more anxiety and depression were reported in the nonvegetarian group. Authors of the study speculate that the higher level of antioxidants in the vegetarian group may account for this finding.

your food arsenal

foods	nutrient	health benefits
broccoli cooking greens figs	calcium	Calcium is vital for normal communication between nerve cells and for muscle contraction.
beans potatoes rice whole grains	complex carbohydrates	Eating foods that are high in complex carbohydrates along with foods high in tryptophan (see below) will help facilitate the proper absorption of the tryptophan.
amaranth avocados sunflower seeds wheat germ	magnesium	Magnesium helps relax muscles.
bananas peas turnips	tryptophan	The brain uses tryptophan to help produce serotonin, a mood-enhancing neurotransmitter.
bananas potatoes	vitamin B$_6$	Vitamin B$_6$ assists in the production of brain chemicals, such as serotonin, which help the body cope with anxiety and stress.

bronchitis

what it is

Bronchitis is swelling and inflammation of the lining of the bronchial tubes of the lungs, caused by an infection or an irritant. This results in narrowed airways, making breathing difficult. Irritation can damage the cells lining the airways. It can also destroy tiny cilia, protective "hairs" that normally trap and sweep away foreign matter; damage to the cilia sets up an environment wherein an accumulation of irritants creates excess mucus, resulting in a heavy, deep cough, shortness of breath, and wheezing.

There are two forms of bronchitis, acute and chronic. Acute bronchitis is more common and it often follows a severe cold or flu (see *Colds & Flu, page 152*), though it can also be triggered by environmental pollutants or a bacterial infection. Though not considered a serious health threat to most people, acute bronchitis may be more dangerous for the very young, the elderly, or people who have a suppressed immune system or suffer from certain conditions such as heart disease or pulmonary disorders such as asthma.

Bronchitis is termed "chronic bronchitis" when symptoms such as excessive mucus production, coughing, and wheezing are experienced regularly for a long period of time (coughing up phlegm most days for at least three months of the year for at least two years in a row). Chronic bronchitis is principally a disease of smokers, and is a potentially life-threatening disease that causes progressive and permanent damage to the lungs. Pneumonia is another complication associated with chronic bronchitis.

what causes it

Smoking is a primary offender and is believed to be responsible for a majority (80 to 90%) of chronic bronchitis cases. Viral infections such as the flu and the common cold, as well as bacterial infections, can also lead to bronchitis.

Other factors that may contribute to bronchitis include exposure to chemical fumes, aerosol products (such as hair sprays, deodorants, and insecticides), dust, smog, and other environmental pollutants.

how food may help

Along with quitting smoking, a diet that includes plenty of fruit and vegetables may help to protect your lungs from free-radical damage. The inflammatory nature of acute bronchitis may be ameliorated by **omega-3 fatty acids,** which are thought to reduce the production of inflammatory compounds. Though scientific evidence is scarce, alternative practitioners feel that **bromelain,** an enzyme found in pineapples, also reduces inflammation in the airways.

Certain foods contain substances that help to protect your lungs from destructive environmental pollutants. For example, **vitamin C**-rich foods may offer antioxidant protection against free radicals in smog and cigarette smoke.

Fundamental for maintaining optimum health, vitamin C may also maintain a robust immune system to help fight off colds and viruses, which are often implicated in the onset of bronchitis. The mineral **zinc** is also instrumental in maintaining the immune system's defenses.

Preliminary studies indicate that the flavonoid **naringin,** found in white grapefruit, appears to shield the lungs from environmental toxins. Foods rich in **vitamin E** may also prevent oxidative damage to the lungs.

recent research

Numerous studies reveal a beneficial association between fruit and vegetable intake and lung function. Results from a large cross-sectional study carried out in 69 counties in rural China indicate that participants who consume foods rich in vitamin C had better lung function and, consequently, a lower risk for developing pulmonary diseases such as bronchitis than those participants with lower intakes of vitamin C.

Interestingly, study participants consumed about 50% more vitamin C per day than the average North American. The authors suggest that the antioxidant properties of vitamin C may protect the lungs from free-radical damage.

your food arsenal

foods	nutrient	health benefits
chia seeds **flaxseeds** **walnuts**	omega-3 fatty acids	Since bronchitis is an inflammatory disorder, consuming foods rich in omega-3 fatty acids may help to protect lungs by lowering the body's production of inflammatory substances.
citrus fruit **kiwifruit** **pineapple** **strawberries**	vitamin C	The antioxidant properties of vitamin C may help to shield the lungs from free radicals produced by environmental pollutants such as smog and cigarette smoke. Further, vitamin C may help your immune system fight off colds and viruses, which often precede bronchitis.
beans **pumpkin seeds**	zinc	The immune-enhancing ability of zinc may protect against viruses that cause colds and flu, which often trigger acute bronchitis.

cancer

what it is

Cancer is a group of more than 100 related diseases caused by an abnormal proliferation of cells that divide continuously. This unregulated cell growth may spread and invade normal tissue, creating malignancy, which can invade surrounding tissues and may spread further. Cancer can strike at any age and can develop in any part of the body. After cardiovascular disease, cancer is the second leading cause of death in the United States.

The good news is that many types of cancer are highly preventable, and with early detection, a great number can be successfully treated. You can reduce your risk for developing cancer through proper medical screening, awareness of symptoms and risk factors, regular self-examination, and a healthy diet and lifestyle. Poor lifestyle decisions may play a substantial role in many cancer cases; it is estimated that at least 18% of all cancers in the United States have a nutritional and/or fitness connection.

what causes it

The development and progression of cancer is a complex, multistep process. Cancer often takes years to develop, and is thought to occur as a result of a combination of factors, including heredity, genetic damage, environment, lifestyle, and diet. The immune system's inability to repair damage caused by outside forces such as cigarette smoke, chemicals, asbestos, radiation (X-rays and ultraviolet sunlight), smog, and other environmental carcinogens, as well as excessive alcohol consumption, can cause normal cells to mutate into precancerous cells. These cells, in turn, may or may not become cancer cells. Repeated exposure to free radicals can cause basic cellular damage and may induce the onset of cancer.

how food may help

Even if you do have some of the risk factors associated with the development of cancer, you can start to tip the odds in your favor by selecting healthful foods (as well as quitting cigarette smoking and starting an exercise program). First and foremost, you should reduce dietary fat. Studies show a reduced incidence of cancer among people who eat a diet that is low in fat. Replacing saturated fats with **monounsaturated fats** such as olive oil can also protect against cancer and other life-threatening conditions; and preliminary research indicates that **omega-3 fatty acids** may provide protective effects against developing various cancers and treatment for existing conditions.

Many other compounds in foods are also under scientific scrutiny for their potential either to prevent the onset of cancer or to prevent cancerous tumors from growing. One piece of fruit, for example, could contain *hundreds* of potentially beneficial phytonutrients. Clearly, the best way to ensure that you are benefitting from a diverse array of cancer-fighting nutrients and phytonutrients is simply to consume a wide variety of fruits and vegetables every day.

your food arsenal

foods	nutrient	health benefits
garlic **onion family**	allium compounds	These compounds, also known as sulfur compounds, may stimulate the immune system's natural defenses against cancer, and they may have the potential to reduce tumor growth.
apples **berries** **cherries** **red grapes & wine**	anthocyanins	Anthocyanins, plant pigments classed as flavonoids, may have antioxidant potential to reduce the risk for developing cancer by neutralizing free radicals.
apricots **carrots** **sweet potatoes**	beta-carotene	Studies suggest that this carotenoid may function as a powerful antioxidant and protect cells from free-radical damage.
dark chocolate **green tea** **pomegranates**	catechins	Green tea contains EGCG, a catechin that may help to fight cancer in three ways: It may reduce the formation of carcinogens in the body, increase the body's natural defenses, and suppress cancer promotion.
apples **berries** **broccoli** **citrus fruits** **onion family**	flavonoids	Many flavonoids act as antioxidants, and some have several other biological anticancer effects, mostly related to altering enzymes of metabolism and cell growth. Flavonoids are also thought to prevent DNA damage to cells.
asparagus **beets** **lentils**	folate	This B vitamin is crucial for normal DNA synthesis and repair; low levels of folate are thought to make cells vulnerable to carcinogenesis.

continued on next page

your food arsenal

foods	nutrient	health benefits
broccoli **brussels sprouts** **cabbage**	glucosinolates	Glucosinolates are transformed into a variety of protective substances, which enhance the immune system's defenses and help to block cancer-promoting enzymes.
apricots **pink & red grapefruit** **tomatoes** **watermelon**	lycopene	As an antioxidant, lycopene may detect and destroy harmful free-radical molecules. Lycopene is thought to help protect against prostate cancer.
avocados **olives/olive oil** **peanuts/peanut oil** **walnuts**	monounsaturated fat	Monounsaturated fat may protect against breast and colon cancer, though how it works is currently unknown and under review.
apples **berries** **green tea** **pomegranates** **turmeric**	phenolic acids	Phenolic acids are a subgroup of plant polyphenols that may have the ability to destroy free radicals as well as activate cancer-fighting enzymes in the body, which can help to reduce tumors early in the cancer process.
flaxseed **legumes** **pomegranates** **soy foods**	phytoestrogens	Phytoestrogens help to block estrogen by attaching themselves to places (receptor sites) where natural estrogen wants to lodge, thus lowering estrogen levels and reducing the risk of developing hormone-related cancers (breast, uterine, as well as prostate).
peanuts **red & purple grapes** **red wine**	resveratrol	Resveratrol may help fight cancer at three different stages: cancer initiation, promotion, and progression.
Brazil nuts **fortified cereals** **mushrooms** **whole-wheat bread**	selenium	Studies suggest that this mineral may help to prevent lung, prostate, and colon cancer, possibly through its antioxidant abilities, though other actions are under review.
broccoli **cabbage family** **cooking greens**	sulforaphane	This powerful isothiocyanate is thought to activate detoxifying enzymes in the body that fight off cancer, and it also may destroy precancerous cells and block carcinogens.
bell peppers **broccoli** **citrus fruits**	vitamin C	Vitamin C may help to prevent cancer cell division and growth, and it also may inhibit carcinogenic nitrosamines.
nuts **olive oil** **sunflower seeds** **super grains**	vitamin E	Antioxidant protection provided by vitamin E may help to guard cells against free radicals. Vitamin E may also play a role in stimulating the immune system's response to cellular changes.

Antioxidant Vitamins and Trace Minerals: Free-radical molecules are produced in the body by cellular reactions between oxygen and glucose. They can also be generated from environmental sources (cigarette smoke, radiation, and smog) and can cause direct damage to cells. This free-radical damage can set off the initiation of the cancer process. Nutrients that behave as antioxidants neutralize free radicals, thus helping to prevent cells from becoming cancerous. Some of the principal antioxidant nutrients include **vitamin C, vitamin E,** and the trace mineral **selenium.**

recent research
Multiple studies show significant benefits of a plant-based diet for cancer survivors in place of a meat-centered diet. As a result, top health organizations recommend cancer survivors follow a plant-based diet in addition to maintaining a healthy weight.

Carotenoids: These plant pigments may help the body's immune system defend against harmful free radicals. Carotenoids are also thought to interrupt the process of uncontrolled abnormal division typical of cancer cells. Studies show that some carotenoids may help to stimulate the immune system's natural killer (NK) cell activity. Natural killer cells attack and neutralize cancer cells. Two carotenoids under continuous review for their cancer-fighting abilities include **beta-carotene** and **lycopene.**

Flavonoids: A large class of phytonutrients (there are thousands of flavonoids), flavonoids can be broken down into numerous categories. Each type of flavonoid functions in a different way, with many flavonoids acting as antioxidants. Flavonoids may also improve the absorption of **vitamin C,** an important antioxidant vitamin. Key flavonoid categories that have been studied for their potential to combat cancer include **anthocyanins, citrus flavonoids, quercetin, isoflavones** (in soy), and **catechins** (in tea).

Glucosinolates: Natural substances found in cruciferous vegetables, such as broccoli and cabbage, glucosinolates are precursors for some potentially vigorous cancer fighters such as **indoles** and **isothiocyanates.** Glucosinolate derivatives are thought to enhance the body's own defenses against cancer.

Phenolic Acids: These compounds may have the ability to destroy free radicals as well as activate cancer-fighting enzymes in the body, and they may also have the ability to block the formation of carcinogens such as nitrosamines in cigarette smoke and cured meats. Notable phenolic acids that may help to battle cancer are **curcumin** and **caffeic, chlorogenic, ferulic,** and **ellagic acids.**

Phytoestrogens: Often referred to as "plant estrogens," phytoestrogens are plant substances that are thought to block estrogens. High levels of estrogen are linked to certain hormone-related types of cancer. There are two main types of phytoestrogens—**isoflavones** such as **genistein** in soy foods and **lignans** in flaxseeds, rye, and sesame seeds.

Sulfur Compounds: Also known as **allium compounds,** sulfur compounds impart pungency to garlic, onions, leeks, chives, and shallots. Sulfur compounds may help to enhance the immune system, may inhibit the growth of cancer cells, and may also prevent the formation of nitrosamines, dangerous carcinogens found in cigarette smoke and cured meat.

cataracts

what it is

The development of cataracts is a gradual, age-related eye disorder that causes the lens of the eye to lose transparency, which impairs vision. When normal proteins in the eye become damaged, they cluster together and become opaque, a process that creates a cloudy area in the lens that, over time, causes blurry and distorted vision. So common is this condition that approximately one in four Americans over age 65, and half over age 75, have cataracts. The good news is that cataracts are treatable and probably more preventable than previously believed.

what causes it

Researchers feel that chronic free-radical damage may be associated with cataract development. Thought to be the cause of a number of age-related conditions, free-radical damage can result from a lifetime of exposure to sunlight's harmful ultraviolet (UV) rays, cigarette smoke, pollution, and other environmental factors. In the case of the eye, free-radical damage can weaken the delicate cell structure in the lens of the eye, which slowly causes development of cataracts. Because most cataracts are age-related, preventive strategies adopted early on may help to delay or prevent them. Diabetes can also cause the development of cataracts.

how food may help

In addition to various lifestyle changes you can make to reduce free-radical damage, such as wearing sunglasses that block UV rays and stopping smoking, certain dietary adjustments can be made that may be beneficial, including consuming a diet rich in fiber and antioxidants. Foods that are high in antioxidants play a significant role in combatting the damage caused by free radicals.

Because **vitamin C** is a potent antioxidant, consuming foods that are high in this nutrient may help protect against cataracts. Studies also show that vitamin C may play a role in preventing the clustering of proteins in the eye, a process associated with cataract formation.

Working hand-in-hand with other important nutrients, such as the mineral selenium, **vitamin E** functions as a powerful antioxidant by shielding cell membranes from harm caused by sunlight. It also protects the vitamin A found in the eye from UV damage.

Studies suggest that the carotenoid **lutein** may act like internal sunglasses by filtering out the sun's harmful ultraviolet rays. Lutein is the yellow substance found inside the macula lutea (the tiny yellow spot in the center of the retina). Lutein absorbs sunlight's harmful waves, thus blocking damage to the delicate structure of the cells in the eyes. A closely related carotenoid compound, **zeaxanthin,** is also thought to defend the lens from free-radical harm incurred from sunlight.

Preliminary research also indicates that **quercetin,** a flavonoid found in a number of foods, may protect against cataracts. Studies suggest that quercetin helps to maintain lens transparency after free-radical damage from sunlight.

recent research

Curcumin, a powerful substance in turmeric (a spice used in Indian curry dishes), may be one of the most effective antioxidants that help to protect against cataracts. Multiple laboratory studies suggest curcumin may protect the lens of the eye from becoming cloudy by enhancing vitamin C and glutathione levels, both potent antioxidants. Curcumin's antioxidant power may protect the eyes from cell damage caused by sunlight's ultraviolet rays and delay the progression of diabetic cataracts.

your food arsenal

foods	nutrient	health benefits
corn kale kiwifruit peas spinach	lutein & zeaxanthin	Lutein may protect the eye from sunlight's dangerous ultraviolet rays by filtering out the light waves that destroy cells in the eye's lens. Zeaxanthin provides antioxidant protection by shielding against free-radical damage.
apples cherries red onions	quercetin	Quercetin may help to protect eyes even after they have been exposed to sunlight's harmful rays.
bell peppers broccoli citrus fruit strawberries	vitamin C	Vitamin C may play a role in preventing the clumping of proteins in the eye, which is linked to cataract formation.
almonds avocados peanut butter sunflower seeds wheat germ	vitamin E	Some studies suggest that vitamin E's antioxidant activities may help prevent cataract formation.

chronic fatigue syndrome

what it is

This elusive condition, clinically known as myalgic encephalomyelitis, is characterized by so many different symptoms that it is often very difficult to diagnose. Many other illnesses have symptoms that mimic those of chronic fatigue syndrome (CFS), and for this reason, your health care practitioner will have to rule out other illnesses and other possible causes of fatigue, such as anemia, depression, fibromyalgia, infection, diabetes, heart disease, thyroid disease, and cancer. Overwhelming and persistent fatigue is the overriding primary symptom of CFS, which is defined as extreme fatigue and malaise not improved with bed rest. Symptoms often last for at least six months and interfere significantly with daily living.

what causes it

Although CFS is recognized as a complex brain disorder, its cause is unknown and, as such, is a conundrum to health care practitioners. Numerous medical theories abound, including proposals that CFS is linked with infections such as Epstein-Barr virus (the virus that also causes mononucleosis), allergies, Lyme disease, impaired metabolic function, low blood pressure, adrenal gland dysfunction, immune abnormalities, neurological disturbances, rheumatic diseases, disorders of the central nervous system, autoimmune disorders, hormonal problems, and certain medications. Although no single virus has been implicated, many patients with CFS nonetheless report having had a flu-like illness that triggered the symptoms. There is no evidence that CFS is contagious.

how food may help

While there is no known cure for this ailment, some nutrient deficiencies appear to affect the severity and progression of the disease. That means certain nutrients in foods may help to improve symptoms. Some of the symptoms of CFS include swollen glands, inflammation of the joints, and other flu-like symptoms, all of which may be temporarily relieved by foods rich in **essential fatty acids (EFAs).** EFAs may help to block the release of inflammatory substances in your body. It is thought that there may be an abnormality in essential fatty acid metabolism in some people with chronic fatigue syndrome. Note, too, that a particular type of EFA, **omega-3 fatty acids,** may also help to fight off depression, which often accompanies CFS.

Because **vitamin B$_{12}$** deficiency is associated with fatigue and depression, it's possible that consuming foods rich in this vitamin could help to minimize the fatigue and depression of CFS. Other B vitamins, such as **thiamin, B$_6$,** and **riboflavin,** are instrumental in fighting fatigue by assisting the body in energy production.

For many people, CFS occurs directly after they have fallen ill from a cold, the flu, or an intestinal infection. Therefore, consume foods rich in **vitamin C,** which help to fortify a weakened immune system (believed by many to be a factor in CFS). **Zinc** promotes the destruction of foreign microorganisms and hinders the growth of viruses such as the common cold (see also *Colds & Flu, page 152*), and also helps to enhance and repair the immune system.

Since a number of people with CFS experience headaches and muscle aches, foods rich in **magnesium** are helpful. To combat the accompanying insomnia that plagues many people with CFS, it may be helpful to eat foods rich in the amino acid **tryptophan,** which is converted by your body into the brain chemical serotonin. Note that **carbohydrate**-rich meals often help to increase serotonin levels.

recent research

While stress is not the root cause of chronic fatigue syndrome, there is quite a bit of evidence showing that stress can trigger or exacerbate existing CFS. One study explored stressful situations associated with CFS symptoms. The researchers identified pregnancy, spousal abuse, eating disorders, car accidents, financial problems, and sleep issues as the top stressors associated with the onset of Chronic Fatigue Syndrome.

your food arsenal

foods	nutrient	health benefits
amaranth avocados quinoa sunflower seeds	magnesium	Magnesium plays a role in the production and transport of energy and it also assists in the contraction and relaxation of muscles, an important function since people with chronic fatigue syndrome often experience muscle tenderness.
bananas peas spirulina wheat germ	tryptophan	Though one of the main symptoms of CFS is fatigue, many people suffering from this condition also have trouble sleeping and experience bouts of insomnia. Tryptophan is converted to serotonin, which helps to make you feel relaxed and sleepy. Note that eating foods high in complex carbohydrates will help in the proper absorption of tryptophan.
almonds beans cashews fortified cereal pumpkin seeds	zinc	Foods rich in the mineral zinc may help to keep the immune system working properly. A robust immune system can help to ward off certain viruses, such as the common cold and flu, conditions that may possibly precede the onset of CFS.

cold sores

what it is

Cold sores (herpes simplex virus), also called fever blisters, are painful, sensitive infections that appear on the lips, the outside of the mouth, and occasionally inside or on the nose. Most people have experienced these uncomfortable blisters, and in fact 90% of all people develop at least one cold sore in their lifetime. Often preceded by a burning, pulsating, itching sensation, a small fluid-filled sore will emerge. Within a day or so, the sore ruptures and a scab forms.

Once you have had a cold sore, the herpes virus that causes it remains with you for the rest of your life. It lies dormant in nerve cells and may re-emerge for a variety of reasons, perhaps when the immune system is supressed or when you are under a lot of stress or don't get enough sleep. For most people who have recurrent cold sores, subsequent sores will appear in the same location as the initial sore and will be less painful. Some people are more prone to getting cold sores, and while almost everyone has had the virus, only some people actually experience symptoms. Cold sores generally last for a week to 10 days.

what causes it

Cold sores are caused by the herpes simplex virus type 1 (not to be confused with herpes simplex virus type 2, which causes sexually transmitted genital herpes). The virus that causes cold sores may be spread by touch from lip sores to other parts of the body, primarily the mucous membranes of the eyes, nose, and, though rare, the genital areas. Careful hand washing, and avoidance of kissing when the sore is in its early stage, are important in preventing its spread. Once it has scabbed over, the cold sore is less contagious.

Certain factors can trigger cold sores, such as being run-down, ultra-violet radiation (too much exposure to the sun), hormonal changes such as menstruation, some medications that reduce your immune system's effectiveness, infections, and emotional stress. Dietary measures can help bolster your immune system's defenses; this is important for the possible prevention and control of cold sores.

how food may help

Some health care providers theorize that a diet high in **lysine** may reduce the recurrence of cold sores. Lysine is an amino acid that is thought to combat the onset of cold sores (or reduce the duration of them) by interfering with the absorption of arginine, an amino acid that is necessary for the herpes virus to reproduce and for a viral infection to progress. So, along with eating foods high in lysine, it may help to avoid foods that contain arginine (see *Foods to Avoid,* right).

Another nutritional strategy to combat and manage cold sores is to regularly eat foods that maintain a strong immune system. Foods rich in **vitamin C** and **zinc** possess antioxidant powers that increase the immune system's ability to help fight off the virus that causes cold sores. Cold sores tend to occur when the body is under stress, which can compromise your immune system (see *Anxiety & Stress, page 138,* for dietary advice).

foods to avoid

Try to stay away from chocolate, peanuts, almonds, seeds, cereal grains, gelatin, carob, beer, and raisins. These foods have an unfavorable arginine-to-lysine ratio, which may make you more susceptible to experiencing a recurrence of cold sores. Some research suggests that arginine-rich foods have specific biochemical actions and proteins that trigger the onset of cold sores.

your food arsenal

foods	nutrient	health benefits
fenugreek seeds spirulina soybeans tofu	lysine	Lysine is an amino acid that may interfere with the absorption of arginine in the intestine, thus preventing the onset of cold sores.
berries citrus fruits kiwifruit melons	vitamin C	A vital nutrient for the body's healing process, vitamin C is also involved in the production of antibodies and white blood cells, which work to ward off infections and viruses.
beans fortified cereals nuts whole grains	zinc	Zinc helps to maintain a strong immune system, so that it can destroy viruses, which often opportunistically attempt to strike when the body is run-down.

colds & flu

what it is

The common cold is something that we have all had, and its presence has plagued mankind from the beginning of time. And it has managed, to date, to elude a cure. The common cold is a highly contagious infection that often starts out as throat irritation and a stuffy nose, and culminates in red, watery eyes, sneezing, coughing, sore throat, runny nose, congestion, mild headache, and general fatigue and malaise. Colds rarely cause serious complications, with the exception of ear infections in children. Colds can, however, exacerbate asthma, and also lead to lower respiratory tract infections such as bronchitis and pneumonia (especially in the elderly, who are often very susceptible to infection). A cold will generally subside after five to 10 days. Americans develop about two to four colds a year.

With more than 20,000 deaths from complications of the flu (influenza) in America annually, the flu virus is certainly more dangerous than the common cold. Flu symptoms include muscle aches, joint pain, high fever, fatigue, headache, sore throat, and sometimes a dry, nonproductive cough. Young children, infants, the elderly, and people with serious medical conditions or who are on immune-suppressing medications are at increased risk for developing complications such as pneumonia and other respiratory infections.

what causes it

Colds and influenza, which are caused by different types of viruses, are both highly contagious: The viruses can be spread through the air and through contact with things such as telephones and doorknobs. Certain factors can predispose one to contracting either infection, including being run-down (immune defenses aren't working efficiently), having an illness, experiencing prolonged stress, being exposed to cigarette smoke, smog, and other environmental pollutants that can damage the cilia (little hairlike structures that clear the airways) as well as inadequate or infrequent hand washing.

how food may help

For both the common cold and the flu, drinking plenty of fluids, getting lots of rest, and eating nutritious foods are important keys to hastening recovery. Establishing a nourishing stockpile of protective foods can also be the main line of defense in the difficult task of preventing a cold or flu.

Luteolin, a flavonoid found in rosemary, sage, thyme, and artichokes, may act as a natural antihistamine by interfering with the release of histamine, a chemical pinpointed as one of the causes of congestion and other respiratory symptoms. Studies show that the flavonoid **quercetin** creates a similar result. Quercetin is also linked to optimal lung health.

To fight off viruses that cause these two illnesses, it is helpful to maintain a strong immune system. Folk medicine advocates the use of **garlic** to help prevent common respiratory infections, though there is currently little scientific evidence to support this notion.

The immune-bolstering properties of **vitamin C** and **zinc** may help your body combat both the common cold as well as the flu. Vitamin C may also function as a natural antihistamine. Try to eat foods rich in the antioxidant mineral **selenium:** Preliminary studies indicate that selenium deficiency may prolong symptoms of the flu, including duration of the illness and lung inflammation.

If you already have caught one of these ailments, cooking with garlic can offer some temporary comfort (see *Home Remedy,* right). And the fiery nature of certain foods, such as chili peppers, ginger, horseradish, and mustard, may offer immediate relief from nasal congestion by perking up the nasal passages and alleviating stuffiness.

home remedy

Adding garlic to your diet every day during cold and flu season may help prevent the onset of viral infections like cold and flu. A systematic review of studies related to the effects of garlic on respiratory viral infections found that garlic has not only antiviral properties but also strong immune-boosting powers. Garlic exerts its protective powers against viruses by blocking the virus from entering cells and by enhancing the immune response. One recent study also confirmed that inhaling the volatile oils released while chopping onions, scallions, or garlic can help relieve the cough, headache, and accumulation of mucus during the early stages of a cold or flu virus.

your food arsenal

foods	nutrient	health benefits
apples **berries** **plums & prunes** **red onions**	quercetin	Some research indicates that this flavonoid may relieve congestion by reducing the release of histamine, which is associated with runny nose, congestion, and watery eyes.
citrus fruit **kiwifruit** **peppers** **strawberries**	vitamin C	Although it will not cure the common cold or influenza, vitamin C, by maintaining a strong immune system, may prevent the onset of these viruses, and it may also reduce the duration of symptoms.
cashews **fortified cereals** **whole grains**	zinc	There is some evidence that zinc may reduce the severity of symptoms and shorten the duration of the common cold.

constipation

what it is

Constipation is typified by infrequent or difficult bowel movements and hard, dry stools. Hard stools often are a result of excess absorption of water from the intestines. This can happen because the muscle of the colon contracts too slowly, causing the stool to pass through too slowly. Drinking lots of water is important in helping to move stool through the colon. Symptoms of constipation are often accompanied by bloating, abdominal distension, straining, and a feeling of incomplete evacuation. Hemorrhoids can result from the pressure of excessive straining.

The frequency of bowel movements among people varies greatly, ranging from three movements a day to three a week. Generally, fewer than three bowel movements a week indicates constipation. A common misconception about constipation is that a bowel movement every day is necessary. Contrary to common belief, frequency is of less importance than the degree of discomfort associated with bowel movements or the absence of an urge to have one. Constipation and irregularity are common, particularly in older adults and children.

what causes it

Numerous factors are linked to constipation. Excluding causes that are associated with specific diseases, the most common causes of constipation include a hereditary component, lack of exercise, certain types of medication, emotional stress, a diet high in animal fats and processed foods, not eating enough foods high in fiber, and not drinking enough water. Poor bowel habits, such as ignoring the urge to have a bowel movement, can cause constipation. Overuse of enemas as well as laxatives can, over time, interfere with the colon's natural ability to contract. Psychological issues are sometimes the cause of constipation in children. Not surprisingly, constipation is one of the most frequently reported gastrointestinal complaints in this country.

how food may help

There are two types of dietary fiber, insoluble and soluble. Often called "roughage," **insoluble fiber** is particularly effective in promoting regular bowel movements by adding bulk and providing mass to the stool. Insoluble fiber also helps to move the waste through your colon, and eases elimination. **Soluble fiber** can help to soften stools by acting as a gel in the intestine, where it helps to increase water content. Both types of dietary fiber are useful for management of constipation. Dried fruit, such as dried apricots, figs, prunes, and pears, is especially rich in fiber as well as other beneficial nutrients.

High-fat and processed foods are typically fiber-poor. Eating too many of them can contribute to constipation by filling you up without providing the gastrointestinal benefits of fiber. When picking high-fiber foods, choose those that are nutritionally rich in other nourishing compounds: Good choices are dried fruit, peas, beans, lentils, broccoli, and sweet potatoes.

As many high-fiber foods tend to produce bloating and gas, it may be a good idea to increase your consumption of these foods gradually so that your system can adjust to the added fiber. Be sure to drink a lot of water to prevent your digestive system from slowing down.

Foods rich in **magnesium** may also offer some relief. Magnesium is thought to have mild laxative properties.

Plums, dried plums (prunes), and prune juice are particularly beneficial in coping with constipation. They are not only rich in both types of fiber but they also contain **sorbitol**—a natural type of sugar that stimulates the digestive system. It may also have a laxative effect.

your food arsenal

foods	nutrient	health benefits
broccoli cabbage family flaxseed sweet potatoes	insoluble fiber	Insoluble fiber (often called "roughage") is particularly useful in promoting regular bowel movements by adding bulk and providing mass to the stool, helping to move the waste through the colon, and easing elimination.
apricots beans figs plums & prunes	soluble fiber	Soluble fiber can help to soften stools due to its ability to act as a gel in the intestine, where it helps to increase water content.

depression

what it is

Depression is a common mood disorder that strikes approximately 16 million Americans each year. An all-encompassing illness affecting body, mood, and thought, depression is a treatable condition that often goes untreated. Symptoms of depression include an oppressive feeling of despair and despondency that simply will not go away. Other symptoms that occur are a sense of hopelessness, feelings of guilt, low energy, difficulty concentrating, restlessness, sleep disturbances (such as insomnia or too much sleep), emptiness, negative and sad thoughts, difficulty maintaining normal relationships, as well as a general lack of interest in life. Proper treatment can offer relief for most people who suffer from this potentially debilitating condition.

what causes it

Many factors are linked to depression. They include hereditary, biological, and environmental factors, and significant life events, such as physical illness, the loss of a loved one, or the loss of a job. Also linked to depression are certain medications, alcohol or drug abuse, diet, and having had a baby (as well as other hormonal fluctuations). The biological causes of depression may be attributed to disturbances in neurotransmitters, chemical messengers in the brain, though much about the biochemical causes has yet to be learned.

how food may help

Certain nutrients may have a beneficial effect on the brain chemicals that are responsible for mood. For example, researchers believe that the essential amino acid **tryptophan** may play an important role in normal brain function because it helps produce the neurotransmitter serotonin, which may help to reduce feelings of depression.

Depressed people sometimes turn to foods rich in **complex carbohydrates** (found in "comfort foods"), which are thought to also have a favorable effect on the production of serotonin. Foods high in complex carbohydrates also help the body absorb tryptophan efficiently.

You can also fight the blues by eating foods high in B vitamins. **Folate** is an important B vitamin that is sometimes deficient in people who are depressed. Preliminary research shows that depressed people may have abnormalities in **vitamin B$_{12}$** status as well. A link may exist between low levels of vitamin B$_{12}$ and folate and impaired metabolism of the brain chemicals associated with mood regulation.

Vitamin B$_{12}$ works with folate and **vitamin B$_6$** to help reduce homocysteine, an amino acid linked to depression. Vitamin B$_{12}$ helps to convert homocysteine into other substances, thus preventing a buildup of homocysteine in the bloodstream. Vitamin B$_6$ may also assist in the manufacture of enzymes responsible for the metabolism of certain mood-regulating brain chemicals such as serotonin and dopamine.

Omega-3 fatty acids, which are lacking in most people's diets in the United States, are abundantly present in the brain and are essential for normal brain function. Though little is currently known about how omega-3 fatty acids regulate mood, recent findings show a correlation between low levels of these compounds and depression.

recent research

An international panel of nutritional psychiatry researchers and experts recently agreed on the use of omega-3 fatty acids to help prevent depression in high-risk populations and treat depression in pregnant women, children, and the elderly.

your food arsenal

foods	nutrient	health benefits
asparagus lentils peas salad greens	folate	There may be a link between folate deficiency and impaired metabolism of brain chemicals associated with mood regulation.
chia seeds flaxseed	omega-3 fatty acids	These fats are vital for optimum brain functioning and are linked to a reduced incidence of depression.
bananas peas	tryptophan	Tryptophan is a precursor of serotonin, a neurotransmitter in the brain that has been shown to be involved in reducing depression.
fortified cereals nutritional yeast	vitamin B$_{12}$	Deficiency of this vitamin has been linked to depression.
bananas peas potatoes	vitamin B$_6$	This B vitamin helps in the manufacture of enzymes responsible for the metabolism of certain mood-regulating nerve chemicals.

diabetes

what it is

Diabetes is characterized by high levels of glucose (a simple sugar that all cells require for energy) in the blood, the result of an impairment in the secretion and/or the action of insulin (the hormone required to utilize glucose). There are two forms of diabetes, type 1 and type 2. Type 2 is the more prevalent form of diabetes and is responsible for about 90% of cases. As opposed to type 1 diabetes, which is usually diagnosed in childhood or adolescence, type 2 diabetes generally afflicts adults; hence, it is also referred to as adult-onset diabetes. Type 2 diabetes develops gradually and usually affects people over the age of 40 who tend to be obese. Symptoms of diabetes mellitus (the full name of both types of the disease) include frequent and excessive urination, excessive thirst, weight loss, fatigue, and increased hunger, as well as recurring infections, such as urinary tract and vaginal yeast infections. Complications associated with either type of diabetes include cardiovascular disease, nerve damage, vision loss, and kidney disease.

what causes it

Diabetes is a complex disorder, the cause of which is not clearly understood, though genetic factors may play a role in both types of diabetes. In type 2 diabetes, in addition to a genetic component, metabolic disturbances and obesity have both been implicated in its onset. Numerous studies show that obesity not only promotes the development of diabetes but it also furthers the progression of heart disease. Pregnant women can develop gestational diabetes, placing them at higher risk for developing diabetes later in life. In the less common form of diabetes, type 1, the immune system mistakenly attacks the body's insulin-producing cells, resulting in insulin deficiency.

how food may help

Before embarking on any type of nutritional plan, people with diabetes need to carefully review any dietary decisions with their healthcare provider. Each person's diet needs to be individually tailored to accommodate insulin needs.

Foods high in **complex carbohydrates** tend to be digested at a rate that allows glucose to be released gradually into the bloodstream, which helps in maintaining normal glucose levels.

The importance of **dietary fiber** lies in its ability to slow the absorption of glucose and promote satiety (feeling full), which is helpful for weight loss. **Soluble fiber** also helps to decrease serum cholesterol levels, which is important since many people with diabetes are at an increased risk for developing coronary vascular disease.

Although findings are inconsistent, some researchers speculate that a low serum **magnesium** level may possibly be a predictor of type 2 diabetes and increasing dietary magnesium may lower the risk. Note that foods rich in magnesium, such as brown rice and whole grains, tend also to be rich in fiber.

Eating heart-healthy foods such as those rich in **monounsaturated fat** is also helpful, particularly when they replace artery-clogging saturated fats.

Because people with diabetes often suffer from vascular problems, a **vitamin C**-rich diet will help to protect veins and connective tissues. Vitamin C also acts as an antioxidant, which is important because some studies show that free-radical oxidation may play a role in the damage to tissues caused by diabetes.

recent research

A recent study followed 55 type 1 and type 2 diabetes patients on a plant-based diet including raw fruits and vegetables with no medication. Of the 21 type 1 patients, 57% had controlled blood glucose after three days. All of the type 2 patients had controlled glucose after three days. The effect was the same in both newly diagnosed patients and those with a long-standing history of the disease. Most of the patients who maintained the diet were able to stay off medications; others were able to reduce their medications.

your food arsenal

foods	nutrient	health benefits
beans potatoes brown rice whole grains	complex carbohydrates	Complex carbohydrates are digested slowly and release glucose gradually into the bloodstream, helping to maintain normal glucose levels.
asparagus beans lentils	dietary fiber	Soluble fiber may help to decrease serum cholesterol levels as well as glucose levels, and it also helps to prevent weight gain.
amaranth brown rice sunflower seeds	magnesium	A low serum magnesium level may possibly be a predictor of type 2 diabetes. Foods rich in magnesium tend also to be rich in fiber.
avocados canola oil nuts olive oil	monounsaturated fat	These beneficial fats may help to lower blood glucose levels and, when replacing saturated fats, are also helpful in managing heart disease and maintaining weight levels.
bell peppers broccoli citrus fruit	vitamin C	Vitamin C helps to protect connective tissues and veins; many people with diabetes suffer from vascular problems.

diarrhea

what it is

Something that we have all experienced at some time in our lives, diarrhea is typified by the frequent passage of unformed, usually watery stools. Often referred to as a "stomach flu" or "a bug," diarrhea can be extremely distressing, and is sometimes accompanied by abdominal pain and severe cramping. Extreme cases of diarrhea can cause dehydration.

If an infant or child develops diarrhea, a health care provider should be consulted since children are more vulnerable and tend to become weak and dehydrated. Also, the elderly and people with immune system disorders and other serious illnesses should receive professional care to manage diarrhea. For many people, however, most bouts of diarrhea are not dangerous, are self-limiting, and don't last more than three days. If you do experience symptoms of diarrhea for more than three days, you should contact your health care provider to determine if there is a more serious problem.

what causes it

The most common form of diarrhea is generally caused by consuming food or drinking water that has been contaminated with certain viruses, bacteria, or parasites (such as cryptosporidium). Foodborne bacteria (*E. coli*, salmonella, and listeria) are also found in raw foods and on improperly cleaned cutting boards, cooking surfaces, and utensils. Wash all food preparation and cooking surfaces with hot soapy water after use.

When traveling abroad, particularly in developing countries, be careful to drink bottled water and avoid unwashed fruit and vegetables; otherwise you may develop what is known as "traveler's diarrhea" which is linked to consuming local water, ice, or raw foods that contain bacteria or parasites.

Proper hygiene practices can help to prevent diarrhea linked to viruses and infections. Diarrhea can be caused by fecal contamination of hands or other objects, which can spread rapidly. Therefore, washing hands thoroughly is essential after using the bathroom or changing diapers. Teach and encourage children to maintain proper hygiene, especially before eating meals.

Other factors that can lead to diarrhea include lactose intolerance, stress, eating foods that contain sorbitol, certain medications, megadoses of vitamin C, or antacids containing magnesium. Inflammatory diarrhea (also called chronic diarrhea) is less common and is usually linked to medical conditions such as colitis, irritable bowel syndrome, and other gastrointestinal disorders.

how food may help

One of the most helpful dietary steps to take if you have diarrhea is to replace fluid loss: Drink lots of water. Though you may not feel hungry, try to eat small amounts of food throughout the day. If diarrhea is severe and you simply cannot bear to eat, at the very least, suck on ice chips and try to sip small amounts of clear liquids such as broth and sports drinks (or seltzer mixed with a small amount of sugar and salt).

Some bland **complex carbohydrate**-rich foods (mashed potatoes, dry toast, or rice) tend to be the least aggravating to the digestive system. Be sure to eat white rice and peeled potatoes, as the bran layers of brown rice and the potato skin contain insoluble fiber that can actually worsen diarrhea.

Foods containing the soluble fiber **pectin,** such as applesauce and bananas, are useful in helping to firm stools. These foods also slow down the transit time of waste in the colon. Bananas are a rich source of potassium, which is often lost in the excessive elimination of fluids.

If you are taking antibiotics, foods containing **probiotics** may help to replenish the healthful bacteria in your colon that are destroyed by the medication. The probiotics (healthful bacteria) in kombucha or tempeh may help to restore a normal balance of bacteria in the intestines.

foods to avoid

During a bout with diarrhea, avoid foods containing caffeine, which can exacerbate symptoms by stimulating colonic activity. Other foods that can make diarrhea worse are prunes, fruit and fruit juices, fatty foods, highly seasoned foods, and alcohol.

Avoid foods high in insoluble fiber (roughage) as they will not absorb excess water in the intestinal tract. Instead, because they are roughage, they will make diarrhea worse by stimulating the colon.

your food arsenal		
foods	nutrient	health benefits
potatoes, peeled white rice	complex carbohydrates	Foods high in complex carbohydrates that tend to be bland and easily digested.
applesauce bananas	pectin	A type of soluble fiber that helps to absorb excess fluid in the digestive tract, pectin also slows down transit time in the digestive tract and adds bulk to stools.

eczema

what it is

An inflammatory, noncontagious skin condition, eczema causes itching, flaking, dryness, and often redness. Sometimes small blisters will form and when they burst, the surface of the skin may be left moist and irritated. Persistent scratching of the skin in affected areas can subsequently result in scaly, rough, and thickened patches. There are various forms of eczema, with atopic dermatitis being the most common (it is estimated that more than 30 million adults and children in the United States suffer from it). Eczema often appears in the folds of the skin where your limbs bend, such as elbows and knees, though it can also appear anywhere on the body. Scratching can worsen eczema and cause it to spread.

what causes it

Those with a family history of allergies to foods, pollen, dust mites, and animal dander are more susceptible to eczema. Disturbances in proper immune response (how the body reacts to irritating or infectious substances) may be a contributing factor: Many eczema sufferers have above-normal levels of histamine, a chemical in the body that triggers an allergic defense reaction in the skin (and resulting in inflammation) when it's released. Eczema, particularly atopic dermatitis, has also been associated with asthma and hay fever, though the exact relationship is unclear. Flare-ups of eczema are also linked to anxiety and stress (see *page 138* for dietary advice that may help with the management of stress), as well as extremes in weather. Those with dry skin are also more vulnerable to eczema outbreaks.

how food may help

One of the triggers (as well as a consequence) of eczema is dryness, which may, in part, be ameliorated by foods rich in beta-carotene, vitamin E, and essential fatty acids. Preliminary studies indicate that **beta-carotene** (a precursor to vitamin A) may protect the skin from free-radical stress. Foods rich in **essential fatty acids** may decrease swelling by helping to generate hormonelike substances called prostaglandins, which reduce inflammation.

Immune system abnormalities have been noted in some people who have eczema, and it is sensible for these people (as well as those with a family history of allergies, asthma, and eczema) to eat immune-enriching foods that are high in **zinc, vitamin C,** and **vitamin E.** Vitamin E's antioxidant properties may shield cells from free-radical damage and help to promote skin healing. Vitamin C may also be instrumental in reducing the release of histamine, an inflammatory compound released by the body in response to allergens. As the immune system's response to allergens triggers release of histamine, consuming foods that function as natural antihistamines, such as those rich in vitamin C as well as the flavonoids **quercetin** and **luteolin,** may inhibit this inflammatory reaction. Vitamins C and E operate as robust antioxidants and help to defend against free-radical damage.

recent research

A recent small study found that children and adolescents with eczema had lower calcium intakes than their peers who did not have eczema. The study authors suggest increasing consumption of calcium-rich foods, including calcium-fortified cereals and dairy substitutes; tofu and other soy products; and kale and other dark leafy greens.

your food arsenal

foods	nutrient	health benefits
brussels sprouts carrots spinach sweet potatoes	beta-carotene	Beta-carotene acts as an antioxidant by neutralizing harmful elements that could damage skin.
chia seeds flaxseed vegetable oils	essential fatty acids	Essential fatty acids may facilitate the release of anti-inflammatory substances in the body; this can help to reduce inflammation that often occurs in eczema.
avocados broccoli sunflower seeds tomato juice	vitamin E	Vitamin E is important for maintenance of the immune system. A healthy immune system can help to promote normal responses to allergens, which are linked to eczema.
beans nuts seeds whole grains	zinc	As immune system abnormalities have been noted in some people who have eczema, it may be beneficial to consume foods that are high in zinc, a mineral that enhances immunity.

fibrocystic breasts

what it is

The term "fibrocystic breast disease" is misleading since it is not a disease, but rather a condition that occurs in a large number of women, generally between the ages of 25 and 50. Fibrocystic changes usually mean breast lumpiness.

Characterized by breast tenderness, pain, a dull, heavy feeling, swelling, and lumps (cysts), symptoms of fibrocystic breasts generally are thought to be hormone-related and tend to occur about a week to 10 days before the onset of menstruation. Symptoms most often improve after the menstrual period and, in fact, there appears to be a strong link between fibrocystic breast changes and premenstrual syndrome (see *page 208*). Fibrocystic breast changes usually disappear after menopause (except if you're on hormone replacement therapy), most likely because of the change in hormonal status.

Although fibrocystic breast lumps are benign and do not increase your risk for breast cancer, they can sometimes complicate diagnosing breast cancer (a mammographic image of fibrocystic breasts can sometimes be difficult for radiologists and breast specialists to decipher). Any lump in your breast should be brought to the attention of your health care practitioner.

what causes it

The cause is not completely understood, though fibrocystic breast changes are thought to be caused by an increased estrogen-to-progesterone ratio. Some research suggests that fibrocystic breast changes may be more pronounced in women with higher peak estrogen levels before ovulation and greater declines in progesterone after ovulation. These hormonal fluctuations may lead to a surplus of prolactin, a lactation hormone that can make the breasts swell and feel tender in non-breastfeeding women. More research is required to shed light on fibrocystic breast changes.

how food may help

Although there seems to be little established information about the relationship between diet and fibrocystic breast changes, some research indicates that foods rich in **essential fatty acids** may possibly help to diminish swelling by lowering the body's production of inflammatory substances.

As there is a possible link between elevated estrogen levels and fibrocystic breast symptoms, consuming a diet rich in soy **isoflavones** and other **phytoestrogens** such as **lignans** (in flaxseeds) may help to reduce estrogen. Phytoestrogens are mildly estrogenic phytonutrients that block estrogen by attaching to areas in the body (so-called receptor sites) that would otherwise be claimed by estrogen.

Preliminary studies suggest that the soy isoflavone **genistein** in particular may have an effect on menstrual cycle patterns and increase cycle length, thus reducing estrogen exposure. This, in turn, may reduce fibrocystic breast changes.

A low-fat, high-fiber diet may be helpful for women with fibrocystic breast disease. Eating foods rich in **fiber** and decreasing the intake of foods high in saturated fat may reduce circulating estrogen, though more studies are required to determine how estrogen levels are affected by a high-fiber diet.

Caffeine does not cause fibrocystic breast changes; however, some women do feel that caffeine (found in coffee, tea, colas and some other soft drinks, and chocolate) exacerbates breast tenderness and discomfort. If your symptoms seem to be reduced by eliminating caffeinated foods from your diet, then it may be prudent to do so. (The same is true for eliminating foods high in salt.)

recent research

Though scientific evidence is scant regarding vitamin E and fibrocystic breast changes, many women nevertheless continue to attest to vitamin E's benefits, such as reduced pain, tenderness, and cyst size.

The problem, however, with dietary vitamin E is that a large segment of the population isn't consuming enough foods rich in this important vitamin. Findings from a survey of more than 16,000 individuals indicate that approximately 30% of adults in America don't get enough vitamin E.

Good sources of this antioxidant vitamin include wheat germ, almonds and other nuts, vegetable oils, olive oil, and green leafy vegetables. It may also be a good idea to consult your health care provider to determine if you should take a vitamin E supplement.

your food arsenal

foods	nutrient	health benefits
edamame flaxseed nuts seeds	essential fatty acids	Essential fatty acids may reduce swelling associated with fibrocystic breasts by lowering the body's production of inflammatory substances.
apples kidney beans lentils whole grains	dietary fiber	Fibrocystic disease may be linked to excess estrogen, and some studies show that when women with fibrocystic breasts are placed on a high-fiber, low-fat diet they experience a decrease in estrogen levels.

gout

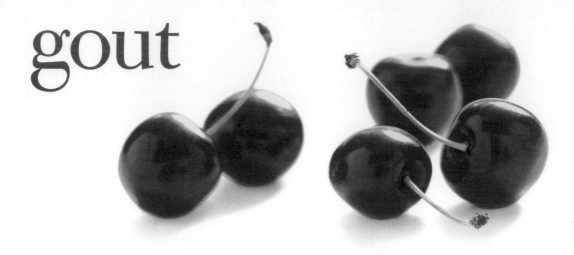

what it is

Often first characterized by sudden, extreme pain and inflammation in a single joint (generally the big toe), gout is a type of arthritis (an inflammation or pain in the joints or muscles) that strikes men more often than women. (The likelihood of women suffering from gout tends to increase after menopause.) Persistent episodes of gout, which occur for years, can potentially affect joints in the knees, elbows, wrists, hands, and feet, as well as other parts of the body.

Elevated blood levels of uric acid, one of the body's waste products, can lead to the accumulation of tiny, painful needlelike crystals in the joints. As a natural reaction to this accumulation, the immune system releases compounds in the body that produce inflammation, causing the joints to become sensitive, inflamed, red, and warm to the touch.

Though gout seems to appear out of nowhere, chances are that a symptom-free buildup of uric acid in the blood has been going on for years. The first attack of gout is usually followed by a complete remission of symptoms; but in untreated cases, many people can expect a recurrence. In fact, if left untreated, gout can lead to other serious conditions, such as kidney stones or other kidney problems, as well as destruction of the affected joint. Considered an intermittent disease, gout may be asymptomatic for years, but then produce a painful attack without warning.

what causes it

Gout occurs when there is either an increased production of uric acid or failure of the body to eliminate it efficiently. Being overweight (see *page 202* for advice on losing weight) and/or having high blood pressure (see *page 174* for dietary advice) or high cholesterol (see *page 176* for dietary advice) are also risk factors for gout. There is also an association with kidney disease, as well as with certain medications that tend to decrease uric acid excretion from the body—e.g., diuretics ("water pills"), immunosuppressive drugs, or low doses of aspirin—thus raising uric acid levels in the blood. Alcohol consumption as well as fasting can also raise uric acid levels. Alcohol not only contains purines (see *Foods to Avoid*, right), but it also intensifies the body's production of uric acid, interferes with the kidneys' ability to excrete uric acid, and dehydrates the body, which can increase uric acid levels.

how food may help

Although gout can't be prevented, there are dietary steps you can take to lessen the symptoms to some extent, starting, clearly, by avoiding purine-rich foods (see *Foods to Avoid*, right). Maintaining a normal weight is very important for people who are susceptible to gout. But note that crash dieting or fasting can increase uric acid levels and can cause an acute gout attack. Be sure to drink an ample amount of water to help remove uric acid crystals from the body.

Home remedies for gout that many people swear by include eating **celery** (and/or celery seeds) and/or a half pound of **black cherries** every day. There is some research offering evidence to support a connection between these foods and the relief of gout; it is possible that they reduce inflammation.

Also, **bromelain,** an enzyme found in pineapples, may reduce inflammation. Eating foods rich in **essential fatty acids** may also help to reduce inflammation.

There is also evidence that eating **tofu and other soy foods** is a better choice than meat-based protein for people suffering from gout.

foods to avoid

Certain foods are high in purines, compounds that are thought to exacerbate an attack of gout in people already with the condition. To play it safe, if you feel that you are predisposed to gout or if you have had gout in the past, be sure to avoid purine-rich foods, such as anchovies, herring, organ meats, and sardines.

your food arsenal

foods	nutrient	health benefits
celery celery seeds	unidentified	Early studies show that celery and celery seeds may have antigout properties due to their anti-inflammatory and antioxidative properties.
cherry juice dark cherries	unidentified	There is some evidence that cherries and cherry juice can reduce uric acid levels in people suffering from gout, which may be helpful in reducing inflammation and pain associated with gout.

heart disease

recipe rx

what it is

The leading cause of death in developed countries, heart disease is actually atherosclerosis—an accumulation of fatty plaque deposits along the inside of artery walls. The plaques impede blood flow throughout the body's blood vessels, and when a delicate artery in the heart clogs and deprives the organ of oxygen and nutrients, a heart attack occurs.

what causes it

Heart disease is often associated with factors related to lifestyle, such as high blood pressure, high cholesterol, obesity, inactivity, stress, and smoking. Declining estrogen levels, diabetes, family history, elevated levels of blood lipids called triglycerides, oxidative damage from free radicals, and increased age also contribute to the development of heart disease.

how food may help

Consuming a low-fat diet with mono- and polyunsaturated fats from olive oil and foods like nuts and avocado can significantly improve cholesterol levels. Olive oil and nuts are especially good sources of **vitamin E,** which may inhibit the oxidation of LDL cholesterol, a critical factor in the formation of artery-clogging plaque.

Consuming plenty of **vitamin C** may protect against heart disease by scavenging harmful free radicals, strengthening blood vessels, and possibly regulating blood pressure. **Flavonoid** phytonutrients are thought to enhance the antioxidant actions of vitamin C, and numerous studies link flavonoids in fruit, vegetables, tea, and red wine to protection against heart attacks. The actions of these powerful antioxidants may delay the breakdown of artery-clogging cholesterol that contributes to heart disease. Researchers believe a unique flavonoid in tomatoes, called **lycopene,** may prevent atherosclerosis by preventing harmful LDL cholesterol from being oxidized. One study of over 1,000 middle-aged men from 10 European countries found those who had the most lycopene in their diet reduced their risk for heart attack by half.

Potent **sulfur phytonutrients** in garlic and the onion family may protect against cardiovascular disease. Research suggests that regular garlic consumption may inhibit, and even shrink, fatty plaques in the arteries. Some experts recommend a half to 1 clove per day.

Though controversial, some data link elevated levels of the amino acid homocysteine to clogged arteries and heart disease. **Folate,** a key B vitamin, appears to team up with **vitamins B$_6$** and **B$_{12}$** to lower homocysteine levels. According to one study, when participants adopted a diet high in folate, average homocysteine levels dropped by an impressive 7%. Avocados and potatoes provide generous amounts of vitamin B$_6$; nutritional yeast is rich in vitamin B$_{12}$.

A diet rich in soy foods and soluble fiber has been shown to improve heart health by reducing harmful LDL cholesterol. **Soy protein** (25 g per day) and the **soluble fiber** in oats (beta-glucan), beans, and psyllium seed husk and flaxseed are especially beneficial.

Because high cholesterol is a major cause of atherosclerosis, and high blood pressure contributes to heart disease, refer to *pages 174–177* for dietary advice on managing these conditions.

recent research

After analyzing data collected from more than 12,000 middle-aged adults followed over a 25-year period, researchers concluded that plant-based diets (those high in plant foods and low in animal foods) are associated with a lower incidence of cardiovascular disease and a lower risk of dying from cardiovascular disease.

your food arsenal

foods	nutrient	health benefits
beans carrots oats	soluble fiber	Soluble fiber is especially beneficial for improving cholesterol levels, which lowers the risk for developing atherosclerosis.
asparagus lentils	folate	Folate helps reduce levels of homocysteine, an amino acid sometimes linked to heart disease.
avocados olive oil	monounsaturated fat	Because they are not easily damaged by oxidation, these fats are less likely to promote clogged arteries and should replace saturated and trans fats whenever possible.
chia seeds flaxseed walnuts	omega-3 fatty acids	These heart-healthy fats may reduce the risk for heart attack by reducing blood clotting, lowering levels of harmful triglycerides, and decreasing the risk for irregular heartbeat.
soy foods	soy protein	Numerous studies have confirmed that 25 g of soy protein per day can improve cholesterol levels, lowering the risk for cardiovascular disease.

heartburn

what it is

The burning discomfort of heartburn, or acid reflux, is familiar to many Americans, some on a daily basis. Heartburn is usually triggered by eating and occurs when stomach acid washes up into the digestive tube (esophagus), burning the back of the throat. The fiery pain may radiate across the chest, traveling from behind the breastbone to the neck. Belching, flatulence, or nausea may accompany acid reflux, and the burning distress may last from one to four hours.

Recurring indigestion (occurring at least twice a week) is medically termed gastroesophageal reflux disease, or GERD, and may be quite severe. Symptoms include painful heartburn, increased salivation, a chronic hoarse voice, and regurgitation. Left untreated, corrosive stomach acid may gradually erode the delicate lining of the esophagus, a process that is linked to esophageal cancer. Fortunately, consuming healing foods and altering eating habits can help quell fiery heartburn.

what causes it

A muscular valve at the bottom of the esophagus, the lower esophageal sphincter (LES), serves as a gatekeeper to the stomach and seals off its contents, blocking backwash into the esophagus. Numerous factors, however, may weaken the LES, or cause it to relax, resulting in heartburn. (Hiatal hernia is another cause of GERD.) Smoking and excess abdominal pressure from pregnancy or obesity may weaken the LES, preventing this valve from closing tightly. Certain foods and medications may relax and open the LES, allowing stomach acid to splash into the esophagus. Additional heartburn triggers include acidic foods (tomatoes and citrus fruits and juices), which may promote excess stomach acid and irritate a damaged esophageal lining; and overeating, tight-fitting clothes, and lying down or bending over after eating, all of which may push stomach contents upward.

how food may help

Several dietary changes are recommended to help prevent heart-burn flare-ups and to minimize irritation to the esophagus.

Though scientific data are scant, simple alterations to eating hab-its, such as eliminating trigger foods, may prevent reflux. Common heartburn triggers include coffee (both decaffeinated and regular), alcohol, peppermint, chocolate, onions, and tomato products. In general, spicy, fatty, or acidic foods frequently lead to heartburn. If irritating foods and beverages must be part of the menu, eat them in very small portions. Drink beverages between meals, instead of with them, to suppress reflux. In addition, remain upright for up to an hour after eating and don't eat for two to three hours before going to bed.

Many experts recommend eating small, low-fat meals each day. Large meals distend the stomach, increasing the chance of reflux. Smaller portions, con-sumed more frequently throughout the day, may be easier to digest, prevent-ing heartburn distress. Eating slowly is important as well, because eating too fast (and too much) can overload the LES muscle, pressuring the valve to open and propel acidic juices into the esophagus. A low-fat diet is thought to prevent heartburn, since high-fat foods may exacerbate acid reflux by prolonging diges-tion and weakening the LES valve.

Studies have linked obesity with an increased incidence of heartburn, so maintaining a healthy weight is important for heartburn prevention. Too much weight around the abdomen appears to stress the LES valve, allowing stomach contents to seep out. **Fiber**-rich foods may assist weight loss by improving feelings of fullness without encouraging overindulgence in extra calories.

Eating a diet rich in high-fiber **complex carbohydrates** may ease digestion and help prevent heartburn. Experts suggest centering meals around such low-fat complex carbohydrates as beans, vegetables, and whole grains.

home remedy

Chewing gum, preferably sugarless, after meals may ease heartburn. Some research suggests that the saliva pro-duced by gum chewing may help neu-tralize and sweep away acidic stomach juices. (Note, however, that excessive gum chewing is not recommended since it increases swallowed air and belching, which can lead to reflux.)

your food arsenal

foods	nutrient	health benefits
beans potatoes brown rice whole grains	complex carbohydrates	Complex carbohydrates may ease heartburn because they are generally bland and gentle on stomach digestion.
beets lentils pomegranates	dietary fiber	By improving satiety, dietary fiber may promote weight loss, which may significantly improve heartburn symptoms.

hemorrhoids

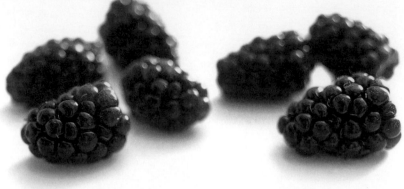

what it is

Varying in symptoms and severity, hemorrhoids are extremely common, affecting most adults at least once in their lifetime. Hemorrhoids, also known as piles, are really varicose veins, or weakened swollen veins, in the anus or rectum. Veins—vessels that transport blood to the heart—are delicate, and veins in the rectum and anus are fragile. Hemorrhoid symptoms include itching, pain, and bleeding. Hemorrhoids are classified as either internal or external and tend to worsen over time if not treated.

what causes it

Pregnancy, obesity, or frequent heavy lifting may lead to hemorrhoids by creating excess pressure on veins, weakening them. Because straining during bowel movements stresses veins, constipation may aggravate hemorrhoids. Bouts of diarrhea and prolonged sitting or standing may also contribute to the condition. A predisposition toward frail veins and poor muscle tone around veins tends to run in families.

how food may help

Regular exercise, a high-fiber diet, and plenty of fluids are key to managing hemorrhoids. Frequent physical activity may help tone muscles around veins, enhancing their ability to propel blood.

Dietary fiber eases elimination and prevents constipation. **Insoluble fiber** promotes regularity and **soluble fiber** softens waste and stimulates intestinal contractions, making stools easier to pass. Research has shown that a high-fiber diet can significantly improve hemorrhoid symptoms, including soreness and bleeding. It is essential to drink at least 8 glasses of water each day when eating a high-fiber diet.

Vitamin C may help fortify vessel walls and reduce swollen veins. Flavonoids are thought to enhance the actions of vitamin C. Preliminary human studies suggest **flavonoids** may improve blood vessel function, possibly strengthening vein tissue. These phytonutrients are potent antioxidants that may combat free-radical damage and reduce blood vessel breakage. The citrus flavonoid **hesperidin** is thought to enhance the actions of vitamin C and may improve blood vessel function. **Diosmin,** a related flavonoid found in rosemary and citrus fruit, may strengthen blood vessels as well. Experimental studies suggest that **rutin,** a flavonoid present in apples and buckwheat, may fortify support cells and connective tissue in blood vessels. The grapefruit flavonoid **naringin** (related to rutin and hesperidin) is thought to bolster blood vessel structure and function.

Laboratory research indicates that **quercetin,** a flavonoid found in red onions, apples, and blueberries, may have powerful anti-inflammatory properties that protect against faulty veins. In addition, scientists believe **tannin compounds** (also known as proanthocyanidins) in blackberries may benefit veins by protecting against damaging free radicals.

The infection-fighting mineral **zinc** is important for the healing process and may help to minimize irritation while hemorrhoid tissue mends.

> ### recent research
>
> A matched case-control study of 47 patients, with and without hemorrhoids, found that people who routinely skipped breakfast had as much as seven times the risk for developing hemorrhoids. Experts believe that breakfast may provide a unique opportunity for bulking up on dietary fiber.

your food arsenal

foods	nutrient	health benefits
flaxseed **prunes** **salad greens** **whole grains**	insoluble fiber	Fiber promotes regularity and minimizes straining during bowel movements, which otherwise pressures veins, contributing to hemorrhoids. Fiber may also help tone muscles around veins.
apples **beans** **carrots** **plums**	soluble fiber	Soluble fiber eases elimination by bulking up the stool and stimulating contractions of the digestive tract.
apples **berries** **citrus fruits** **grapes**	flavonoids	Experimental research suggests flavonoids may bolster blood vessels by reducing fragility and permeability. Preliminary human studies indicate flavonoids may improve blood vessel function and relieve hemorrhoid symptoms.
citrus fruits **kiwifruit** **peppers** **strawberries**	vitamin C	Vitamin C may help fortify blood vessel walls and may protect against free radicals that can undermine blood vessel strength.
fortified cereals **legumes** **seeds** **wheat germ**	zinc	Zinc may enhance the healing of hemorrhoids.

high blood pressure

what it is

Blood pressure is technically the force of blood as it pushes against artery walls during circulation. High blood pressure, or hypertension, is labeled "the silent killer," because symptoms don't emerge until damage has already been done. The Centers for Disease Control and Prevention (CDC) estimates almost half of American adults suffer from hypertension. Statistically, high blood pressure is defined as at least 140 (systolic)/90 (diastolic), recorded at two separate times.

what causes it

For the majority of high blood pressure cases, the cause is unknown, and this is referred to as essential or primary hypertension. Factors that increase the risk for hypertension include obesity, smoking, gender (male), race (African American), family history, stress, and a high-sodium diet.

how food may help

To control blood pressure, experts recommend consuming a diet low in saturated fat and rich in a variety of fresh produce, whole grains, and nuts. An array of healing nutrients, including **calcium, dietary fiber, magnesium, potassium,** and **vitamin C,** are plentiful in a diet that includes many of these delicious, nourishing foods and can substantially lower blood pressure.

Heart-healthy fats, **monounsaturated** and **omega-3s,** may lower blood pressure and are recommended in place of harmful saturated and trans fats. These unhealthy fats are found primarily in animal-based foods and commercially prepared foods, and can contribute to clogged arteries, raising blood pressure.

Observational studies indicate that moderate amounts of **protein,** particularly from plants, are linked to healthy blood pressure. Legumes, soy foods, and grains, such as amaranth and quinoa, offer ample protein without saturated fat.

Arginine, a protein building block, is thought to benefit hypertension by increasing amounts of nitric oxide, a substance involved in blood vessel dilation. Nuts, whole grains, and soy products provide generous amounts of arginine.

A wealth of disease-fighting phytochemicals have been suggested for blood pressure control. Epidemiological data link a flavonoid-rich diet (plenty of fruits and vegetables) with healthy blood pressure; scientists believe **flavonoids** may relax blood vessels, lowering pressure.

Pungent, robust **sulfur compounds** in garlic and onions may assist in blood vessel dilation and help reduce both diastolic and systolic blood pressure in some people, as shown in several studies.

A phytonutrient found in celery seed, **phthalide (3-n-butyl phthalide),** has shown promise in reducing blood pressure, possibly by reducing levels of stress hormones, which constrict blood vessels.

Multiple studies suggest that beet juice, celery juice, and hibiscus tea can significatnly lower high blood pressure. If you are taking medication to reduce your blood pressure, however, speak with your doctor before adding the beverages to your diet.

foods to avoid

Most researchers advise a sodium-restricted diet to help lower blood pressure. A portion of the population, including African Americans, older people, and individuals suffering from diabetes, appears to be particularly sensitive to sodium, and may benefit significantly from eating low-sodium foods. Many experts recommend less than 2,400 mg of sodium each day for healthy individuals. The best way to reduce sodium intake is to avoid adding salt to food at the table, omit salt when cooking, and avoid most processed foods, which are usually loaded with sodium.

your food arsenal

foods	nutrient	health benefits
broccoli cooking greens figs tofu	calcium	According to population studies, low levels of calcium are related to a higher risk for elevated blood pressure, particularly in sodium-sensitive individuals, the elderly, and African Americans.
asparagus lentils pomegranates	dietary fiber	Observational studies demonstrate a beneficial association between generous fiber intake and reduced blood pressure.
amaranth quinoa seeds	magnesium	Observational dietary studies link high magnesium intake with reduced blood pressure.
chia seeds flaxseed walnuts	omega-3 fatty acids	Research indicates that these cardioprotective fats may help blood to circulate more freely, lowering blood pressure.
avocados bananas potatoes quinoa	potassium	Findings from the Dietary Approaches to Stop Hypertension (DASH) study support previous research that indicates a potassium-rich diet may improve blood pressure, and may be just as important as a low-sodium diet.
berries broccoli citrus fruits peppers	vitamin C	Population-based and preliminary clinical studies suggest that vitamin C may have a benefit by widening blood vessels and promoting excretion of environmental toxins, such as lead, which can contribute to high blood pressure.

high cholesterol

what it is

Cholesterol, a fatlike substance, circulates in the blood primarily in two forms. LDL cholesterol (the "bad" cholesterol) can clog arteries and contribute to cardiovascular disease. HDL (the "good" cholesterol) sweeps harmful cholesterol out of the arteries. Medical experts recommend that total cholesterol levels be no higher than 200 mg/dl and that HDL levels be no lower than 40 mg/dl.

what causes it

You need some cholesterol to stay healthy, and your liver produces as much cholesterol as your body needs from fats, sugars, and proteins circulating in your bloodstream. A diet high in saturated fat and trans fatty acids is associated with increasing your cholesterol levels. Genetic factors, smoking, inactivity, and obesity raise your risk of having unhealthy cholesterol levels.

how food may help

Although it has been shown that dietary cholesterol does not generally contribute to cardiovascular disease, foods that are high in cholesterol (such as animal products and processed foods) are usually high in saturated fats as well. Saturated fats (and trans fats) can raise cholesterol levels and are associated with heart disease. Substitute heart-healthy **monounsaturated** for saturated and trans fats as often as possible.

Long maligned as a fatty food, **nuts** are rich in unsaturated fat that benefits the heart, according to numerous studies. One large-scale study found that women who ate 5 ounces of nuts per week reduced their risk for heart disease by one-third. In another study, people who consumed 8 to 11 walnuts each day in place of other fats significantly cut their LDL ("bad") cholesterol.

Foods high in **soluble fiber** are useful for lowering LDL cholesterol. Studies show that soluble fiber in oats, carrots, and psyllium (available in health-food stores) is particularly beneficial. Research has found that 3 g of **beta-glucan** (a soluble fiber in oats) can lower cholesterol by 5% when consumed regularly.

Foods high in **flavonoids,** including **lycopene,** may help moderate cholesterol levels, according to research. Some evidence suggests that drinking orange juice, which is brimming with flavonoids, can also improve cholesterol levels.

Several studies found that the fiber in **shiitake mushrooms** significantly reduces cholesterol. Shiitakes are rich in several heart-healthy phytonutrients, including **eritadenine,** and enhance the excretion of cholesterol before it is absorbed into the bloodstream.

Evidence indicates that plant protein, such as **soy protein,** helps reduce cholesterol. A recent meta-analysis of 46 clinical trials on adult men and women found that approximately 25 mg of soy protein daily reduced total and LDL cholesterol in those with blood levels ranging between 110 and 201 mg/dl. (Optimal blood levels of LDL cholesterol are below 100 mg/dl.)

your food arsenal

foods	nutrient	health benefits
apples **citrus fruits** **onions**	flavonoids	There is growing evidence that anti-inflammatory, antioxidant, flavonoid-rich foods contribute to healthy cholesterol levels.
apricots **tomatoes** **watermelon**	lycopene	Studies have found that this carotenoid may help lower LDL cholesterol by interfering with cholesterol synthesis in the body.
avocados **olive oil**	monounsaturated fat	Replacing harmful saturated and trans fats with monounsaturated fats helps lower dangerous LDL cholesterol levels in the blood.
beans **carrots** **flaxseed** **oats**	soluble fiber	By forming a gel-like mass around food particles in the digestive tract, soluble fiber helps prevent cholesterol from being absorbed and promotes its excretion from the body.
soy foods	soy protein	Numerous clinical studies have confirmed that consuming 25 to 50 g of soy protein each day can significantly lower LDL cholesterol.
garlic **onions**	sulfur compounds	Some studies suggest that individuals who consume diets rich in onions and garlic have lower cholesterol levels.

hyperthyroidism

recipe rx

what it is

Rapid heartbeat, insomnia, weight loss, and sweating are hallmarks of an over-active thyroid. The condition occurs when excess thyroid hormone is manufac-tured and released by the butterfly-shaped thyroid gland, which surrounds part of the windpipe. This vital gland maintains a delicate balance of energy-regulat-ing thyroid hormone in the blood that influences metabolism. A surplus of hor-mone accelerates energy metabolism, speeding up body processes. Women are far more likely to suffer from hyperthyroidism than men. With proper treat-ment (including prescription drugs), the condition is quite manageable.

what causes it

An overactive thyroid may have one of several origins. In Graves' disease (a form of hyperthyroidism), an autoimmune disorder leads to an overproduction of thyroid hormone. Excess thyroid hormone may also be caused by abnormal nodules present in the thyroid gland or by inflammation of the gland. In rare instances, a cancerous growth or a dysfunctional pituitary gland, which influ-ences thyroid hormone synthesis, may lead to hyperthyroidism.

how food may help

To maintain adequate energy and weight, an individual with hyperthyroidism may need to consume 15% to 20% more calories than a healthy person. Once prescription drugs take effect, this additional caloric requirement may diminish. Protein and nutrient-dense foods are recommended to protect body muscle stores from being depleted by an accelerated metabolism.

Iodine is an essential component of thyroid hormone, and limiting this mineral is believed to suppress the synthesis and secretion of thyroid hormone.

Experimental research suggests that the antioxidant **vitamins E** and **C** may possibly combat oxidative damage linked to hyperthyroidism. An accelerated metabolism may speed up the generation of destructive free radicals. In addition, foods high in the healing nutrient **beta-carotene,** such as carrots, pumpkin, and sweet potatoes, may benefit individuals with an overactive thyroid; beta-carotene is converted to vitamin A, which is believed to modify iodine utilization in the body.

Evidence is accumulating that an overactive thyroid may alter calcium metabolism in the skeleton. An always-changing tissue, bone is in a constant state of being remodeled, and excess thyroid hormone appears to reduce bone mass through this process, raising the risk for bone-thinning osteoporosis. A **calcium**-rich diet may help combat this risk by improving bone density. And **vitamin D** promotes bone strength by enhancing calcium absorption.

Other nutrients important for bone strength include **vitamin K** (in leafy greens such as kale); **omega-3 fatty acids** (in flaxseeds and walnuts); and minerals such as **magnesium, manganese,** and **potassium** (in fruits and vegetables). **Vitamin C,** in addition to improving bone density, is essential for the connective tissue (collagen) matrix that holds bones together. Researchers believe that estrogenlike plant compounds, **isoflavones** (in soy) and **lignans** (in flaxseed), promote bone strength as well, staving off fractures.

Digestive disturbances, particularly diarrhea, often accompany an overactive thyroid. (For advice on managing *Diarrhea*, see *page 160*.)

recent research

New research suggests that excess thyroid hormone may increase the risk for bone-thinning osteoporosis. In a preliminary study, women with a history of an overactive thyroid had double the risk for hip fracture, compared with healthy women. Scientists believe elevated thyroid hormone hastens bone turnover, thus weakening bones. (For dietary advice on *Osteoporosis*, see *page 200*.)

your food arsenal

foods	nutrient	health benefits
broccoli cooking greens figs	calcium	A calcium-rich diet is important, because hyperthyroidism often spurs calcium loss from bones.
berries citrus fruits melons peppers	vitamin C	Experimental research links hyperthyroidism with reduced blood levels of vitamin C, which is thought to improve symptoms of the condition.
avocados nuts seeds whole grains	vitamin E	Animal research indicates that this antioxidant vitamin may protect against oxidative damage associated with hyperthyroidism.

hypothyroidism

what it is

A healthy thyroid gland successfully regulates energy metabolism by synthesizing and releasing sufficient amounts of thyroid hormone. In hypothyroidism, too little thyroid hormone is manufactured or released, causing a slowdown in body processes. The drop in thyroid hormone depresses energy levels, compromises nutrient absorption, and promotes weight gain. Constipation, depression, goiter (enlargement of the thyroid), dry skin, fatigue, and sensitivity to cold frequently accompany an inactive thyroid. Research indicates that people who suffer from the disorder have an elevated risk for heart disease because they can develop high levels of artery-clogging cholesterol.

Experts estimate that almost 5 out of 100 Americans may be afflicted with some form of hypothyroidism; the condition is most prevalent among those over 60 and, for unknown reasons, women are much more likely than men to have an underactive thyroid.

what causes it

The most common cause of hypothyroidism is an autoimmune disease called Hashimoto's thyroiditis in which immune cells accumulate in thyroid tissue and reduce thyroid hormone synthesis. Treatment for *hyper*thyroidism, surgery on the thyroid gland, radiation, a hormonal imbalance elsewhere in the body, medication, or genetic factors may also lead to an inactive thyroid. In some instances, insufficient amounts of the mineral iodine—a major constituent of thyroid hormone—can cause hypothyroidism.

Note that iodine deficiency is rare in developed countries because iodine is abundant in the food supply, particularly in iodized salt. Substances that interfere with iodine absorption, called goitrogens, are found in some foods and are believed to possibly contribute to hypothyroidism (see *Foods to Avoid,* right).

how food may help

Because of their sluggish metabolism, people with hypothyroidism may require only half the calories of a healthy adult, at least until their prescription medication becomes effective, normalizing metabolism. Opting for fiber-rich, nutrient-dense foods cuts calories and satisfies the appetite, helping to stave off the weight gain frequently associated with hypothyroidism. A plant-based diet high in **complex carbohydrates** may ease depression symptoms linked with hypothyroidism and supports weight loss (when eaten in moderation).

Though iodine deficiency is rare in the United States and other developed nations, a deficiency of the mineral may result in hypothyroidism. The thyroid gland uses **iodine** to create thyroid hormone, and when the mineral is lacking, the thyroid gland swells to what is known as a goiter, to more effectively capture iodine. Note that the human requirement for iodine is very small, but extremely important since thyroid hormone regulates energy production.

Several vitamins and minerals are essential for normal thyroid function, including **zinc,** which teams up with **vitamin E** to assist in the synthesis of thyroid hormone. Research suggests that low levels of zinc may possibly be linked to an elevated risk for hypothyroidism, particularly in the elderly. Important plant sources of zinc include beans and fortified cereals, and vitamin E is found in sunflower seeds and wheat germ. **Vitamin B₆,** plentiful in bananas and soybeans, is also required for thyroid hormone synthesis and proper iodine absorption. The mineral **selenium,** present in nuts and whole grains, is thought to activate thyroid hormone.

Cholesterol levels are often elevated among people with hypothyroidism. Substituting healthy fats for harmful fats is a key to managing cholesterol, but there are other dietary measures that help. (See *High Cholesterol, page 176.*)

To combat constipation, which typically accompanies hypothyroidism, drink plenty of water and eat a diet plentiful in both insoluble and soluble fiber. (For more information, see *Constipation, page 154.*)

foods to avoid

Because raw goitrogens may interfere with the body's absorption of iodine and synthesis of thyroid hormone, it may be advisable for people with hypothyroidism to avoid certain foods containing goitrogens, including raw cruciferous vegetables, peanuts, pine nuts, and soybeans. Cooking inactivates goitrogens.

your food arsenal

foods	nutrient	health benefits
beans beets lentils pomegranates	dietary fiber	Both insoluble and soluble fiber help alleviate constipation, which often accompanies hypothyroidism. In addition, fiber may protect against high cholesterol and weight gain, both of which are frequently associated with hypothyroidism.
fruits and vegetables iodized salt seaweed	iodine	This mineral is essential for the manufacture of thyroid hormone. Note that excess iodine can be detrimental.

immune deficiency

what it is

Each day our bodies face an endless barrage of infectious agents, and the immune system mounts an aggressive defense against these foreign invaders. Its army includes macrophages, killer T-cells, and B-cells. An overburdened immune system or a deficiency in its arsenal may compromise the body's ability to fend off illness.

what causes it

There are more than 200 types of primary immune deficiency diseases. A suppressed immune system may stem from poor diet, stress, genetic factors, age, insufficient rest, obesity, medications, chemotherapy, short-term infections, or chronic illness. Oxidative damage from free radicals may undermine immune cell potency as well.

how food may help

Researchers are uncovering powerful links between a nourishing diet and strong immunity. Adequate **protein** and calories are vital for maintaining the immune system, since all immune cells are composed of protein. A low-fat diet with little saturated fat is thought to limit destructive free radicals that can progressively damage and compromise immune cells. Healthful **essential fatty acids** are believed to enhance immunity.

A wealth of nutrients, including **iron, zinc,** and **vitamins C** and **E,** strengthen infection-fighting cells and may revitalize an aging immune system. (Note, however, that excessive intake of iron and zinc can reduce immunity.) **B vitamins**—found in complex carbohydrates, nutritional yeast, and leafy greens—help maintain immunity, including antibody production.

Studies indicate that healthful **probiotic bacteria** in fermented foods may combat pathogens by crowding them out of the body; beneficial bacteria may also manufacture infection-fighting compounds.

Garlic and onions may stimulate the fighting power of macrophages and T-cells because of their powerful **sulfur compounds,** which may also block enzymes that allow organisms to invade healthy tissue.

Eating **shiitake mushrooms** may enhance immunity because researchers believe healing compounds, including **lentinan,** may stimulate the body's production of immune cells.

Preliminary research indicates that **CAY-1,** a substance in cayenne, may ward off microbes that cause pneumonia and yeast infections.

Experts believe **flavonoid** phytonutrients abundant in whole grains and produce, such as pomegranates, may elevate the potency of immune cells and may damage the genetic machinery in germs that allows them to multiply.

Studies suggest that a diet low in **carotenoids,** such as lycopene and beta-carotene, may weaken resistance. Carrots and sweet potatoes are rich in **beta-carotene,** and tomato products contain abundant amounts of **lycopene,** which has shown promise in protecting lymphocytes from oxidative stress that can compromise their infection-fighting power.

recent research

Although research into the association between the gut microbiome and immunity is in its early stages, and mostly in animal models, a review of the current literature concluded that prebiotics and probiotics have positive effects on immune function and may be especially helpful as we age.

your food arsenal

foods	nutrient	health benefits
carrots **sweet potatoes** **tomatoes**	carotenoids	Research suggests that the antioxidant properties of carotenoids may protect immune cells from destructive free radicals.
nuts **seeds**	essential fatty acids	These fats are vital for wound healing and optimal functioning of T-cells.
beans **lentils** **tofu**	iron	Adequate amounts of this mineral are required for the manufacture of B-cells and T-cells.
kimchi **kombucha** **tempeh**	probiotics	Evidence is accumulating that these friendly bacteria improve immune responses against viruses and cancer cells.
berries **citrus fruits** **peppers**	vitamin C	In addition to protecting against oxidative damage, this vitamin may enhance the function of immune cells.
avocados **olive oil** **seeds**	vitamin E	According to studies, vitamin E may enhance T-cell activity and assist in the production of antibodies.
beans **nuts** **whole grains**	zinc	This mineral works with enzymes to heal wounds and may possibly bolster the body's resistance against cold viruses.

infertility
& impotence

what it is

Infertility—an inability to conceive a child after at least one year of regular unprotected intercourse—affects an estimated 12% to 15% of couples in the United States. Repeated miscarriages are considered to be a form of infertility as well. Impotence (also called erectile dysfunction, or ED) is the persistent inability to attain or maintain an erection, and is particularly prevalent in males over age 50.

what causes it

A woman's inability to conceive may result from hormonal imbalances, ovulation problems, weight fluctuations, intense exercise, stress, thyroid disease, or possibly smoking. Male infertility is attributed to defective or an insufficient number of sperm, or impaired reproductive glands. The most common cause of impotence is restricted blood flow to the penis.

how food may help

The B vitamin **folate,** typically recommended for women before conception and during pregnancy, may be vital for male reproduction as well. According to new research, deficient sperm counts are significantly associated with low folate in healthy men. The vitamin's reproductive role in men is unclear, but scientists believe normalizing folate levels through a diet rich in this B vitamin may possibly offset diminished sperm levels.

The antioxidant mineral **selenium** may team up with **vitamin E** to defend against oxidative damage in reproductive organs. Selenium helps ensure normal sperm function, and low levels of this mineral in women have been associated with miscarriages.

Vitamin B$_{12}$ and **iron** may protect against infertility as well. Some evidence suggests vitamin B$_{12}$ may improve sperm count and motility, even in men who are not B$_{12}$ deficient. In rare instances, men and women may be B$_{12}$ deficient (suffering from pernicious anemia), which hinders fertility and can lead to sterility. Low levels of the blood-nourishing mineral iron may impede conception in women.

Since atherosclerosis is a frequent underlying cause of impotence, reducing fat buildup in the arteries may improve blood flow to the penis, thus preventing impotence. **Vitamin C** is important for blood vessel health and may promote uninhibited circulation that allows blood vessels in the penis to enlarge and accommodate blood. **Flavonoids** are believed to enhance vitamin C actions and may fortify blood vessel structure, as well as prevent hardening of the arteries. Decreasing saturated and trans fats in the diet and substituting unsaturated fat, particularly the monounsaturated type, can help prevent the buildup of fatty plaques in arteries.

your food arsenal

foods	nutrient	health benefits
asparagus beans salad greens spinach	folate	Early research links low folate levels in healthy men with reduced sperm count. In addition, low levels of folate may be associated with repeated miscarriages and diminished fertility in women.
guava tomatoes watermelon	lycopene	Preliminary studies suggest that this carotenoid, which is concentrated in the testes, may improve sperm count and motility, particularly in men with low blood levels of lycopene.
Brazil nuts seeds whole grains	selenium	Deficiencies in this antioxidant mineral have been associated with fertility problems, including miscarriages. Scientists believe this mineral is also part of an important structural component in sperm.
berries broccoli citrus fruits peppers	vitamin C	This antioxidant vitamin may shield against oxidative damage, which can reduce sperm count and quality. Vitamin C is also thought to help maintain blood vessels and improve blood flow diminished by atherosclerosis, a frequent underlying cause of impotence.
avocado nuts olive oil seeds	vitamin E	Animal research suggests this vitamin may delay age-associated infertility in women. Vitamin E may protect sperm membranes against oxidative damage and, according to lab research, may help facilitate fertilization.
beans nuts seeds	zinc	This vital mineral is essential for ovulation, development and maturity of sperm, and fertilization.

insomnia

what it is

Insomnia is one of the most widespread health complaints today; sleepless, restless nights are common to more than one-third of the adult population worldwide. Insomnia is waking earlier than planned or having difficulty falling asleep or remaining asleep, and is not a disease itself, but rather a symptom of an underlying health or emotional problem. Daytime fatigue and irritability are consequences of sleep deprivation. For many of us, insomnia is only a temporary annoyance, but chronic sleep debt may mortgage health, since sufficient rest is vital for physical and mental well-being. A variety of diet and lifestyle factors may improve sleep habits, diminishing insomnia and its impact.

what causes it

Like a nagging cough or a fever, insomnia stems from an underlying condition. Stress, anxiety, and depression are the leading causes of temporary sleeplessness. Brief bouts of insomnia commonly result from an erratic sleep schedule, short-term illness (such as bronchitis cough), pain, or environmental factors, such as noise. Medications and serious chronic health conditions can disrupt sleep as well. Also as you age, sleep patterns change. Additional insomnia triggers include vigorous nighttime exercise, pregnancy, heartburn, alcohol, and too much caffeine.

how food may help

A nutritional formula to induce sleep has not yet been discovered, but a variety of nutrients are important for sleep and may help remedy insomnia.

When eaten along with starchy foods, the amino acid **tryptophan,** found in many high-protein foods, may promote drowsiness by fueling the production of serotonin, a brain chemical that fosters relaxation and feelings of well-being (or calm). **Vitamin B_6** and the mineral **magnesium** help convert tryptophan to serotonin. Vitamin B_6 assists in the production of additional brain chemicals that regulate sleep and mood, including melatonin and dopamine. Bananas and potatoes are good sources of vitamin B_6 and magnesium. Though the mechanism is unclear, mild **calcium** deficiencies may be associated with sleep disturbances as well.

Complex carbohydrates may promote restful sleep because they enhance the brain's absorption of sleep-inducing tryptophan. Complex carbohydrates may also ease heartburn-related insomnia. Eating too much or too close to bedtime frequently causes heartburn, an underlying cause of sleep disturbances for many Americans. Eating plenty of bland carbohydrates may prevent heartburn. **Thiamin** (vitamin B_1) helps transform complex carbohydrates into useful energy for the body and is essential for healthy nerve function. Low levels of this B vitamin are thought to interfere with a good night's sleep.

Eating foods rich in B vitamins may help fight the blues, a common cause of insomnia. B vitamins foster the production of the brain's neurotransmitters, essential for restful sleep and a peaceful mood. A deficiency of **folate** and **vitamin B_{12}** is sometimes found in people who are depressed. Folate is abundant in lentils and asparagus, and vitamin B_{12} can be found in nutritional yeast. In addition, there is growing evidence that folate and vitamin B_{12} team up with vitamin B_6 to lower levels of the amino acid homocysteine, which may be associated with depression. **Niacin,** present in grains, nuts, and legumes, is thought to be useful for relieving depression-related insomnia as well, though clinical evidence is lacking.

Evidence is emerging that **omega-3 fatty acids,** such as those present in chia seeds, flaxseed, and walnuts, play a key role in optimal mental activity, which may influence mood and insomnia. Some findings suggest depression may be related in part to inadequate intake of these healthful fats.

Easing the symptoms of menopause may relieve insomnia, as declining hormone levels are frequently connected to sleep disturbances. Studies suggest that consuming foods high in **phytoestrogens,** plantlike estrogen compounds, helps relieve the severity of menopause symptoms, including hot flashes. Findings from population studies indicate that women who regularly consume isoflavones (phytoestrogens in soy foods) tend to suffer far less from unpleasant menopause symptoms.

home remedy

Researchers have established a connection between sleep quality and the gut microbiome. Probiotic and prebiotic foods such as fermented vegetables, kimchi, kombucha, onions, garlic, asparagus, and bananas help balance gut flora and ensure a healthier microbiome.

your food arsenal

foods	nutrient	health benefits
beans **potatoes** **whole grains**	complex carbohydrates	Foods high in complex carbohydrates may promote drowsiness by enhancing tryptophan absorption.
leafy greens **pumpkin seeds**	tryptophan	The body converts this amino acid into the sleep-inducing brain chemical serotonin.

irritable bowel syndrome

what it is

At some point in their lives, nearly 20% of adults experience alternating bouts of constipation and diarrhea characteristic of irritable bowel syndrome (IBS). The most common gastrointestinal disorder in America, IBS occurs when the muscles of the intestinal tract contract in abnormal, uncoordinated spasms. Abdominal pain, bloating, flatulence, and mucus in the stool frequently accompany IBS. Some people have either constipation or diarrhea predominantly, while others suffer from both. Symptoms of the disorder range from mild to debilitating, but IBS is not life-threatening, nor does it lead to or signal more serious conditions such as colon cancer.

what causes it

A single cause for IBS has not yet been established, though experts have proposed many potential triggers. Possible offenders that may overstimulate the nervous and digestive systems include stress and overuse of antibiotics. Researchers believe stress aggravates symptoms, regardless of the underlying reason for the disorder. Because it may have a variety of causes and symptoms, IBS is usually diagnosed by eliminating ailments with similar symptoms, and then devising a strategy to alleviate IBS discomfort. This may include stress management techniques, prescription drugs, and diet modifications.

how food may help

To relieve IBS symptoms, experts recommend eating small, frequent meals since large volumes of food distend the stomach and may lead to gastrointestinal distress. It is equally important to eat slowly; eating too quickly may increase swallowed air, which promotes irritating intestinal gas. Chew foods thoroughly to slow eating and to ensure optimal nutrient absorption in the digestive tract. Sipping peppermint or ginger tea may help settle an uneasy digestive system. Low-fat, high-fiber meals are generally suggested since fatty, greasy food may encourage uncomfortable bowel contractions. Note that IBS sufferers with diarrhea may experience increased symptoms with foods high in insoluble fiber.

Dietary fiber enhances digestive function, promoting regular, rhythmic intestinal contractions. In particular, **insoluble fiber** helps to bulk up feces and ease elimination, relieving IBS-associated constipation. Foods high in **soluble fiber,** on the other hand, absorb water and are especially beneficial for bouts of diarrhea. Clinical studies indicate that psyllium, a type of dietary fiber, may ameliorate IBS for some people. Psyllium bulks up the stool and absorbs water in the digestive tract, alleviating intestinal spasms and promoting regular bowel movements without increasing abdominal cramping or flatulence. To reduce intestinal discomfort, gradually increase fiber in your diet and drink at least 8 glasses of water each day.

Because a bout of IBS-related diarrhea may diminish beneficial bacteria in the colon, **probiotic bacteria** may be useful by replenishing friendly flora. Preliminary research suggests that **fructooligosaccharides (FOS),** sugar molecules in foods such as bananas, may foster the growth of beneficial bacteria. While other foods may contain FOS, bananas appear to be one of the least irritating to the digestive tract.

To quell flatulence associated with IBS, soak gassy foods, including broccoli and cauliflower, before cooking. Drain and rinse foods such as beans and then cook in fresh water. Steaming gassy vegetables may also reduce flatulence.

Food intolerances, particularly lactose intolerance, commonly trigger and worsen IBS symptoms, so determining such food sensitivities may ease symptoms. It is important to keep a food diary and be aware of foods that may trigger symptoms. Work with a doctor or dietitian to determine if food intolerances or allergies play a role in IBS symptoms and what you can do about it.

foods to avoid

Alcohol, caffeine, fat, and sorbitol (a type of sugar present in high amounts in prunes and some commercially prepared foods) can irritate the intestines, exacerbating IBS symptoms. In addition, to minimize IBS discomfort, experts advise testing for intolerances to the milk sugar lactose and possibly fructose sugars (found in fruits and fruit-based foods). Some gas-producing foods, such as broccoli, cauliflower, and onions, may also aggravate IBS symptoms.

your food arsenal

foods	nutrient	health benefits
fermented foods kimchi	probiotics	Research suggests these healthful bacteria enhance the growth of friendly flora in the intestines that may be reduced in individuals suffering from irritable bowel syndrome.
bulgur salad greens sweet potatoes	insoluble fiber	Increasing insoluble fiber intake is useful for combatting constipation associated with irritable bowel syndrome.
oats carrots	soluble fiber	This type of fiber may relieve bouts of diarrhea, associated with irritable bowel syndrome.

kidney stones

what it is

More than half a million Americans end up in the emergency room each year because of kidney stones (or renal calculi), which occur when stone-forming compounds from the urine accumulate in the kidney and start to crystallize. The stones are typically composed of calcium, combined with phosphate or oxalate. (Less common are so-called struvite stones, which can result from kidney or chronic urinary tract infection; and even less frequently, gout-related uric acid stones may form.) Passing one kidney stone dramatically increases the chance of having another stone, but experts believe these odds can be improved through exercise and diet alterations.

what causes it

Heredity and chronic dehydration seem to contribute to kidney stone formation, but the specific cause is unknown. Certain factors and conditions may predispose individuals to kidney stones, including a sedentary lifestyle and being Caucasian or Asian. Some people tend to have higher concentrations of calcium in their urine, which promotes crystal formation and accounts for the majority of stones. Additional risk factors include kidney disease, chronic bowel inflammation, intestinal surgery, and medications such as diuretics. Scientists do not believe that eating any specific food causes stones to form in people who are *not* susceptible. Research suggests, however, that for those who *are* susceptible, oxalates and purines may fuel stone formation.

how food may help

Drinking plenty of fluids, especially water, is perhaps the most important dietary advice for the prevention and management of kidney stones. Water dilutes the urine, making it difficult for salts to crystallize and stones to form. Note that diluted urine should not be darker than pale yellow, and fluid intake should be adjusted accordingly. Experts recommend twelve 8-ounce glasses (3 quarts) of water a day to avoid kidney stones.

Research suggests that drinking orange, grapefruit, and apple juices and sugar-free lemonade may effectively help prevent kidney stones. In addition to the beneficial water content of lemonade and juice, alkaline substances called **citrates** in some of these juices may help neutralize stone-forming acids, inhibiting the formation of certain calcium-based kidney stones. Incidentally, the valuable mineral **potassium,** also found in juice and lemonade, may be useful since potassium is linked to a reduced risk for kidney stones. To help prevent struvite kidney stones, eat **tannin**-rich blueberries. (Although cranberries have tannins, they should be avoided because they are high in oxalates.)

Studies have shown that people who follow a high plant-protein diet are at less risk of developing kidney stones than those whose diets rely on animal protein, which is thought to elevate the concentration of stone-forming calcium and oxalates in the urine.

Because urinary calcium and oxalates contribute to kidney stones, foods high in **insoluble fiber** (but low in oxalates) may help by binding excess oxalates and calcium in the digestive tract, preventing their accumulation in the urine. **Magnesium** may be beneficial as well, because it may bind oxalates in the intestines. It is important to check with your doctor before substantially increasing fiber consumption, because reducing calcium levels may raise the risk for bone-thinning osteoporosis.

Despite the evidence that dietary calcium raises urinary calcium, and urinary calcium encourages kidney stones, two powerful observational studies found that people who ate the most calcium-rich foods were significantly less likely to suffer from calcium-based kidney stones. Researchers surmise that dietary calcium may block the body's absorption of harmful oxalates. (Note that the study subjects who consumed the most dietary calcium also consumed the most fluids, potassium, magnesium, and phosphate.) However, calcium consumed in supplement form may actually increase the risk for stones.

foods to avoid

Because they may increase the chance of kidney stones, certain foods should be limited or completely avoided by people at risk for the condition. These foods include refined carbohydrates, salty foods, alcohol, foods high in animal protein, purine-rich foods, and oxalate-rich foods. Purine-rich foods include organ meats, anchovies, sardines, and herring. Foods high in oxalates include beets and beet greens, chocolate, chard, cranberries, dandelion greens, nuts, parsley, rhubarb, spinach, strawberries, tea, and wheat bran.

your food arsenal

foods	nutrient	health benefits
broccoli peas	insoluble fiber	Generous amounts of insoluble fiber are thought to bind stone-forming oxalates and calcium.
avocados quinoa	magnesium	This valuable mineral may lower levels of harmful oxalates, a major component of many kidney stones.
bananas potatoes	potassium	Research links high potassium intake with a reduced risk for kidney stones.
blueberries	tannins	By protecting against urinary tract infections, tannins may prevent struvite kidney stones, which are associated with chronic UTIs.

macular degeneration

what it is

The leading cause of blindness in the elderly, macular degeneration (often referred to as age-related macular degeneration, or AMD) affects one out of three people over the age of 75. The disease impairs the macula, which is the central part of the retina and is important for clear, sharp vision. As the disease progresses, blank spots gradually appear in the central field of vision. Approximately 90% of macular degeneration sufferers have the "dry" form, and the more serious "wet" form accounts for the remainder of macular degeneration cases.

what causes it

Experts believe that harmful free radicals—unstable oxygen molecules—cause damage to the retina, leading to macular degeneration. It's thought that age-related changes and genetics contribute to the condition as well. Sunlight exposure, pollution, cigarette smoke, and a high-fat diet can increase the amount of destructive free radicals in the eye. Having cardiovascular disease or diabetes may elevate the risk for the disease as well by restricting blood flow to the eye.

how food may help

A natural protective pigment in the macula helps filter out the damaging light rays that contribute to macular degeneration. **Lutein** and **zeaxanthin,** carotenoids abundant in vegetable pigments, are highly concentrated in macular pigment and in the retina. Studies link diets rich in lutein and zeaxanthin with a reduced risk for macular degeneration, and the progression of the disease may even be slowed by this pair. Consumption of dark green, carotenoid-rich, leafy vegetables, particularly spinach and collard greens, has been associated with a reduced risk for macular degeneration, suggesting that carotenoids such as lutein and zeaxanthin (as well as **beta-carotene**) are protective agents.

Another carotenoid, **lycopene,** may protect against macular degeneration because its unique structure and biochemistry make it especially adept at combatting harmful oxidative damage. Preliminary human studies have found that low levels of lycopene are associated with an elevated risk for macular degeneration.

Scientists believe a diet rich in antioxidant vitamins and minerals, such as **vitamins C** and **E, selenium,** and **zinc,** may also defend against macular degeneration by scavenging free radicals in the retina. Vitamin C is particularly concentrated in the eye. Evidence is accumulating that these nutrients are essential for eye health, and deficiencies may increase the risk for macular degeneration.

recent research

Multiple studies have concluded that vitamin D status is associated with the risk of developing age-related macular degeneration (AMD). Researchers have noted that high blood concentration of vitamin D may be associated with lower risk of developing AMD.

your food arsenal

foods	nutrient	health benefits
carrots **spinach** **winter squash**	beta-carotene	Carotenoids such as beta-carotene, found in orange vegetables and dark leafy greens, are linked to a reduced risk for macular degeneration.
collard greens **peppers** **spinach** **sweet potatoes**	lutein & zeaxanthin	These antioxidant pigments are concentrated in the macula and retina, which suggests they may protect vision cells from oxidative damage. Observational studies associate a lower risk for macular degeneration with diets rich in lutein and zeaxanthin.
apricots **tomatoes** **watermelon**	lycopene	According to preliminary research, people with low levels of this antioxidant carotenoid may have as much as twice the risk for macular degeneration.
barley **Brazil nuts** **brown rice** **lentils**	selenium	Some observational studies indicate that individuals who consume a diet abundant in antioxidant minerals, such as selenium, may be less likely to develop macular degeneration.
berries **broccoli** **citrus fruits** **peppers**	vitamin C	Epidemiologic evidence suggests that a diet plentiful in vitamin C may help stave off macular degeneration. Vitamin C is thought to combat free-radical damage in the eye, which can lead to macular degeneration.
avocado **nuts** **olive oil**	vitamin E	High blood levels of tocopherols (vitamin E compounds) may be related to a reduced risk for early-onset macular degeneration.
beans **green peas** **nuts** **whole grains**	zinc	According to preliminary evidence, depressed levels of zinc may be tied to macular degeneration. Zinc is critical to the metabolic function of enzymes important to the retina.

memory loss

what it is

Mild lapses in memory—forgetting names and misplacing objects—are common with age as elements of the cognitive network may falter. Some forgetfulness is to be expected with age and is relatively benign. Profound memory loss is a universal symptom of dementia, and Alzheimer's disease is one form of dementia.

what causes it

Benign age-related memory loss may result from shrinkage of the brain's nerves, diminished production of brain chemicals, or restricted blood flow to brain tissue. Genetic factors, head injuries, viruses, and cardiovascular disease may contribute to Alzheimer's disease.

how food may help

Exercise and a sound diet are instrumental in preserving brain longevity and sustaining memory. Protective brain nutrients include **complex carbohydrates** and **B vitamins,** which help ensure healthy nerve transmission and sufficient quantities of neurotransmitters. In a study of healthy elderly people, memory significantly improved after consuming 1¾ ounces of either potatoes or barley, both complex carbohydrates. B vitamins help convert food, such as complex carbohydrates, into brain fuel. In addition, some epidemiological evidence associates low levels of **vitamin B_6, vitamin B_{12},** and **folate** with Alzheimer's disease.

Scientists believe the blood-nourishing mineral **iron** may be important for neurotransmitter activity, and some research suggests depressed levels of iron can impair memory function. In one study of nonanemic adolescent girls, mild iron deficiency was associated with slightly impaired short-term memory and poorer performance on a test of verbal learning, compared to girls with adequate iron intake.

Blueberries show promise in fighting age-related memory decline; preliminary studies link blueberries with improved cognitive function. The exact mechanism has not yet been clearly established, but the antioxidant actions of **flavonoids** in blueberries, especially the pigment anthocyanin, are thought to reverse some parameters of age-related memory loss by defending against harmful free radicals, which can accumulate in brain cells and compromise memory function. Flavonoids may enhance blood flow to brain tissue involved with memory as well. Additional antioxidant and anti-inflammatory nutrients, including **beta-carotene, isoflavones,** and **vitamins E and C,** may also help preserve memory.

Unobstructed blood flow to the brain is essential for mental fitness, since brain cells require continuous nourishment and accessible communication with supporting systems in the body. Fatty deposits in the arteries frequently impede blood flow to the brain, impairing memory. The risk for arterial plaques may be reduced by consuming **monounsaturated fat** in place of trans fatty acids and saturated fat; population research has found that a diet high in monounsaturated fat protects against age-related cognitive decline. Additional cardioprotective nutrients, such as **soluble fiber,** maintain unclogged blood vessels. Another heart-healthy fat, **DHA,** is a building block for brain tissue, and low levels have been associated with age-related dementia, including Alzheimer's disease.

your food arsenal

foods	nutrient	health benefits
beans potatoes brown rice whole grains	complex carbohydrates	Through glucose metabolism, complex carbohydrates may elevate production of neurotransmitters or influence proteins in the digestive tract, which signal brain cells and enhance memory.
blueberries strawberries	flavonoids	Experimental research suggests that flavonoids in blueberries (and possibly strawberries) may slow age-related decline in mental function, including neuron deterioration.
soy products	isoflavones	According to preliminary evidence, soy isoflavones may protect against Alzheimer's by hindering protein changes that contribute to the disease.
avocados olive oil	monounsaturated fat	Scientists hypothesize that cardioprotective nutrients such as monounsaturated fat may preserve memory by maintaining blood flow to the brain.
avocados seeds	vitamin E	This powerful antioxidant is under review for its potential to enhance memory and slow the progression of Alzheimer's disease.

migraine

what it is

The classic manifestation of a migraine is a throbbing, acutely painful head-ache, beginning usually near one eye or temple (the word migraine is derived from the Greek word *hemikrania*, meaning "half of the head"). Pain can extend throughout one or both sides of the head, and, if the migraine is untreated, it can sometimes last for up to three days. Pain is usually worsened by physical activity. Early warning signs of an impending migraine may include an aura (seeing a bright light) and other visual disturbances such as blind spots and temporary loss of peripheral vision. Other warning signs include temporary nausea, weakness, and sensitivity to noise and bright or flashing lights.

what causes it

Though the exact cause of migraines is currently unknown, there are certain factors that are associated with this type of headache. During a migraine attack, blood vessels in the brain undergo spasms, which cause constriction and then rapid dilation. This triggers the release of brain chemicals that cause inflamma-tion and throbbing pain. A strong hereditary factor is also a component of this affliction, which occurs more often in women than in men.

Caffeine withdrawal, exposure to bright or flashing lights, oral contraceptives, vasodilating medication, dehydration, changes in sleep patterns, stress, hor-monal changes, and consumption of foods that contain certain chemicals can trigger migraines. Preliminary research suggests that an imbalance of the brain neurotransmitter serotonin may also play a role in the onset of this debilitating type of headache.

how food may help

Generally speaking, there is some evidence that low blood sugar can con-tribute to the onset of migraines. Eating regularly, without skipping meals, is important to prevent low blood sugar.

A drop in magnesium levels before or during a migraine attack has been noted in some people with migraines; it's also been noted that migraine sufferers are lacking in this mineral. Therefore, foods rich in **magnesium** may help diminish the severity of migraine pain.

Some migraine sufferers are thought to have low energy, and **riboflavin** helps to increase energy reserves by releasing energy from carbohydrates and producing red blood cells.

Some studies indicate that migraine sufferers have reduced levels of the mood-regulating neurotransmitter serotonin. Foods rich in **tryptophan,** an amino acid that boosts serotonin levels in the brain, may offer some relief of symptoms. Make sure to eat foods rich in complex carbohydrates to increase absorption of tryptophan.

To help reduce inflammation, a diet rich in **omega-3 fatty acids** may aid in migraine management. If you are experiencing nausea, try consuming foods seasoned with **ginger,** a spice thought to help alleviate stomach distress.

Because certain substances in food may induce a migraine attack, some people find it helpful to maintain a daily record of food and beverage intake, as well as a specific record of any migraine attacks, to help identify and avoid suspected migraine triggers (see *Foods to Avoid,* right). Maintaining a daily food record helps isolate and identify specific foods that might play a role in provoking a migraine. It may be useful to eliminate the suspected food from your diet for a few weeks, then reintroduce it, to determine if a migraine attack correlates with intake of the targeted food. Most of the information on dietary migraine triggers is based on anecdotal reports and very small inconclusive studies, rather than hard science. If you feel that a certain food or foods are migraine triggers, it is advisable to eliminate that food from your diet.

foods to avoid

Several compounds may be implicated in the onset of migraines. They are: nitrites (found in bacon, hot dogs, and cured meats), tyramine (found in pepperoni, red wine, chicken livers, active yeast preparations, and aged cheeses), tannins (found in nuts, apple juice, grapes, berries, coffee, red wine, and tea), and sulfites (used as preservatives in wine and dried fruits).

Monosodium glutamate (MSG)—a common ingredient in food served in Asian restaurants and also contained in many commercial products including seasonings (read labels carefully)—might also be a migraine trigger. The artificial sweetener aspartame is also a likely suspect.

Though chocolate is a possible trigger food, research is conflicting, and some studies show that chocolate is more benign than previously believed.

your food arsenal

foods	nutrient	health benefits
amaranth avocados rice winter squash	magnesium	People with migraines tend to have impaired magnesium metabolism as well as low levels of this important mineral. Note that although nuts are a good source of magnesium, it is not advisable to eat them, since they contain tannins, which could trigger migraines.
broccoli mushrooms quinoa	riboflavin	Riboflavin has the potential to increase energy reserves in brain cells, which are often reduced in some people who suffer from migraines.

osteoarthritis

what it is

Decades of use stress cartilage, the spongy, protective cushions located at the ends of bones. With age, damaged cartilage does not repair itself as effectively as it once did and may progressively deteriorate into osteoarthritis, or degenerative joint disease. The initial symptoms of the condition, joint stiffness and discomfort, are usually mild; but, eventually, once-cushioned bones begin to rub together, creating friction, tenderness, and gnarled joints.

Any joint is vulnerable to osteoarthritis, but it usually occurs in the ankles, feet, fingers, hips, knees, neck, or spine. The pain and stiffness of osteoarthritis most frequently affect the weight-bearing joints, and diseased joints may become knobby and deformed. If joint stiffness restricts movement, nearby muscles may become weaker, which contributes to even greater joint pain and stiffness. A very common age-related ailment, osteoarthritis affects more than 32.5 million American adults over the age of 50 and the condition is most prevalent among the elderly.

what causes it

Years of use gradually break down cartilage and its supporting structural tissue. Cartilage and related tissue-repair mechanisms gradually become deficient as a person ages, contributing to osteoarthritis. In addition, excess body weight, a genetic predisposition, defects in joints or cartilage, joint injuries, or repetitive joint motions associated with physical activity can lead to osteoarthritis.

how food may help

Several nutrients may benefit osteoarthritis, alleviating joint pain and inflammation as well as promoting cartilage repair. Research suggests that **vitamin C** may minimize cartilage loss and slow the progression of osteoarthritis. Another powerful antioxidant, **vitamin E,** may relieve osteoarthritis symptoms, according to preliminary clinical research.

Population studies link low levels of **vitamin D** with an elevated risk for osteoarthritis. Vitamin D's partner, **calcium,** may help bolster weight-bearing joints damaged by osteoarthritis and also stave off osteoporosis.

Some clinical evidence suggests that consuming **omega-3 fatty acids** and **shogaols** and **gingerols** (healing substances in ginger) may help relieve the tenderness and swelling of osteoarthritis. These compounds exhibit potent anti-inflammatory properties.

Though scientific data are limited, some experts believe consuming pineapple may defend against osteoarthritis and possibly improve symptoms. The pineapple enzyme **bromelain** is thought to alleviate swelling associated with osteoarthritis, because this compound has demonstrated anti-inflammatory activity in laboratory research.

Because osteoarthritis is more prevalent among women, some experimental evidence suggests that certain forms of estrogen may worsen the disease. So, scientists believe that **phytoestrogens** (estrogenlike plant compounds) may block the possible influence of natural estrogen on osteoarthritis. Phytoestrogens are plentiful in soy foods.

recent research

Observational research has found that older people who consumed inadequate amounts of vitamin D, and who had low levels of this bone-strengthening vitamin in their blood, had a substantially higher risk for progressively worsening osteoarthritis of the knee. Another study suggests that elderly women with low blood levels of vitamin D may have an elevated risk for osteoarthritis in the hip.

your food arsenal

foods	nutrient	health benefits
chia seeds flaxseed walnuts	omega-3 fatty acids	According to clinical research, these anti-inflammatory fats may improve the symptoms of arthritis, including morning stiffness, joint tenderness, and fatigue.
ginger	shogaols & gingerols	Phytonutrients in ginger may help ameliorate the pain and swelling of arthritis by interfering with the synthesis of inflammatory compounds.
berries broccoli cantaloupe peppers	vitamin C	Research suggests that this nutrient may minimize cartilage loss and slow the progression of osteoarthritis. Vitamin C seems to squelch harmful free radicals and enhance tissue repair.
fortified milk substitutes mushrooms	vitamin D	This vitamin has been shown to hinder the breakdown of bone and the progression of osteoarthritis. Population studies link low levels of vitamin D with an elevated risk for osteoarthritis.
avocados nuts olive oil seeds	vitamin E	Experimental data suggest that vitamin E may foster the growth of healthy cartilage. Vitamin E has demonstrated a benefit in preliminary clinical research involving osteoarthritis patients.

osteoporosis

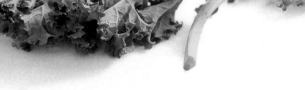

what it is

Aptly named for the Latin phrase "porous bones," osteoporosis is a debilitating, progressive skeletal disease that silently robs bones of their mineral density and strength. More than 1.4 million Americans, mostly women, are afflicted with or are at high risk for this bone-thinning disease, which leads to fractures and collapsed vertebrae.

what causes it

A lack of hormones (usually estrogen), exercise, and/or calcium may deplete bone mass and impair bone structure, weakening bones. Estrogen levels decline after menopause, leaving women, particularly those who are small-boned or underweight, with a heightened risk for the disease. An unbalanced diet, genetic predisposition, steroid use, cigarette smoking, and low testosterone levels (in men) may also contribute to the disease.

how food may help

A lifelong, high-quality diet rich in **calcium** nourishes and strengthens bones. Most of the body's calcium is stored in the skeleton, where this mineral provides a sturdy foundation for bone tissue. Consuming plenty of calcium and maintaining sufficient levels of vitamin D throughout childhood and early adulthood help build peak bone mass, which may offset bone loss later in life. During adulthood, daily calcium intake may bolster bone density.

A complex mix of nutrients in foods—including **isoflavone** and **lignan** phytoestrogens, and **vitamins C, D,** and **K**—helps promote and preserve bone strength as well, staving off fractures. The trace mineral **manganese,** plentiful in pineapple, is thought to improve the body's absorption of other bone-building minerals. Research suggests that **omega-3 fatty acids** may also help preserve bone mass in older women.

Because elevated levels of homocysteine have been implicated in osteoporosis, the B vitamins **folate, B₆,** and **B₁₂** may be useful by converting this amino acid to a less harmful substance. Lentils and greens are high in folate, bananas and rice contain vitamin B₆.

Evidence is accumulating that a diet rich in fruits and vegetables may protect against osteoporosis. Observational studies indicate that men and women who consume the most fruits and vegetables have higher bone-mineral density, an important defense against fractures. Well-known bone-building vitamins and minerals are plentiful in produce, and even **potassium** and **magnesium** in fruits and vegetables may preserve bone strength. Research links these minerals to a slower decline in bone-mineral density. Foods rich in potassium may also help reduce high blood pressure, which scientists believe promotes calcium excretion, thus raising the risk for the bone-thinning disease.

Eating **plant protein** (in vegetables, soy foods, and grains such as quinoa) instead of animal protein, and consuming a diet that is not excessive in any type of protein, are recommended. Preliminary research suggests that over time, eating plant protein may reduce the risk for osteoporosis-related fractures.

recent research

A large-scale, 10-year study of middle-aged women found that participants with the highest vitamin K consumption from foods had a 30% reduced risk for hip fracture. The richest sources of dietary vitamin K include kale, brussels sprouts, lettuce, broccoli, and spinach. Kale is a leading source of the bone-strengthening vitamin.

your food arsenal

foods	nutrient	health benefits
cooking greens sesame seeds	calcium	The cornerstone of healthy bones, calcium raises bone density, an important measure of how well bones resist fractures.
lentils soy foods	isoflavones	Researchers believe these estrogenlike compounds promote bone density. Studies indicate isoflavones may conserve bone mass, particularly during peri- and menopause.
flaxseed	lignans	A study of healthy postmenopausal women (not on hormone replacement therapy) suggests that flaxseed, which is high in lignans, may retain bone mass, elevate antioxidant status, and help prevent urinary loss of calcium.
berries citrus fruits peppers	vitamin C	In addition to enhancing bone density, vitamin C helps form the connective tissue (collagen) matrix that holds bones together.
fortified milk substitutes mushrooms	vitamin D	Necessary for optimal calcium absorption, vitamin D enhances bone strength.
kale spinach	vitamin K	This vitamin may strengthen bone by stimulating osteocalcin, a protein essential for bone strength.

overweight

what it is

Health experts warn that being overweight—defined as weighing more than 20% over the recommended ideal for your height—is a medical concern. Adults 30 to 40 pounds over a healthy weight range (which is significantly more than 20% overweight)—are particularly susceptible to disease. Virtually every population group is becoming increasingly heavier and scientific evidence links the epidemic of excessive weight to a higher risk for diabetes, certain cancers, high blood pressure, heart disease, and various chronic conditions, including varicose veins and arthritis.

what causes it

Consuming too many calories and not expending enough energy lead to weight gain. A sedentary lifestyle, a calorie-dense diet, and genetics are major contributors to obesity.

how food may help

Adopting a healthy eating style and increasing physical activity are critical for balancing energy expenditure. For permanent weight loss, most experts agree that a gradual, realistic weight loss, without mortgaging overall health, is most successful. In addition to learning to cook delicious, healthful food, it's important to listen to hunger cues, learn to limit portions, and avoid calorie-laden convenience foods. Swapping spice for salt and limiting alcohol may improve weight loss efforts as well. Since there is a tendency to overeat when eating fast, slow down—it takes about 20 minutes for the stomach to signal the brain that it is full. Counting total calories is important, but note that there is some evidence that the body stores dietary fat more readily than it does protein or carbohydrate, which can contribute to weight gain.

Preliminary evidence suggests that **calcium** may stimulate fat loss by suppressing hormones that cause us to store, rather than burn, excess fat. Some research among significantly overweight men found that a high-calcium diet assisted weight loss. **Vitamin D** is essential for proper calcium absorption and research findings suggest that it may be particularly important for obese people to consume enough of this vitamin. Scientists suspect obese individuals may have reduced levels of bioavailable vitamin D. Excess body fat stores this fat-soluble vitamin, making it unavailable for its healthful activities, including strengthening the skeleton.

> ### recent research
>
> A recent study found that a calorie-adjusted diet based on high-fiber carbohydrates, that is also low in total and saturated fat, not only helps facilitate weight loss but may also prevent diabetes in at-risk individuals.

Several studies suggest that diets centered around low-fat **complex carbohydrates**—fruits, vegetables, and whole grains—help maintain healthy weight loss and prevent weight gain. Complex carbohydrates are rich in fiber and nutrients. Experts recommend at least five servings of fruits and vegetables each day to stave off extra pounds. Fruits and vegetables provide an abundance of nourishment and volume for their calorie content. A 5-ounce baked potato (with skin) has about 60% fewer calories and far more fiber than a medium 3½-ounce serving of french fries.

Because they satisfy the appetite sooner and usually take longer to eat, foods high in **dietary fiber** are believed to aid in weight loss. Dietary fiber may slow the rate of digestion in the stomach as well. Filling up on high-fiber foods leaves less room for high-fat, calorie-dense foods. Some evidence suggests **soluble fiber** may assist in regulating blood sugar levels, thus controlling hunger pangs. In addition, research suggests that a high-fiber diet may slow fat absorption, helping you to feel fuller more quickly, while acquiring fewer fat calories. In one study, individuals consumed as much as 36 g of fiber each day and absorbed up to 130 fewer calories, translating to a potentially significant weight loss.

According to preliminary research, green tea **catechins** may benefit energy expenditure and weight loss. In combination with the caffeine in green tea, catechins may be especially helpful for maintaining a healthy weight after weight loss.

your food arsenal

foods	nutrient	health benefits
broccoli cooking greens figs tofu	calcium	Experimental research indicates that this indispensable mineral may promote the burning of calories rather than their storage as body fat.
beans brown rice whole grains	complex carbohydrates	Diets rich in low-fat complex carbohydrates have been associated with healthy body weight.
asparagus beets lentils	dietary fiber	High-fiber foods may prompt feelings of fullness with fewer calories.

perimenopause & menopause

what it is

Well before menstruation ceases, a woman's hormone levels may fluctuate for up to 10 years, during a phase known as perimenopause. A woman in perimenopause still menstruates, but experiences symptoms of diminished hormone levels. During menopause, a woman's body produces fewer reproductive hormones and no longer releases eggs or menstruates. Perimenopause and menopause symptoms include hot flashes, mood swings, night sweats, insomnia, and vaginal dryness.

what causes it

Perimenopause occurs as the ovaries gradually produce smaller quantities of the female hormones estrogen and progesterone. A lack of ovarian hormones during menopause, or as a result of surgical removal of the uterus and ovaries, halts ovulation (the release of an egg for fertilization) and ends menstruation. A woman has completed menopause after not having a period for 6 to 12 consecutive months.

how food may help

Consuming foods high in **phytoestrogens** (natural estrogenlike compounds in plant foods) may ease both perimenopause and menopause symptoms. Phytoestrogens are similar in structure to human estrogen but have milder estrogenic properties. Some evidence suggests that **isoflavones,** a type of phytoestrogen in soy foods, may relieve hot flashes, vaginal dryness, and mood changes associated with perimenopause and menopause. Epidemiological data indicate that women who consume soy phytoestrogens as a part of their daily diet—for example in such countries as China and Japan—tend to suffer far less from unpleasant menopause symptoms. In one six-year study of about 1,000 Japanese women between the ages of 35 and 54, researchers found that women who consumed the most soy products experienced significantly fewer hot flashes.

Researchers believe soy isoflavones may also help reduce the risk for heart disease, a major killer among postmenopausal women. After menopause, a woman's risk for heart attack increases tenfold because of declining estrogen levels. To combat this increased risk, a heart-healthy diet is recommended, which emphasizes plant-based meals full of cholesterol-lowering **soluble fiber,** monounsaturated fats, and omega-3 fatty acids. Replacing saturated and trans fats with **monounsaturated fat** helps reduce cholesterol levels and protect against clogged arteries. Several studies have found that eating **omega-3 fatty acids,** which are plentiful in chia seeds, flaxseed, and walnuts, may help prevent heart attacks and stroke as well.

Diminishing estrogen levels during perimenopause and menopause predispose women to osteoporosis. To protect against this bone-thinning disease, consume plenty of bone-building **calcium** and **vitamin D,** the cornerstones of sturdy bones. Studies show that postmenopausal women with the highest intakes of calcium and vitamin D have the lowest risk for osteoporosis-related bone loss and fractures.

To ease the feelings of insomnia and mild depression that frequently accompany menopause, consume foods high in **tryptophan,** such as legumes and nuts. This amino acid is converted into the brain chemical serotonin, which promotes relaxation and rest. Tryptophan may also help reduce feelings of mild depression. **Complex carbohydrates,** such as beans, potatoes, and grains, may be helpful as well because they are believed to enhance the bioavailability of tryptophan in the brain.

Eating foods rich in **B vitamins** may help fight the blues; low levels of these vitamins may be linked to depression. B vitamins also foster the production of certain brain neurotransmitters required for restful sleep and a peaceful mood.

> ### recent research
>
> In a six-week study, perimenopausal women (age 45 to 55) who consumed 20 g of soy protein (containing 34 mg of phytoestrogens) experienced a significant decrease in LDL ("bad") and total cholesterol, blood pressure, and severity of menopause symptoms, including hot flashes. Some experts estimate that about 6 to 8 ounces of tofu (or 60 mg of isoflavones) consumed daily may ease menopause symptoms.

your food arsenal

foods	nutrient	health benefits
broccoli **sesame tahini**	calcium	Postmenopausal women are particularly vulnerable to bone-thinning osteoporosis, which calcium helps to prevent.
edamame **flaxseed** **seaweed**	omega-3 fatty acids	Because a woman's risk for cardiovascular disease dramatically increases after menopause, these healthful fats are recommended to help prevent heart disease and stroke.
flaxseed **soy foods**	phytoestrogens	These estrogenlike plant compounds may ease symptoms of perimenopause and menopause.
fortified dairy substitutes **mushrooms**	vitamin D	By improving calcium absorption, this fat-soluble vitamin helps to strengthen bones.

pregnancy

how food may help

Certain lifestyle decisions (such as eating healthful foods) can help improve pregnancy outcome. While it is important to maintain a healthy diet throughout pregnancy (the fetus requires essential nutrients at every stage of development), good nutrition during the first trimester of pregnancy is particularly vital because rapid growth of the spinal cord, heart, brain, and most fetal tissues occurs during this period.

In fact, improving diet before conception will help to build up nutritional reserves of vitamins and minerals (folate, iron, calcium, and vitamin B_{12}, for example) and other compounds in foods required by the fetus for proper growth. Accumulating nutrients prior to pregnancy will allow the fetus to draw upon them without depleting the mother's supply.

The changing physiological demands of pregnancy require a wide range of nutrients that will help the body to prepare for and sustain a healthy full-term pregnancy, labor, delivery, and breastfeeding. Daily food choices should include ample amounts of whole grains, vegetables, legumes, fruit, low-fat sources of protein, about six to eight 8-ounce glasses of water, and a minimum of sweets and saturated fats. Generally, most pregnant women need to increase their daily caloric intake by only 300 calories.

Calcium is particularly important because the fetus uses it for tooth, bone, and skeletal development. If a woman doesn't consume enough calcium, the fetus will take what is needed from her supply, so plentiful amounts of calcium are important to help preserve the mother's bone density. And for women who are planning on breastfeeding, calcium is vital for lactation.

Pregnant women need **iron** to replenish their red blood cell supply and to accommodate the demand created by increased blood volume. A pregnant woman's blood supply increases in order to provide nutrition to the growing fetus; adequate iron is required to help both the mother and baby transport oxygen through the body. The fetus also accumulates iron for use during early life. Foods high in **vitamin C** will facilitate iron absorption, and these foods are also rich in other beneficial substances. To achieve adequate iron levels, iron supplements may be recommended by a health care provider.

Folate is a B vitamin that is instrumental in preventing birth defects such as spina bifida and brain malformations, which can develop within the first month after conception. To ensure optimal levels of this important vitamin, experts recommend women take folic acid (the synthetic form of folate) supplements three months prior to conception. And because about half of all pregnancies are unplanned, a daily intake of folate is suggested for all women of childbearing age.

Protein is needed for the placenta and for the cellular development of the fetus. Tempeh, tofu, beans, and quinoa are excellent sources of plant protein. Exact protein needs should be discussed with a health care provider.

Complex carbohydrates can help the woman meet energy demands, and they will also supply glucose needed by the fetus for proper nervous system development. These foods are also chock-full of nourishing vitamins, minerals, and fiber.

Eating small meals and avoiding long periods without food may alleviate nausea that is caused by hormonal changes within the first trimester. In addition, try eating soda crackers or dry toast upon waking and at bedtime. Snack on nutrient-dense, high-protein foods and avoid foods high in salt or fat. **Ginger,** as well as foods rich in **vitamin B$_6$,** can serve as natural antinausea agents. To prevent constipation (a common problem in pregnancy), select nourishing fiber-rich foods such as fresh fruits and vegetables, legumes, whole grains, dried fruits, and flaxseeds.

recent research

A recent review of studies measuring the effects of vegetarian and vegan diets during pregnancy concluded that a well-balanced, strict plant-based diet is safe for pregnancy and lactation, as long as calorie and nutrient needs are met.

your food arsenal

foods	nutrient	health benefits
broccoli cooking greens fortified dairy substitutes tofu	calcium	Optimal intake of calcium is vital since a woman's body will "rob" calcium from its own bones to give it to the fetus if the mineral is in short supply. The fetus requires this bone-nourishing mineral for skeletal development.
asparagus beets lentils	folate	This important B vitamin helps to prevent neural tube defects that can develop within the first four weeks after conception.
amaranth cashews quinoa tofu	iron	Pregnant women require extra iron to replenish their red blood supply and to accommodate the demand created by increased blood volume. The fetus accumulates iron for use during early life.

premenstrual syndrome

what it is

As many as 75% of menstruating women can identify with the physical and emotional symptoms of premenstrual syndrome (PMS). A highly individualized experience, PMS is characterized by a constellation of symptoms, including moodiness, tearfulness, irritability, bloating (water retention), insomnia, fatigue, food cravings, headaches (sometimes migraines), breast tenderness, and depression. Symptoms generally start a week or a few days before menstruation and continue into the first few days. Very severe symptoms may indicate premenstrual dysphoric disorder (PMDD). If symptoms become disruptive and impair daily life, it would be prudent to seek medical treatment.

what causes it

The exact cause of PMS is currently unknown, though theories suggest that PMS may result from an imbalance of hormones. This imbalance can cause mood fluctuations and food cravings. Preliminary studies indicate a possible link between PMS and abnormal metabolism of prostaglandins (hormonelike substances) or the hormone progesterone. Also, PMS may be associated with decreased levels of the brain chemical serotonin, which is instrumental in the regulation of mood, appetite, and feelings of well-being.

how food may help

Although food doesn't prevent PMS, certain substances in food may offer relief from some of the distressing symptoms of PMS.

Calcium may help to reduce mood disturbances, abdominal cramping, bloating, and muscular contractions resulting from PMS. Calcium may help regulate brain chemicals and hormones that affect mood.

Foods high in **complex carbohydrates** can be helpful in that they increase the production of serotonin, a brain chemical that regulates mood and appetite. Foods rich in complex carbohydrates also help to regulate glucose levels, which are thought to fluctuate in women with PMS.

Women who experience PMS often have low **magnesium** levels, which may predispose them to PMS-induced headaches.

Many studies show that foods rich in **vitamin B$_6$** may help relieve both the physical and psychological symptoms caused by PMS. Also, vitamin B$_6$ may help to increase the accumulation of magnesium in the body's cells.

One of the reasons that PMS is less common in Asian countries may be the high consumption of soy foods in those cultures. Soy isoflavones such as **genistein** (as well as **lignans** in flaxseeds) are phytoestrogens that may help to balance hormonal fluctuations by reducing high estrogen levels, believed to play a role in PMS.

Eating foods that are rich in **omega-3 fatty acids,** such as flaxseed and nuts, may decrease menstrual pain by promoting the production of anti-inflammatory prostaglandins. Omega-3 fatty acids may also reduce depression (see *page 156*), which is one of the many symptoms of PMS.

In addition to adding foods to the diet to help manage PMS, there are also some foods to be avoided. Reducing caffeine intake as well as sodium may help to reduce PMS symptoms.

recent research

A recent study indicates that whole-grain foods may be helpful in relieving symptoms of PMS. It found that women who replaced at least four servings of refined-grain bread with whole-grain bread on a daily basis had a significant reduction of PMS symptoms compared to the control group that continued to consume refined grains. The whole-grain group had a notable decrease in physical, mood, and behavioral symptoms.

your food arsenal

foods	nutrient	health benefits
kale sesame seeds tofu	calcium	Studies indicate that this mineral may help to reduce mood disturbances, cramping, and bloating resulting from PMS.
beans brown rice potatoes turnips whole grains	complex carbohydrates	By lowering the rate at which glucose enters the bloodstream, foods high in complex carbohydrates may offer satisfaction for those women plagued by PMS-induced food cravings. Further, complex carbohydrates are thought to increase levels of the brain chemical serotonin, which helps to regulate mood.
amaranth avocados quinoa sunflower seeds	magnesium	Some studies show that women suffering from PMS have low levels of magnesium.
acorn squash avocados bananas potatoes	vitamin B$_6$	This vitamin is believed to reduce anxiety and depression by increasing serotonin and other brain chemicals involved with mood.

prostate problems

what it is

"Prostate problems" generally translate into either benign prostatic hyperplasia (BPH) or prostate cancer. Though there are other types of prostate problems, such as prostatitis, BPH and prostate cancer are the most prevalent. Since these prostate problems have similar symptoms, it is vital to consult with a health care provider to seek proper testing and care.

Benign prostatic hyperplasia, also known as enlarged prostate, is one of the most common health problems facing men over the age of 60. In BPH the prostate gland enlarges and eventually places pressure on the urethra. Symptoms of BPH include difficulty with urination (stopping and starting), bladder irritation, a frequent urge to urinate (particularly during the night), dribbling, and a sensation of not emptying the bladder.

Prostate cancer is the most commonly diagnosed male cancer and the second leading cause of male cancer deaths in the United States after lung cancer. Checkups are advisable, particularly for men who experience painful or difficult urination, blood in the urine, painful ejaculation, impotence, or pain in the lower back.

what causes it

A common part of aging, BPH develops slowly over time. It is possible that a hormonal component may be associated with BPH. Prostate cancer may be linked to a hormonal cause, though research is still in the early stages. There is a genetic component, with men who have a family history of the disease being at higher risk compared with men who have no relatives with prostate cancer. Environmental factors also play a role in prostate cancer.

how food may help

Although more research is required in this area, some evidence does show a relationship between nutritional factors and prostate health.

Studies indicate that the antioxidant mineral **selenium** may protect against BPH, and it also may reduce the risk for developing prostate cancer, possibly by preventing oxidative damage to cells in the prostate gland. Selenium may protect against prostate cancer initiation, and it also may play a role in reducing prostate tumor growth by inducing apoptosis (cancer cell death).

Vitamin E teams up with selenium to confer antioxidant protection against free-radical damage to the prostate. Preliminary research also shows that vitamin E may decrease serum androgen concentrations, which are believed to be hormonal factors associated with prostate cancer.

The isoflavone **genistein,** found in soy foods, may help to protect against prostate cancer as well as possibly reducing tumor growth.

Research suggests that **lycopene** may help to decrease DNA damage to cells in prostate tissue, and it may play a role in initiating cancer cell death.

Research also shows that the flavonoid **quercetin** may help to prevent and treat prostate cancer. Quercetin interferes with processes that allow cancer to progress and spread. Quecertin may also help aid in anti-androgen (antitestosterone) therapies that are used to treat prostate cancer by making cancer cells less resistant to therapy. Studies indicate that quercetin may also reduce symptoms of prostatitis.

recent research

One study found a compelling link between lycopene and prostate cancer prevention. The study examined other carotenoids but only lycopene emerged as having protective effects.

Men who ate more than 10 servings of lycopene-rich tomato-based foods showed a 35% decreased risk for developing prostate cancer compared with those who ate fewer than 1.5 servings of tomato-based foods per week.

Early studies show that lycopene may also help treat chronic prostatitis. More research in humans is necessary before recommendations can be made.

your food arsenal		
foods	**nutrient**	**health benefits**
soy foods	genistein	Studies show that this isoflavone may reduce prostate cancer cell growth, possibly through hormonal actions.
pomegranates tomatoes watermelon	lycopene	Lycopene has been linked to the prevention of prostate cancer, possibly through its antioxidant properties.
Brazil nuts legumes whole grains	selenium	This mineral may slow down the course of prostate cancer by inducing cancer cell death without harming healthy cells.
almonds sunflower seeds wheat germ	vitamin E	Vitamin E may protect the prostate gland, possibly through its antioxidant abilities.

psoriasis

what it is

Healthy skin cells gradually divide and migrate to the top layer of skin, replacing old cells. In psoriasis, however, skin growth is accelerated; skin cells multiply too quickly and, instead of being shed from the skin's surface, accumulate in thick patches. The plaques of raised pink skin typically occur in small areas on the scalp, elbows, knees, or lower back. The rash is not contagious and is typically not painful or very itchy.

About 15% of psoriasis sufferers have a widespread rash that interferes with daily activities. Debilitating joint pain and inflammation, similar to arthritis symptoms, affect at least 5% of people with the disorder. Psoriasis is chronic and commonly emerges between the ages of 10 and 30, affecting men and women equally.

what causes it

Experts are unsure of the exact cause of psoriasis, but they suspect a number of factors, including an inherited predisposition and underlying inflammatory condition. The condition tends to run in families, particularly among fair-skinned people, and several genetic determinants have been discovered that make some people more susceptible.

Evidence is accumulating that many of the steps leading to the condition originate from an overzealous immune response—an army of infection-fighting cells invades healthy skin tissue, triggering inflammation. Researchers believe there may be a genetic basis for this immune reaction, and they have found an unusually high number of immune cells in psoriasis plaques. Emotional stress and certain drugs, such as ibuprofen, may precipitate psoriasis flare-ups. Additional triggers include poor diet, skin injuries, sunburn, hormones, illness, alcohol, and cold dry weather.

how food may help

Although research on how nutrition can help this complex skin disorder has not yielded a wealth of information, what we do know is that an overall healthy diet that emphasizes **antioxidant**-rich fruits and vegetables is beneficial for general skin health, as the antioxidants neutralize harmful elements that could damage skin. Foods high in **vitamin C** have antioxidant properties that protect against free-radical damage to the skin caused by environmental toxins.

Low levels of **selenium, zinc,** and **vitamin A** have been reported in people with psoriasis. Foods rich in these substances may have a general beneficial effect upon skin health. **Beta-carotene** is converted by the body to vitamin A, which is vital for maximum skin health. The beta-carotene and selenium act as antioxidants. Dietary zinc not only builds the immune system but it is also important for speeding up the healing of the skin.

Consuming foods rich in **omega-3 fatty acids** may reduce the inflammatory aspect of psoriasis. Some studies show that people with psoriasis may have abnormal levels of inflammatory agents called leukotrienes, which are thought to be involved in the development and progression of psoriasis.

Low serum levels of **vitamin D** have been associated with psoriasis. Food sources of vitamin D include mushrooms and fortified foods such as breakfast cereals and plant-based dairy substitutes. Sunshine initiates natural synthesis of vitamin D just under the surface of the skin.

Preliminary studies suggest that some psoriasis patients with co-existing celiac disease may benefit from a gluten-free diet, though it would be wise to consult a nutritionist or a dermatologist before altering your diet. Total caloric intake may be important as well; some studies show a correlation between being overweight and the incidence of psoriasis.

recent research

One study that examined the relationship between nutrition and psoriasis suggests that a diet rich in carrots, tomatoes, and fresh fruits seems to have a beneficial effect upon study participants with psoriasis.

The authors of the study speculate that the protective substances in the foods may be carotenoids, as well as vitamins that have antioxidant properties. Note that foods containing high levels of antioxidants tend to contain phytonutrients that offer a wide range of benefits.

your food arsenal

foods	nutrient	health benefits
broccoli **carrots** **sweet potatoes** **tomatoes**	antioxidants	Antioxidants such as beta-carotene, vitamins C and E, and the mineral selenium are important defenders against free radicals that may harm the skin.
chia seeds **flaxseeds** **soy foods**	omega-3 fatty acids	It is believed that omega-3 fatty acids help to counteract the formation of inflammatory agents called leukotrienes.

rheumatoid arthritis

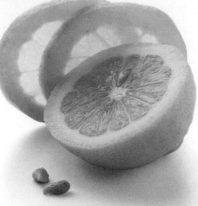

what it is

This chronic inflammatory disease of the joints is the most serious form of arthritis and can affect the entire body. Fever, loss of appetite, and a general ill feeling frequently accompany inflamed, stiff joints.

what causes it

A type of autoimmune disease, rheumatoid arthritis stems from an abnormal immune response in which the body's own immune cells attack and invade the protective linings of joints and sometimes internal organs, causing inflammation. Researchers suspect viruses and hormonal, genetic, and dietary factors as causes of the condition.

how food may help

Scientific studies suggest that consuming a diet high in unprocessed foods—fruits, vegetables, and whole grains—lowers the risk for debilitating rheumatoid arthritis; and a plant-based diet has been linked with pain relief among sufferers. Decreasing both total fat and calories is believed to further ameliorate symptoms.

A diet rich in healing vitamins and minerals, most notably **vitamins C** and **E,** may help prevent and manage rheumatoid arthritis. **Selenium** may enhance the antioxidant actions of vitamin E and helps support an important inflammation-fighting enzyme, glutathione peroxidase. Low levels of selenium, as well as zinc and beta-carotene, have been associated with rheumatoid arthritis.

Some preliminary evidence suggests that **zinc** may help alleviate symptoms of rheumatoid arthritis. Along with its own antioxidant properties, zinc is integral to the body's attack on free radicals.

Because some drugs prescribed for rheumatoid arthritis deplete the important B vitamin **folate,** some experts advise consuming folate-rich foods.

Several studies link low antioxidant status with an increased risk for the disorder, so a diet filled with antioxidant flavonoids, including those found in **green tea,** may be helpful. Epidemiological data link high green tea consumption with reduced rates of rheumatoid arthritis, and preliminary laboratory research using the equivalent of 4 cups of green tea supports this finding. Protection is attributed to the powerful antioxidant polyphenols in green tea.

Some evidence suggests that powerful antioxidants in **turmeric** (the spice responsible for the bright yellow color of curry powder) may modify inflammatory compounds and activate the body's own anti-inflammatory actions.

The anti-inflammatory actions of **bromelain, omega-3 fatty acids,** and **ginger** may ameliorate the condition as well. Researchers believe omega-3s may inhibit the production of inflammatory compounds called prostaglandins and leukotrienes, both of which contribute to joint inflammation. One small clinical study found that 5 g of fresh ginger per day provided significant relief from rheumatoid arthritis symptoms.

recent research

An anti-inflammatory diet similar to a Mediterranean-style diet may help ease symptoms of rheumatoid arthritis, according to a recent stydy of 50 patients who followed the diet for 10 weeks. An anti-inflammatory diet features high-fiber whole grains, legumes, nuts, seeds, and fresh fruits and vegetables, plus sources of omega-3 fatty acids, probiotics, and spices such as ginger and turmeric.

your food arsenal

foods	nutrient	health benefits
pineapple	bromelain	The pineapple enzyme bromelain has been reported to decrease inflammation associated with rheumatoid arthritis, possibly by blocking the formation of inflammatory compounds.
apples berries citrus fruits onions	flavonoids	Because they may support connective tissue and quell inflammation, flavonoids may help relieve symptoms of rheumatoid arthritis.
chia seeds edamame walnuts	omega-3 fatty acids	Clinical studies demonstrate a beneficial effect of these fats on arthritis symptoms, including joint stiffness, tenderness, and fatigue.
ginger	shogaols & gingerols	Ginger exhibits potent antioxidant activity and is thought to suppress the development of inflammatory compounds.
citrus fruits peppers strawberries	vitamin C	This healing nutrient supports connective tissue in the joints, provides valuable antioxidant activity, and may inhibit inflammation.
avocados nuts seeds whole grains	vitamin E	Preliminary clinical findings suggest this potent antioxidant may help relieve the pain and stiffness of rheumatoid arthritis.

rosacea

what it is

Rosacea is a chronic, inflammatory, vascular skin condition that affects approximately 16 million American adults. The disorder is typified by prolonged redness and the occurrence of acnelike bumps on the cheeks, forehead, nose, chin, or eyes. Rosacea can affect anyone but is most common among fair-skinned women between the ages of 30 and 60.

In the early stages of rosacea, sporadic occurrences of blushing, flushing, and redness of the face take place, and are often mistaken for simple blushing. If left untreated, tiny blood vessels swell and become larger, and facial redness can become permanent. If untreated, men with rosacea often develop rhinophyma, which causes the nose to become enlarged, red, and bulbous. Because of the redness (as well as the rhinophyma), rosacea is sometimes unfairly attributed to alcoholism.

If you suspect that you may have rosacea, it is important to seek treatment as soon as possible, because proper treatment can reduce symptoms and help to prevent the disorder from getting worse.

what causes it

Though a single cause has not yet been identified, certain people may have a hereditary tendency to develop rosacea. Some scientists suspect that rosacea may result from an overabundance of microscopic mites that normally live in human skin. These tiny organisms may block the sebaceous gland openings, thus promoting inflammation.

Other potential causes include immune system abnormalities and systemic inflammation. Also, anecdotal reports show a connection between stress and the exacerbation of rosacea. Hormonal changes caused by menopause may also be a factor in its onset. Histamines, chemicals released by the body as a natural response to allergens, cause inflammation and may also trigger rosacea. A common rosacea trigger, facial flushing may be brought on by blushing, stress, heat, sun, wind, cold, spicy foods, or certain medications. More research is required to identify the causes of this skin disorder.

how food may help

Although research on how diet may help rosacea is currently lacking, certain foods may help to promote general optimal skin health. Foods rich in **beta-carotene** and **vitamin E** may be helpful for general skin health because they act as antioxidants by neutralizing harmful elements that could damage skin.

To offset stress that may trigger or aggravate rosacea, it may be helpful to eat foods that are rich in **vitamin B$_6$,** which assists in the production of certain brain chemicals that help to regulate mood.

Rosacea is believed to be a disorder linked to swollen blood vessels, so it may be useful to eat foods high in **essential fatty acids,** which are thought to have anti-inflammatory properties.

Eating foods high in antioxidant-rich, immune-building **vitamin C** may help to protect the skin from free-radical damage as well as inflammation caused by histamines. Foods containing vitamin C are also useful for protecting veins. Foods rich in **zinc** help to promote healing and enhance the functioning of the immune system.

foods to avoid

Although the exact cause of rosacea is currently unknown, we do know that certain foods may trigger the characteristic flushing and redness. For example, people with rosacea should try to avoid spicy foods, hot drinks, and alcoholic beverages. You may not have to give up hot coffee or tea altogether—just allow them to cool a little bit before drinking them. There is no common ingredient at the root of these triggers.

It might be helpful to keep a diary of foods and episodes of flushing and redness to try to determine which foods may be triggers for the condition.

your food arsenal

foods	nutrient	health benefits
chia seeds **flaxseed** **pumpkin seeds**	essential fatty acids	As inflammation of the skin occurs in rosacea, it may be useful to eat foods rich in essential fatty acids, which help to reduce swelling by generating substances in the body that can reduce inflammation.
berries **broccoli** **citrus fruits** **kiwifruit**	vitamin C	The antioxidant properties of vitamin C may help to protect the skin from free-radical damage caused by pollution and the sun's harmful rays. Vitamin C may inhibit the release of histamine, a substance that is thought to cause inflammation as the immune system's response to allergens.

sinusitis

what it is

One of the most common ailments in the United States, sinusitis is an infection of the lining of one or more of the sinus cavities, causing inflammation. There are two types of sinusitis: acute, which lasts for three weeks or less, and chronic, which often lasts for three to eight weeks but can continue even longer. Nearly 29 million Americans are diagnosed with sinusitis every year. Both types of sinusitis are extremely uncomfortable and symptoms can range from intense pain to a general malaise.

In sinusitis, tissues swell and cells produce thick mucus, which is unable to drain properly through the small sinus channels and openings. What results is a heavy pressure that builds up, causing a sinus headache, congestion, persistent cough, fatigue, tender cheekbones, and pain around the sinus areas. A typical sinus headache tends to be mild in the morning and gets worse during the day. It is also sometimes accompanied by fever, runny nose, congestion, irritation, and general fatigue and weakness.

what causes it

Both acute and chronic sinusitis often develop after an upper-respiratory infection (a cold or flu) spreads to the sinus cavities. Blockage of the sinus passages caused by allergies, the flu, or the common cold may lead to the development of bacterial infections that can lead to acute sinusitis. It is thought that some forms of chronic sinusitis result from an immune system response to naturally occurring fungi in the nose. Studies suggest an association between asthma and sinusitis.

Other potential causes of sinusitis may include allergies; bacteria that cause infections of the mouth, gums, or teeth; exposure to airborne or environmental irritants such as tobacco smoke, smog, mold spores, or dust; and polyps inside the nasal cavities.

how food may help

Sinusitis often follows a cold or the flu, so it is important to maintain a strong immune system to avoid these infections. Foods containing the antioxidant **vitamin C** can help to bolster your immune system by stimulating the activity of antibodies and immune system cells. Dietary **zinc** is also an important defender against invading viruses and infections, and it may also have anti-inflammatory properties.

One of the symptoms of sinusitis is inflammation along the nasal passages caused by allergens. These allergens initiate an immune response, which releases histamines and other chemicals that are thought to cause congestion. The anti-inflammatory actions of certain flavonoids such as **luteolin** and **quercetin** may decrease congestion by reducing the body's release of histamine.

It may also be useful to eat pineapple, which contains the enzyme **bromelain.** Preliminary studies indicate that this substance may have anti-inflammatory properties. Note that pineapple is also a good source of vitamin C, which may also dampen inflammation.

A hot cup of tea soothes the soul and may also help to reduce congestion. Not only does the steam help to temporarily open up the nasal passages, but tea also contains **theophylline,** a compound believed to ease breathing by relaxing the smooth muscles in the walls of the airways.

Eating spicy foods, such as horseradish, mustard, and ginger, can provide temporary relief by reducing congestion. **Allyl isothiocyanate,** a pungent substance in horseradish and mustard, helps to thin mucus. Be sure to also drink plenty of water and fluids to keep mucus thin.

home remedy

For temporary relief of congestion from sinusitis, try cooking with chili peppers. Chili peppers as well as cayenne pepper contain capsaicin, a powerful and fiery compound that acts as a mucolytic agent by breaking up mucus and promoting mucus flow, offering temporary relief from pressure in the sinuses.

your food arsenal

foods	nutrient	health benefits
berries **citrus fruits** **peppers** **pineapple**	vitamin C	Vitamin C helps to maintain a strong immune system, and it works to fight off colds—a common antecedent to sinusitis. Vitamin C may also help to minimize the inflammation and swelling of mucous membranes lining the sinuses by preventing the release of histamine.
beans **fortified cereals** **nuts** **wheat germ**	zinc	The immune-fortifying capability of zinc may help to ward off viruses that are often implicated in the onset of sinus problems.

sprains & strains

what it is

Sprains and strains can afflict young and old, couch potatoes and professional athletes. A sprain is an injury to a ligament, which links bone to bone and supports a joint. It is usually the result of a ligament being stretched too far or being torn. A strain, on the other hand, is an injury to a tendon (which connects muscle to bone) or a muscle. The time it takes sprains and strains to heal depends on their severity, but relatively speaking a strain usually takes longer since the damaged fibers in muscles require more time to mend.

Both sprains and strains vary in severity and levels of discomfort, and, depending upon how serious the damage is, both types of injury can cause sharp pain as well as impairment of power and movement. Ankles are the joints most vulnerable to sprains, while the back and hamstring muscle (back of the thigh) are the most common strains. Swelling occurs in both sprains and strains.

what causes it

Often the result of a sudden force, typically a twisting motion, sprains and strains sometimes occur during jogging, running, or playing basketball. Lifting a heavy object or weight, or extending and stretching muscles and tendons too far (for example, when swinging a golf club or a tennis racket) can all cause injury. Overweight people and sedentary people are especially vulnerable to sprains or strains.

how food may help

Clearly, what you eat will not prevent a sprain or a strain; however, diet certainly has an effect on overall health and weight. Maintaining a healthy weight is key, as excess pounds place stress on joints and increase the risk for injuries to muscles and ligaments.

Muscles require glycogen (derived from glucose) for optimum exertion for athletic events. To ensure that muscles receive enough fuel, you should eat foods rich in **complex carbohydrates.** Glucose from complex carbohydrates is metabolized slowly, and supplies the required energy for a sustained level of exertion.

Protein is required for muscle and joint health. Low-fat sources of protein, such as soy foods and certain grains such as amaranth and quinoa, are excellent plant-based alternatives to meat protein.

Vitamin C is helpful in keeping ligaments and tendons strong. It also helps to repair tissue.

Omega-3 fatty acids are particularly beneficial in that they may help to accelerate the healing of ligaments injured by sprains. Also, omega-3s may have an anti-inflammatory effect, which can relieve discomfort from swelling in joints.

Though more research is necessary, early studies indicate that **bromelain** may also reduce swelling. Bromelain is an anti-inflammatory enzyme found in pineapple (pineapples are also a good source of vitamin C, which is important for the production of collagen).

Certain minerals are needed for bone, ligament, and muscle health. For example, **magnesium, calcium,** and **phosphorus** form bones; and **manganese** is required for the formation of cartilage and connective tissue. **Zinc** promotes tissue repair and growth.

The "sunshine vitamin," **vitamin D,** assists in regulating blood levels of calcium and phosphorus and is essential for the maintenance of healthy cartilage and bones. The body also needs vitamin D to help properly absorb calcium from food. Vitamin D is produced by the body and also found in fortified dairy substitutes and juices.

recent research

Results of a laboratory study on the effect of omega-3 fatty acids suggest that they speed up the healing of ligament cells. The experimental study compared arachidonic acid (an omega-6 fatty acid), eicosapentaenoic acid (an omega-3 fatty acid), and a third substance that served as a control. The researchers compared the cells of the ligaments treated with each compound and examined the rate at which the ligament cells healed over a 72-hour period.

While both the arachidonic acid and the eicosapentaenoic acid revealed the ability to heal the cells, the omega-3 showed a significantly greater ability to enhance the entry of new cells into the wound area and to speed up collagen synthesis. This experiment suggests that omega-3 fatty acid in foods may have the ability to speed up the healing of ligament injuries that occur in sprains.

your food arsenal

foods	nutrient	health benefits
beans potatoes rice whole grains	complex carbohydrates	Complex carbohydrates provide fuel and, as they take longer to digest than simple carbohydrates, are useful for sustained energy.
amaranth legumes quinoa soy foods	protein	Important for muscle and joint health as well as tissue repair, protein can be found in numerous low-fat foods that also confer a wide range of other nutritional benefits.
berries citrus fruits kiwifruit pineapple	vitamin C	This vitamin helps to build and maintain collagen, the fibers that make up the tissue between tendons, ligaments, bones, and cartilage.

stroke

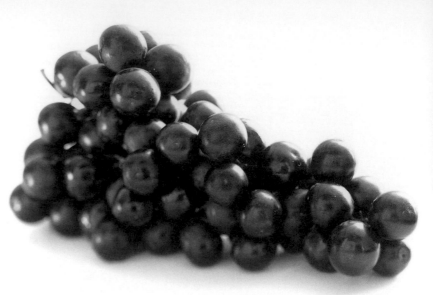

recipe rx

what it is

A stroke occurs when a blocked or ruptured artery suddenly deprives the brain of oxygen-rich blood, potentially leading to permanent detrimental effects on physical and emotional well-being. Speech, vision, movement, and sensation are most commonly compromised by a stroke.

what causes it

The most common type of stroke, ischemic stroke, is caused by a blood clot that blocks blood flow to the brain. A clot usually forms as a result of fatty plaque buildup that narrows arteries near or in the brain and impedes circulation. A clot may also form in another part of the body, travel, and lodge in a blood vessel that nourishes the brain. Hemorrhagic strokes, caused by a ruptured, bleeding artery in the brain, are less common.

how food may help

Numerous studies indicate that eating a low-fat diet rich in fruits and vegetables significantly protects against stroke. One study found that people who ate vegetables six to seven days per week cut their risk for stroke by over 50%. Eating plenty of whole grains is important for stroke protection as well since data suggest a whole-grain diet may reduce risk for the condition. Several nutrients and phytonutrients plentiful in produce and whole grains—**calcium, flavonoids, fiber, magnesium, omega-3 fatty acids, potassium, resveratrol,** and **vitamin C**—have shown promise in protecting against the condition.

Scientific evidence is accumulating that free-radical-fighting antioxidants, such as resveratrol and **selenium,** may protect against ischemic stroke. Researchers believe **vitamin E** may protect against stroke by squelching free radicals and inhibiting oxidation of LDL ("bad") cholesterol, which can clog arteries and contribute to stroke.

There is growing evidence that elevated levels of the amino acid homocysteine, long linked to heart attacks, may also increase the risk for stroke: As levels of homocysteine increase, stroke risk tends to increase as well. The B vitamins **folate, vitamin B$_6$,** and **vitamin B$_{12}$** appear to team up to lower homocysteine levels. According to one study, when participants adopted a high-folate diet, average homocysteine levels dropped by an impressive 7%. Citrus fruit and lentils are excellent sources of folate, potatoes and avocados are high in B$_6$, and nutritional yeast is rich in B$_{12}$.

Since elevated blood pressure and high cholesterol increase the risk for stroke, see pages 174–177 for advice on managing blood pressure and cholesterol.

recent research

A recent analysis of 20 studies involving a total of more than 682,000 people found that sticking to a Mediterranean-style diet is associated with lower risk of both ischemic and hemorrhagic strokes for both Mediterranean and non-Mediterranean populations. A Mediterranean-style diet features nutrient-rich vegetables, fruits, legumes, whole grains, nuts and seeds, and extra-virgin olive oil.

your food arsenal

foods	nutrient	health benefits
broccoli figs fortified dairy substitutes	calcium	A meta-analysis of 42 studies found that calcium has a small but significant benefit on blood pressure. Calcium is thought to inhibit blood clots that lead to a stroke.
green peas lentils winter squash	dietary fiber	Studies link a high-fiber intake from fruits and vegetables with a reduced risk for stroke. Soluble fiber in particular is believed to interfere with atherosclerosis and blood clots, which can lead to an ischemic stroke.
apples berries onions	flavonoids	Population-based studies suggest that dietary flavonoids, particularly quercetin, may reduce fat deposits in arteries that can block blood flow to the brain.
chia seeds edamame flaxseed seaweed soy foods walnuts	omega-3 fatty acids	Studies find the importance of including many vegetable sources of alpha-linolenic acid (ALA), which is converted in the body to omega-3 fatty acids, in order to meet the guidelines for cardiovascular disease prevention.
bananas orange juice potatoes	potassium	By contributing to lower blood pressure and possibly diminishing blood clots, potassium may decrease stroke risk.
peanuts red grapes red wine	resveratrol	Preliminary evidence suggests this phytonutrient may inhibit blood clots and also help to relax blood vessels.
citrus fruits kiwifruit melons	vitamin C	A population-based study found that individuals with the lowest levels of vitamin C in their blood had a 70% increased risk for stroke. The protective effects of vitamin C may extend beyond its antioxidant properties, according to researchers.

tooth & mouth conditions

what it is

Gum disease, dental caries (cavities), canker sores, and bad breath (halitosis) all fall into the category of tooth and mouth conditions. Gum disease (gingivitis) develops when bacteria infect the crevices between gums and teeth. Gums typically become red and swollen and, when left untreated, could lead to tooth loss.

One of the major causes of tooth loss is dental caries, which can be traced to tooth-coating plaque. Bacteria, food debris, saliva, and acid combine to form plaque. Gradually, the corrosive acids dissolve tooth enamel, creating pits in the grooved surfaces on teeth. Canker sores are small shallow white ulcers that can suddenly flare up on the gums, tongue, soft palate, or inside the cheeks. Bad breath is a frequent consequence of poor dental hygiene, dry mouth, infrequent eating or drinking, or lingering food smells (e.g., garlic or onions).

what causes it

Poor dental hygiene—a lack of brushing, flossing, or rinsing—frequently leads to gum disease, cavities, or bad breath. Increasing age and a genetic predisposition may leave some people more prone to poor dental health as well. A multitude of additional factors, including odor-causing and infectious bacteria, stress, smoking, a poor or high-sugar diet, and chronic illness, may contribute to tooth and mouth conditions.

how food may help

Population studies have found that a high consumption of sweet, sticky ("cariogenic") foods—such as juice, soda, and candy—increases risk for dental decay. To reduce risk, experts advise limiting sugar intake and minimizing the amount of time that teeth are exposed to sugary and sticky foods and drinks.

On the other hand, there is a wealth of foods that can improve dental health. For example, there are several anticariogenic foods that are believed to inhibit plaque formation (thus protecting against cavities and gum disease). Nuts, popcorn, tea, and fibrous vegetables, such as celery, may help prevent tooth decay.

Preliminary research on green tea suggests that its powerful **catechin, EGCG,** may prevent *Streptococcus mutans*, a major culprit in tooth decay, from sticking to tooth enamel and initiating cavities.

Some evidence suggests a carbohydrate-like component in **shiitake mushrooms** may reduce plaque formation, though research is very preliminary. Chewing sugar-free, xylitol-sweetened gum may prevent cavities by inhibiting growth of decay-causing bacteria and reduce the amount of plaque.

Calcium is the cornerstone of solid, sturdy teeth and may protect against gum disease. Research has found that adults, particularly between the ages of 20 and 40, with the lowest calcium intakes (below 500 mg daily) have twice the risk for gum disease. Scientists believe that one way in which calcium may improve resistance against infection is by strengthening the jawbone and maintaining tooth structure.

Foods high in **insoluble fiber** may help by removing food particles from between teeth and in gum pockets. Crunchy, fibrous foods, such as carrot sticks, may cleanse teeth, as well as stimulate gum tissue.

Vitamin C is essential for healthy gums and may enhance the healing of cuts and sores in the mouth. Some experts believe low levels of **vitamin B$_{12}$, zinc, folate,** or **iron** contribute to canker sores.

home remedy

To freshen bad breath, create a home-made herbal mouthwash with parsley and cloves. In a heatproof bowl, combine several sprigs of coarsely chopped parsley with 2 cups of boiling water. Next add ¼ teaspoon of cloves or 2 whole cloves. Let cool to room temperature (with occasional stirring), strain, and use as a mouthwash, gargling several times a day. (Store it in the refrigerator.) Parsley's chlorophyll content and the eugenol (a type of phytonutrient) in cloves are thought to neutralize bad breath.

your food arsenal

foods	nutrient	health benefits
almonds broccoli cooking greens	calcium	This bone-building mineral is essential for sturdy teeth, and research suggests that adults with low calcium intakes have a significantly increased risk for gum disease.
green tea pomegranates	catechins	These powerful green tea polyphenols, particularly EGCG, may prevent cavity-causing bacteria from adhering to teeth.
broccoli celery salad greens	insoluble fiber	This type of dietary fiber may dislodge food particles from between teeth and gums.
beans citrus fruits	folate	Canker sores have been associated with a deficiency of this B vitamin.
berries citrus fruits peppers	vitamin C	In addition to promoting healing in the mouth, this vitamin is a vital component of connective tissue of teeth and bones.

urinary tract infection

what it is

Urinary tract infections (UTIs) are among the most common bacterial infections and are characterized by a frequent urge to urinate and a painful burning sensation during urination. Symptoms may also include mild fever, back pain, abdominal cramps, and blood in the urine. The infection typically affects the bladder or the urethra, the tube that carries urine away from the bladder out of the body. Because of a shorter urethra (which makes it easier for bacteria to migrate up to the bladder), women are far more likely to suffer from a UTI than men. UTIs often recur, and if an infection is left untreated, it can lead to a serious kidney infection.

what causes it

UTIs are caused by bacteria that migrate into the urethra. Urine is usually free of germs, but bacteria from the genital area or rectal area may travel into the urinary tract through the urethra and, most commonly, up to the bladder, where they attach to the bladder lining, multiply, and cause an infection. Ignoring the urge to urinate increases the risk for a UTI. Other causes include not drinking enough fluids, improper hygiene (wiping should be front to back), pregnancy, and sexual activity.

how food may help

Because a UTI may rapidly progress into a dangerous infection, it is best to immediately consult a physician if you are suffering from symptoms.

To improve urine flow during an infection, drink at least one 8-oounce glass of water each hour to wash harmful germs out of the urinary tract. Regularly consuming plenty of water may help prevent infectious bacteria from taking hold in the urinary tract in the first place. Folk healers often recommend parsley to help flush out a UTI. Compounds in parsley, such as **myristicin** and **apigenin,** may act as diuretics, increasing urine flow.

Conventional science has begun to confirm another traditional folk remedy for urinary tract infections—drinking **cranberry juice**. A clinical trial of 153 elderly women found that women who drank 10 ounces of low-calorie cranberry juice each day had 50% fewer bacteria in their urine. The cranberry drinkers were also 25% less likely to have infected urine from month to month.

Researchers have isolated tannin compounds in cranberry juice and have found that these substances may be highly protective against UTIs. It's thought that the tannin compounds may combat UTIs by preventing bacteria from attaching to the bladder and kidney walls, multiplying unrestrained, and causing an infection. The bacteria are instead flushed out in the urine.

Cranberries are also thought to acidify urine, making the urinary tract a less hospitable environment for harmful bacteria to thrive. And **vitamin C** (in addition to fortifying the body's immune defenses) may also acidify urine, making it more difficult for infectious bacteria to colonize.

If infectious bacteria in the genital area are allowed to multiply unrestrained, they may travel from the genitals into the urethra, causing a UTI. But consuming **probiotics** (beneficial bacteria) can be helpful, since this promotes the growth of healthy bacteria in the body. These bacteria crowd out harmful microbes and may even secrete anti-infective substances. More human studies are required to determine which beneficial bacteria are most likely to be successful in treating UTIs.

recent research

Like cranberry juice, blueberry juice may wash harmful bacteria out of the urinary tract, because blueberries have protective tannin compounds similar to those found in cranberries.

your food arsenal

foods	nutrient	health benefits
kimchi kombucha	probiotics	Though clinical data are scant, beneficial bacteria may inhibit the growth of microorganisms that can cause UTIs. These beneficial bacteria are also thought to foster the growth of friendly flora in the body, which may be reduced by antibiotic therapy.
blueberries cranberries	tannins	Research suggests that these phytonutrients, plentiful in berries, inhibit bacteria from sticking to the lining of the urinary tract, thus preventing infection.
berries broccoli citrus fruits peppers	vitamin C	This indispensable vitamin reinforces the body's immune defenses against infection.

varicose veins

what it is

Typically an unsightly cosmetic problem in the legs and feet, varicose veins look like swollen bluish cords just beneath the skin's surface. Sore, achy legs may accompany varicose veins, though pain and tenderness are usually mild. Lumpy skin frequently surrounds bulging veins and small patches of flooded capillaries—superficial spider veins—may cluster in the area or appear on the ankles and thighs. Blood clots may occasionally develop in varicose veins, but clots in these superficial veins are generally not considered life-threatening. Women are at least twice as likely as men to have varicose veins, and diet and lifestyle factors may play an important role in preventing and managing the condition.

what causes it

Weak vessel walls or faulty valves inside veins may hamper circulation, causing blood to pool and distend veins. Less frequently, phlebitis (inflammation of a vein) or inherited abnormal vein structure may result in varicose and spider veins. The condition tends to run in families, and hormones, obesity, pregnancy, lack of exercise, increasing age, and heavy lifting may also lead to varicose veins. Constipation, tight clothing, leg crossing, and prolonged sitting and standing may increase the risk for the disorder by unduly pressuring veins.

how food may help

Insoluble fiber promotes regularity and reduces straining during bowel movements. This is important, because straining contributes to varicose veins by increasing abdominal pressure and blocking blood flow from the legs. **Soluble fibers** such as pectin, gum, and psyllium are particularly useful in easing elimination by bulking up waste and promoting contractions of the digestive tract.

Vitamin C is thought to benefit varicose veins by teaming up with antioxidant flavonoids to fortify vessel walls and fend off oxidative damage, which may compromise vein strength. A host of **flavonoids,** especially those abundant in citrus fruit, may bolster vein structure by reducing blood vessel frailty and leakiness. The citrus flavonoid **hesperidin** is thought to enhance the actions of vitamin C and may be required for optimal capillary function. **Diosmin,** a flavonoid found in rosemary and citrus fruit, may prevent blood vessel fragility, which can lead to varicose veins. A flavonoid in white grapefruit called **naringin** may also enhance blood vessel health. According to preliminary research, **rutin,** a flavonoid present in apples and buckwheat, may promote blood vessel health by bolstering cell membrane support cells and structural tissue. In laboratory studies, the highly active flavonoid **quercetin** (closely related to rutin, hesperidin, and diosmin and found in red onions and blueberries) has exhibited potent anti-inflammatory properties, which may protect against varicose veins.

Additional antioxidants are under review for their benefit to vein health, including **green tea** polyphenols and **vitamin E** (a potent antioxidant found in avocados and olive oil), which may be important for blood vessel health by improving vessel function and strengthening capillaries. And finally, researchers believe **tannin compounds** (also known as proanthocyanidins) may benefit varicose veins because these antioxidants are incorporated into cell membranes, where they are thought to protect against damaging free radicals.

recent research

One recent study of 150 patients with varicose veins found that those who eat a mostly plant-based diet and were no more than slightly overweight had improved quality of life and significantly decreased symptoms after minimally invasive treatment.

your food arsenal

foods	nutrient	health benefits
beans **beets** **lentils** **whole grains**	dietary fiber	Dietary fiber decreases pressure on blood vessels in the legs by promoting regular bowel movements and reducing strain during bowel movements.
apples **berries** **citrus fruits** **grapes** **whole grains**	flavonoids	Experimental research suggests flavonoids may team up with vitamin C to fortify blood vessel membranes and to enhance vessel function by reducing breakage, free-radical damage, and permeability.
berries	tannins	These antioxidant compounds (also known as proanthocyanidins) may help reduce blood vessel leakage and protect vessels against free-radical damage.
berries **broccoli** **citrus fruits** **peppers**	vitamin C	This vitamin may strengthen blood vessels and defend membranes against damaging free radicals. A deficiency in vitamin C leads to blood vessel frailty.

yeast infection

The irritating discharge and uncomfortable burning of a vaginal yeast infection afflict most women at some point in their lives. Infrequently, men may develop a genital yeast infection, though they may not display any apparent symptoms.

Normally, small numbers of harmless microorganisms live harmoniously in the linings of the vagina, digestive tract, and skin. These friendly germs assist with digestion, combat invading pathogens, and help manufacture essential nutrients. The vagina is an ideal warm, moist environment for many fungi, especially yeast, to thrive. So when the balance of vaginal flora is upset, an infectious overgrowth of yeast organisms, usually *Candida albicans*, may occur. As yeast multiplies unrestrained, an unpleasant white, lumpy, cottage cheese-like discharge is secreted and the external genital area frequently becomes inflamed and itchy and may cause burning or pain during intercourse.

what causes it

Benign vaginal yeast may grow unchecked when pH (acid/base) levels or the balance of bacteria and yeast in the vagina is disturbed. Hormonal changes from pregnancy or birth control pills frequently change vaginal pH levels, leading to yeast infections. Antibiotic therapy for any condition commonly causes yeast infections by depleting the friendly bacteria that usually prevent vaginal yeast from multiplying out of control.

A yeast infection may also be symptomatic of a suppressed immune system overburdened from stress, sleep deprivation, chemotherapy, or illness, including HIV and diabetes. In addition, wearing nylon underwear, tight jeans, or using spermicides, deodorant tampons, or douches may increase risk for infection.

An overabundance of simple carbohydrates (sugars) in the diet upsets the balance of vaginal flora and causes yeast-like fungi that increase the likelihood of yeast infections and inflammation. Excessive dietary fat can raise vaginal pH and increase the risk of bacterial infection.

how food may help

Increasing the body's levels of healthful **probiotic bacteria** may prevent overgrowth of infectious vaginal yeast. These friendly flora help crowd out infectious yeast and maintain an acidic environment that prevents these irritating fungi from multiplying unchecked. Confirming the folk medicine belief in these healthful microbes, some clinical evidence suggests that consuming sufficient quantities of yogurt with live bacteria cultures, including *Lactobacillus acidophilus*, may alleviate symptoms of a yeast infection and lower the risk for repeated infections.

Since probiotic bacteria thrive on nondigested sugars from plant foods such as asparagus, artichoke, and banana known as **fructooligosaccharides (FOS),** consuming more FOS compounds may foster the growth of beneficial bacteria. These compounds are believed to nourish friendly flora, enhancing and sustaining their growth in the body.

Garlic may be a natural anti-yeast agent, because laboratory studies have demonstrated this bulb's ability to inhibit the growth of *Candida albicans*, the organism commonly responsible for vaginal yeast infections. The highly active substance **allicin,** which gives garlic its pungent odor and bite, is thought to be responsible for garlic's antifungal activity.

By enhancing immunity, **vitamin C** may protect against yeast infections. This vitamin, abundant in citrus fruit and peppers, is believed to galvanize infection-fighting white blood cells, which may fortify immune defenses.

your food arsenal

foods	nutrient	health benefits
garlic	allicin	Laboratory experiments have demonstrated garlic's antifungal activities, attributed to the pungent phytonutrient allicin.
kimchi kombucha sauerkraut	probiotics	Some research suggests that these healthful bacteria may suppress the growth of *Candida albicans*, the fungus responsible for yeast infections.
artichokes onion family	fructooligosaccharides (FOS)	These indigestible carbohydrate compounds may promote the growth of friendly vaginal bacteria, which protect against the growth of yeast.

recipe rx

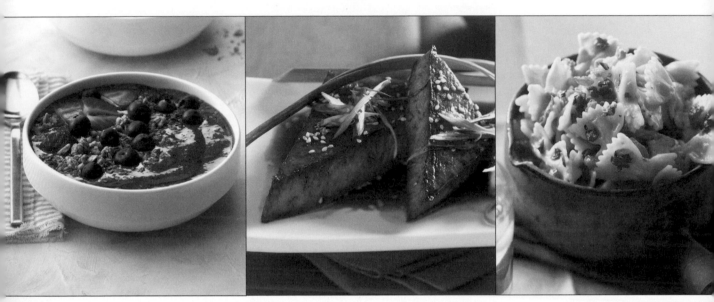

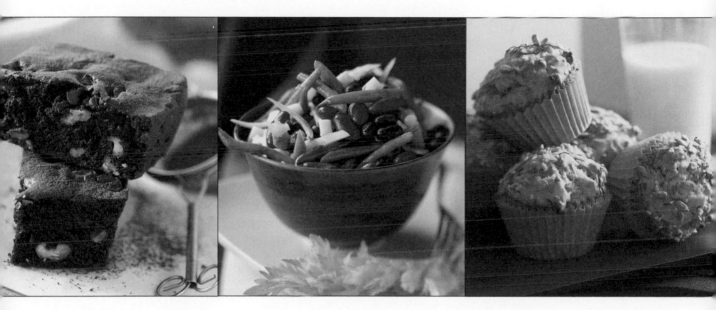

Delicious Dishes

That Maximize the Healing

Power of Plant Foods

mango-berry shake

If you purchase an unsweetened soy milk, you may need to increase the honey.

- 1 LARGE MANGO, PEELED, PITTED, AND CUT INTO WEDGES (2 CUPS)
- 2 CUPS CANTALOUPE CHUNKS
- 12 OUNCES FROZEN UNSWEETENED RASPBERRIES
- 1½ CUPS SOY MILK
- 2 TABLESPOONS FRESH LIME JUICE
- 2 TABLESPOONS HONEY
- 1 TEASPOON VANILLA EXTRACT
- 1 TEASPOON GROUND GINGER

Working in 2 batches, combine the mango, cantaloupe, raspberries, soy milk, lime juice, honey, vanilla, and ginger in a blender. Blend until smooth.

Makes 4 servings. Per serving: 217 calories, 2.7 g total fat (0% saturated), 6 g protein, 47 g carbohydrate, 1.5 g fiber, 0 mg cholesterol, 52 mg sodium

warm pineapple-ginger punch

This hot and spicy punch is a nice change from mulled cider. It's also a good source of bromelain.

- 4 CUPS PINEAPPLE JUICE
- 1 CUP SLICED FRESH GINGER (NO NEED TO PEEL)
- 1 TABLESPOON HONEY
- 1 CINNAMON STICK, SPLIT LENGTHWISE
- 8 WHOLE CLOVES
- ¼ TEASPOON PEPPER

In a medium saucepan, combine the pineapple juice, ginger, honey, cinnamon, cloves, and pepper; bring to a boil. Reduce to a simmer and cook for 10 minutes. Strain and serve warm.

Makes 4 servings. Per serving: 152 calories, 0.2 g total fat (0% saturated), 1 g protein, 38 g carbohydrate, 0 g fiber, 0 mg cholesterol, 4 mg sodium

mexican-spiced hot cocoa

Spiced with cinnamon and nutmeg, this Mexican-style cocoa is rich in calcium and magnesium.

- 1 TABLESPOON UNSWEETENED COCOA POWDER
- 2 TEASPOONS DARK BROWN SUGAR
- ¼ TEASPOON CINNAMON
- ⅛ TEASPOON NUTMEG
- 1 TABLESPOON BOILING WATER
- 1 CUP OAT MILK
- ½ TEASPOON VANILLA EXTRACT
- ⅛ TEASPOON ALMOND EXTRACT

1 In a large mug, stir together the cocoa powder, brown sugar, cinnamon, and nutmeg until well combined. Add the boiling water, and stir until completely moistened and smooth.

2 In a small saucepan, heat the milk for 3 minutes over low heat, or until hot. Stir the milk into the cocoa mixture until well combined. Stir in the vanilla and almond extracts and serve.

Makes 1 serving. Per serving: 190 calories, 1.9 g total fat (11% saturated), 10 g protein, 43 g carbohydrate, 3.1 g fiber, 0 mg cholesterol, 16 mg sodium

banana-peanut smoothie

The soy milk provides isoflavones while the banana contributes a healthy amount of potassium.

- 1 CUP SOY MILK
- 1 MEDIUM BANANA
- 2 TEASPOONS CREAMY PEANUT BUTTER
- 2 TEASPOONS HONEY
- 2 ICE CUBES

In a blender, combine the soy milk, banana, peanut butter, honey, and ice cubes. Blend for 1 minute, or until thick and smooth.

Makes 1 serving. Per serving: 341 calories, 9.8 g total fat (11% saturated), 14 g protein, 53 g carbohydrate, 2.4 g fiber, 0 mg cholesterol, 166 mg sodium

warm pineapple-ginger punch ▶

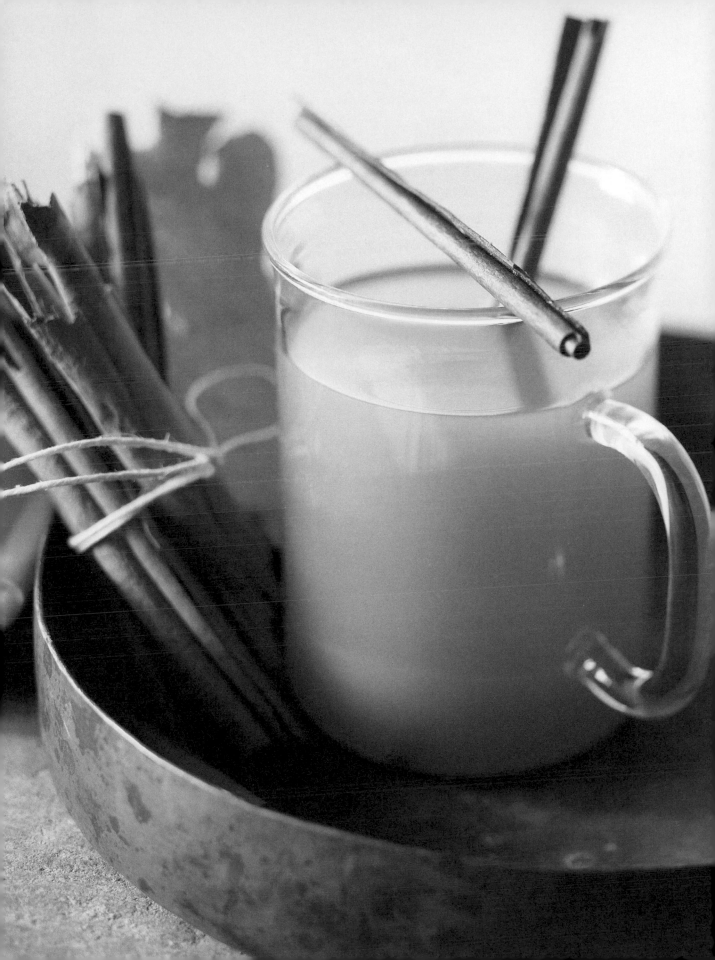

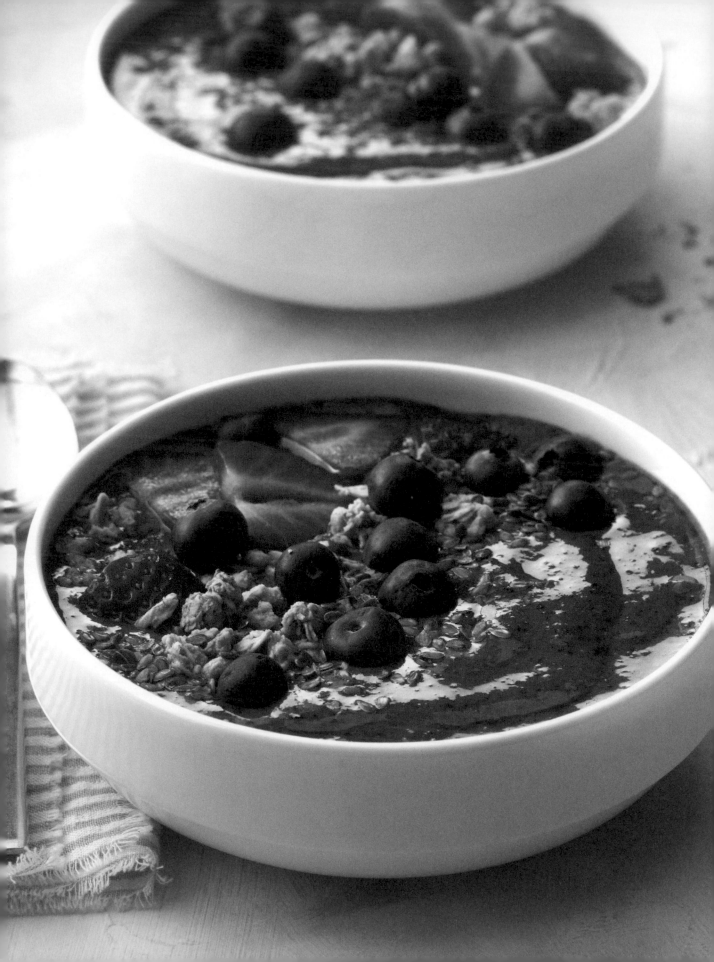

power berry smoothie bowl

There are many plant-based yogurts available, including ones made from oat, soy, almond, and coconut milk. Check the label to select one with the least amount of sugar.

½ CUP POMEGRANATE JUICE

½ CUP ORANGE JUICE

1 CONTAINER (5.3 OUNCES) BERRY PLANT-BASED YOGURT

1 CUP FROZEN UNSWEETENED STRAWBERRIES

1 CUP FRESH BABY SPINACH

½ MEDIUM RIPE FROZEN BANANA, SLICED

½ CUP FROZEN UNSWEETENED BLUEBERRIES

2 TABLESPOONS GROUND FLAXSEED

SLICED FRESH STRAWBERRIES, FRESH BLUEBERRIES, FLAXSEED, AND GRANOLA FOR TOPPING

In a blender, combine the juices, yogurt, strawberries, spinach, banana, blueberries, and flaxseed. Cover and process for 30 seconds or until smooth. Pour into chilled bowls; top with the strawberries, blueberries, flaxseed, and granola. Serve immediately.

Makes 3 servings. *Per serving: 172 calories, 3 g total fat (0% saturated), 5 g protein, 35 g carbohydrate, 4 g fiber, 0 mg cholesterol, 47 mg sodium*

apple-cranberry breakfast grains

Bursting with phytonutrients, antioxidants, and fiber, this recipe is a warm and hearty start to the day. Makes a great weekend breakfast or brunch dish. Refrigerate leftovers for up to 4 days for a quick breakfast when reheated in the microwave.

2 MEDIUM APPLES, PEELED AND CHOPPED

1 CUP PACKED BROWN SUGAR

1 CUP FRESH CRANBERRIES

½ CUP WHEAT BERRIES

½ CUP QUINOA, RINSED

½ CUP OAT BRAN

½ CUP MEDIUM PEARL BARLEY

½ CUP CHOPPED WALNUTS

1½ TEASPOONS GROUND CINNAMON

6 CUPS WATER

DAIRY-FREE MILK FOR SERVING

In a 3-quart slow cooker, combine the apples, sugar, cranberries, wheat berries, quinoa, oat bran, barley, walnuts, cinnamon, and water. Cover and cook on high for 2 hours or on low for 4 to 5 hours until the grains are tender. Serve with the milk.

Makes 10 servings. *Per serving: 167 calories, 4 g total fat (13% saturated), 4 g protein, 31 g carbohydrate, 4.9 g fiber, 0 mg cholesterol, 562 mg sodium*

◀ **power berry smoothie bowl**

cherry baked oatmeal

A great way to start your day, the cherries in this dish are a good source of the phytonutrient perillyl alcohol and the oatmeal is packed with fiber and nutrients that help reduce cholesterol.

- 2 CUPS SOY, ALMOND, OR OAT MILK
- 1 CUP OLD-FASHIONED OATS
- ½ CUP CHUNKY APPLESAUCE
- ¼ CUP DRIED CHERRIES
- 1 TABLESPOON BROWN SUGAR
- ¼ TEASPOON ALMOND EXTRACT
- 2 TABLESPOONS SLICED ALMONDS

1 Preheat the oven to 350°F. Coat a 3-cup baking dish with cooking spray.

2 In a large bowl, combine the milk, oats, applesauce, cherries, sugar, and almond extract. Transfer to the prepared dish and sprinkle with the almonds.

3 Bake, uncovered, for 45 to 50 minutes or until set.

Makes 3 servings. Per serving: 259 calories, 4 g total fat (25% saturated fat), 10 g protein, 48 g carbohydrate, 4 g fiber, 3 mg cholesterol, 73 mg sodium

loaded quinoa breakfast bowl

Goji berries or cranberries add a tangy undertone to this hearty dish and provide anthocyanins, ellagic acid, and quercetin.

- ¼ CUP TRI-COLORED QUINOA, RINSED
- 2 TABLESPOONS DRIED GOJI BERRIES OR DRIED CRANBERRIES
- 1 SMALL BANANA
- ¼ CUP UNSWEETENED ALMOND MILK
- 1 TABLESPOON MAPLE SYRUP
- ⅛ TEASPOON GROUND CINNAMON
- ⅛ TEASPOON VANILLA EXTRACT
- ¼ CUP FRESH OR FROZEN UNSWEETENED BLUEBERRIES
- 1 TABLESPOON CHOPPED WALNUTS
- 1 TABLESPOON SLIVERED ALMONDS
- 1 TABLESPOON FRESH PUMPKIN SEEDS

1 In a small saucepan, bring ½ cup of water to a boil. Add the quinoa. Reduce to a simmer; cover and cook for 12 to 15 minutes or until the liquid is absorbed.

2 Meanwhile, soak the berries in ¼ cup water for 10 minutes; drain. Halve the banana crosswise. Slice 1 banana half; mash the other half.

3 Remove the quinoa from heat and fluff with a fork. Stir in the mashed banana, almond milk, maple syrup, cinnamon, and vanilla. Transfer to a bowl; add the blueberries, walnuts, almonds, pumpkin seeds, banana slices, and the drained goji berries.

Makes 1 serving. Per serving: 475 calories, 13 g total fat (8% saturated), 13 g protein, 83 g carbohydrate, 10 g fiber, 0 mg cholesterol, 85 mg sodium

loaded quinoa breakfast bowl ▶

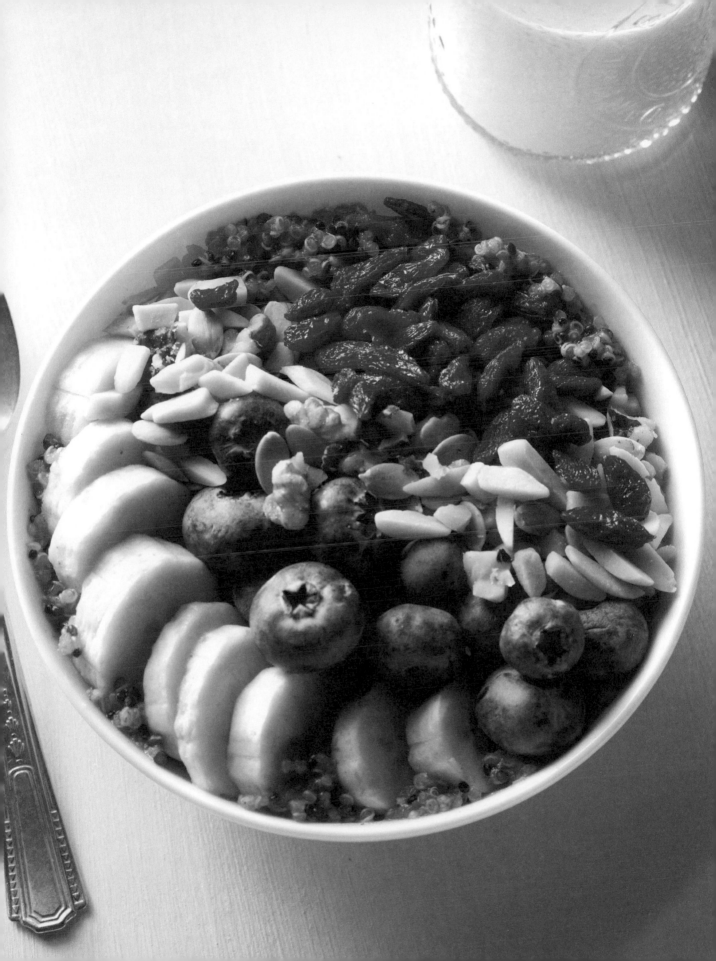

hot & spicy tomato-apple gazpacho

Tomato juice, packed full of lycopene, provides the base for this take on a traditional gazpacho. Both spicy and sweet, this is a refreshing summer soup.

- 3 CUPS TOMATO JUICE
- 3 TABLESPOONS TOMATO PASTE
- 1 LARGE APPLE, CUT INTO CHUNKS
- ¾ CUP FINELY CHOPPED RED ONION (ABOUT 1 MEDIUM)
- 2 CLOVES GARLIC, PEELED
- ⅓ CUP NATURAL ALMONDS
- ¼ CUP RED WINE VINEGAR
- 2 TEASPOONS LOUISIANA-STYLE RED PEPPER SAUCE
- 1 TEASPOON CHILI POWDER
- ¾ TEASPOON GROUND CORIANDER
- ¼ TEASPOON SALT
- 4 PLUM TOMATOES, CUT INTO ½-INCH CHUNKS
- 1 HASS AVOCADO, CUT INTO ½-INCH CHUNKS

1 In a blender, combine the tomato juice, tomato paste, apple, ½ cup of the onion, the garlic, almonds, vinegar, red pepper sauce, chili powder, coriander, and salt; process until blended but not pureed (it should still have a chunky texture).

2 Pour the gazpacho into a serving bowl and stir in ½ cup of water and the tomato chunks; chill.

3 Serve the soup topped with the remaining ¼ cup onion and the avocado.

Makes 4 servings. Per serving: 213 calories, 12 g total fat (12% saturated), 6 g protein, 26 g carbohydrate, 5.4 g fiber, 0 mg cholesterol, 985 mg sodium

spiced moroccan carrot soup

Warm Moroccan spices, tempered by the sweetness of carrots, carrot juice, and tomato paste, add complexity to this thick, creamy soup. The garnish of cilantro, a typical Moroccan seasoning, provides this beta-carotene-packed soup with a fresh, clean finish.

- 1 TABLESPOON OLIVE OIL
- 1 MEDIUM ONION, THINLY SLICED
- 3 CLOVES GARLIC, THINLY SLICED
- 1 POUND CARROTS, THINLY SLICED
- ¾ TEASPOON CINNAMON
- ¾ TEASPOON GROUND GINGER
- ¾ TEASPOON TURMERIC
- ½ TEASPOON PAPRIKA
- 1 CUP CARROT JUICE
- 2 TABLESPOONS TOMATO PASTE
- 3 TABLESPOONS WHITE RICE
- ¾ TEASPOON SALT
- ½ TEASPOON PEPPER
- ½ CUP CHOPPED CILANTRO

1 In a medium saucepan, heat the oil over medium heat. Add the onion and garlic, and cook, stirring frequently for 5 minutes, or until the onion is golden.

2 Stir in the carrots, cinnamon, ginger, turmeric, and paprika, and cook for 1 minute. Stir in the carrot juice, tomato paste, rice, salt, pepper, and 2 cups of water; bring to a boil. Reduce to a simmer; cover and cook for 20 minutes, or until the carrots and rice are tender.

3 Transfer the mixture to a food processor and puree until smooth. Sprinkle the soup with the cilantro when serving.

Makes 4 servings. Per serving: 167 calories, 4 g total fat (13% saturated), 4 g protein, 31 g carbohydrate, 4.9 g fiber, 0 mg cholesterol, 562 mg sodium

black bean& pumpkin chili

Orange-fleshed pumpkin and bold red peppers fill this dish with beta-carotene, lutein, and vitamin C. Serve with a scoop of quinoa and these nutrients will enhance the iron in the quinoa.

2 TABLESPOONS OLIVE OIL

1 MEDIUM ONION, COARSELY CHOPPED

1 MEDIUM RED BELL PEPPER, COARSELY CHOPPED

3 CLOVES GARLIC, MINCED

2 CANS (15 OUNCES EACH) LOW-SODIUM BLACK BEANS, DRAINED AND RINSED

1 CAN (15 OUNCES) SOLID-PACK PUMPKIN

1 CAN (14.5 OUNCES) DICED TOMATOES, UNDRAINED

3 CUPS LOW-SODIUM VEGETABLE BROTH

2 TEASPOONS DRIED PARSLEY FLAKES

2 TEASPOONS CHILI POWDER

1½ TEASPOONS GROUND CUMIN

1½ TEASPOONS DRIED OREGANO

1 In a large skillet, heat the oil over medium-high heat. Add the onion and pepper; cook, stirring frequently for 5 minutes or until the vegetables are tender.
Add the garlic and cook for 1 minute.

2 Transfer to a 5-quart slow cooker; stir in the beans, pumpkin, tomatoes, broth, parsley, chili powder, cumin, and oregano. Cover and cook on low 4 to 5 hours.

Makes 6 servings. Per serving: 282 calories, 9 g total fat (11% saturated), 12 g protein, 42 g carbohydrate, 14 g fiber, 0 mg cholesterol, 441 mg sodium

sweet potato kale soup

This dish—ready in just 30 minutes—boasts a trifecta of the superfoods kale, sweet potatoes, and beans, providing an abundance of beta-carotene, lutein, zeaxanthin, and fiber.

2 TEASPOONS OLIVE OIL

1 LARGE ONION, CHOPPED

1 TABLESPOON ITALIAN SEASONING

2 CONTAINERS (32 OUNCES EACH) LOW-SODIUM VEGETABLE BROTH

1 CAN (15 OUNCES EACH) LOW-SODIUM CANNELLINI BEANS, DRAINED AND RINSED

1 POUND SWEET POTATOES, PEELED AND CUT INTO 1-INCH CHUNKS

5 CUPS CHOPPED FRESH KALE

6 CLOVES GARLIC, MINCED

¼ TEASPOON PEPPER

1 In a large saucepan or Dutch oven, heat the oil over medium-high heat. Add the onion and Italian seasoning; cook, stirring frequently for 5 minutes or until the onion is tender.

2 Stir in the broth, beans, sweet potatoes, kale, garlic, and pepper. Bring to a boil. Reduce to a simmer; cook, uncovered, for 20 minutes or until the potatoes are tender.

Makes 4 servings. Per serving: 315 calories, 4 g total fat (0% saturated), 12 g protein, 46 g carbohydrate, 10 g fiber, 0 mg cholesterol, 478 mg sodium

summer vegetable soup

The fresh flavors of summer are highlighted in this light, delicious soup. The anti-inflammatory properties of turmeric boost the health benefits of the vegetables.

- 1 TABLESPOON OLIVE OIL
- 1 SMALL ONION, QUARTERED AND THINLY SLICED
- 4 CUPS REDUCED-SODIUM VEGETABLE BROTH
- 1 CUP CUBED ZUCCHINI
- 1 CAN (15 OUNCES) NAVY BEANS, DRAINED AND RINSED
- ½ CUP CUBED RED POTATO
- ½ CUP CUT FRESH GREEN BEANS (2-INCH PIECES)
- ½ CUP CHOPPED PEELED TOMATO
- ½ TEASPOON GROUND TURMERIC
- ¼ TEASPOON PEPPER
- ¼ CUP CHOPPED CELERY LEAVES
- 2 TABLESPOONS TOMATO PASTE

1 In a large saucepan, heat the oil over medium-high heat. Add the onion and cook, stirring frequently for 3 minutes or until tender. Add the broth, zucchini, beans, potato, green beans, tomato, turmeric, and pepper. Bring to a boil. Reduce to a simmer; cover and cook for 25 minutes or until the vegetables are tender.

2 Stir in the celery leaves and tomato paste. Cover and let stand for 5 minutes before serving.

Makes 4 servings. Per serving: 210 calories, 4 g total fat (25% saturated), 13 g protein, 32 g carbohydrate, 8 g fiber, 0 mg cholesterol, 591 mg sodium

spiced cream of butternut squash soup

Curry powder and ginger lend a decidedly Indian feel to this nutrient-packed soup. Not only is it soothing, but it also provides a hefty amount of beta-carotene as well as potassium, calcium, and magnesium.

- 2 TEASPOONS OLIVE OIL
- 1 LARGE ONION, FINELY CHOPPED
- 4 RED APPLES
- 2 POUNDS BUTTERNUT SQUASH, PEELED AND THINLY SLICED (ABOUT 6 CUPS)
- 1 LARGE BAKING POTATO, PEELED AND THINLY SLICED
- 2 TEASPOONS CURRY POWDER
- 1 TEASPOON GROUND GINGER
- 1 TEASPOON SALT
- ½ TEASPOON CINNAMON
- 1 CUP UNSWEETENED SOY MILK
- ¼ CUP ROASTED CASHEWS, COARSELY CHOPPED

1 In a large saucepan, heat the oil over medium heat. Add the onion, and cook, stirring frequently for 5 minutes, or until golden brown.

2 Peel, core, and slice 3½ of the apples. Add to the pan along with the butternut squash, potato, curry powder, ginger, salt, and cinnamon, and stir to combine. Add 3 cups of water; cover and simmer for 30 minutes, or until the squash is tender.

3 Transfer to a food processor and process until smooth. Return the mixture to the pan, add the milk, and whisk to combine. Cook over low heat until heated through.

4 Meanwhile, thinly slice the remaining ½ apple (unpeeled). Spoon the soup into 4 mugs or soup bowls and top with the cashews and apple slices.

Makes 4 servings. Per serving: 298 calories, 7 g total fat (20% saturated), 7 g protein, 58 g carbohydrate, 8.1 g fiber, 0 mg cholesterol, 599 mg sodium

spiced cream of butternut squash soup ▶

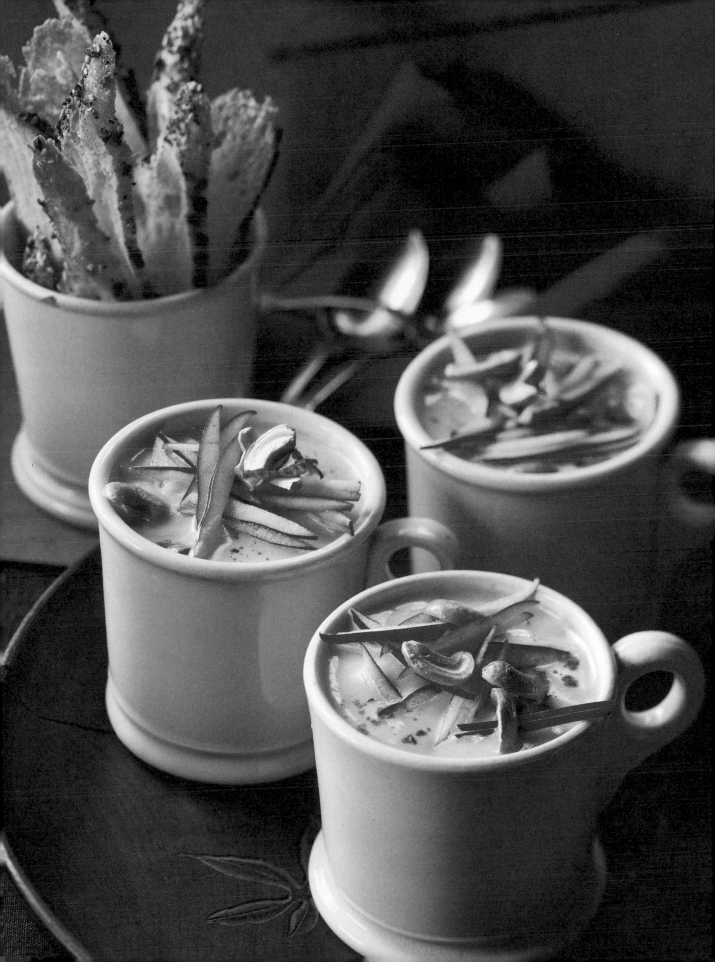

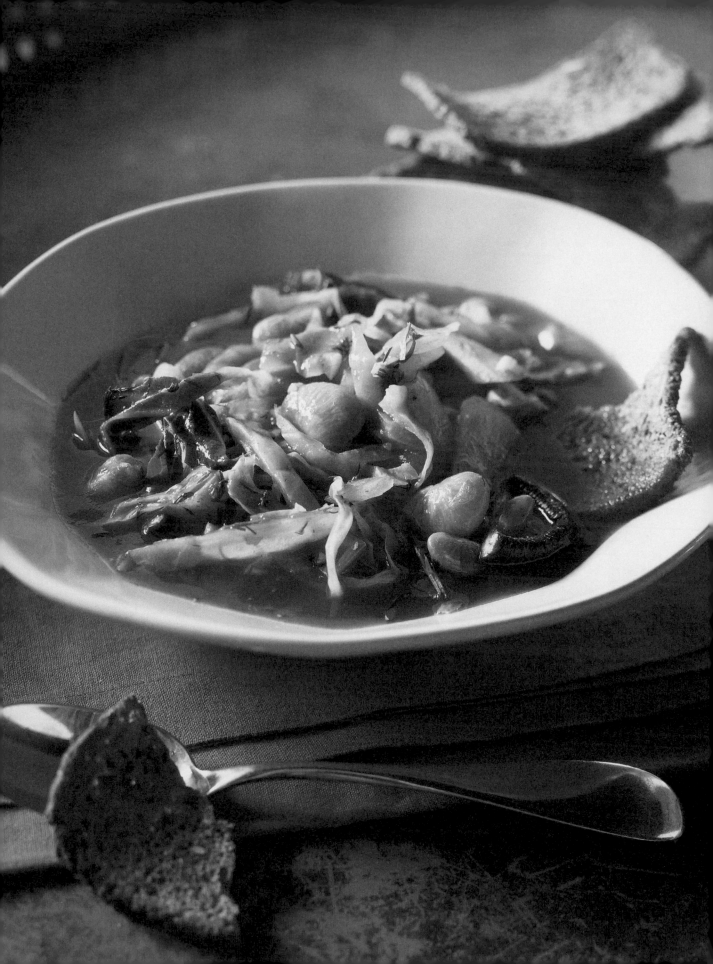

mushroom & winter vegetable soup

Cabbage and mushrooms, two phytonutrient-rich foods, team up in this hearty winter soup. Serve with thin dark rye or pumpernickel toast.

½ CUP DRIED SHIITAKE MUSHROOMS

1½ CUPS BOILING WATER

2 TABLESPOONS OLIVE OIL

1 LARGE ONION, FINELY CHOPPED

4 CLOVES GARLIC, MINCED

1 LARGE CARROT, THINLY SLICED

1 LARGE PARSNIP (8 OUNCES), THINLY SLICED

1 SMALL HEAD GREEN CABBAGE (1½ POUNDS), SHREDDED (ABOUT 8 CUPS)

1¼ CUPS FROZEN BABY LIMA BEANS

⅓ CUP CHOPPED FRESH DILL

⅓ CUP TOMATO PASTE

¼ CUP RED WINE VINEGAR

¾ TEASPOON SALT

1 In a small bowl, combine the shiitake mushrooms and boiling water. Let stand for 20 minutes, or until softened. With your fingers, remove the mushrooms from the soaking liquid, reserving the liquid. Trim any stems from the mushrooms and coarsely chop the caps. Strain the reserved liquid through a fine-meshed sieve or coffee filter; set aside.

2 Meanwhile, in a large saucepan or Dutch oven, heat the oil over medium heat. Add the onion and garlic, and cook for 5 minutes, or until the onion is light golden. Add the carrot and parsnip, and cook for 5 minutes, or until the carrot is crisp-tender.

3 Stir in the cabbage. Cover and cook for 5 minutes, or until the cabbage begins to wilt. Stir in the mushrooms and reserved liquid, the lima beans, dill, tomato paste, vinegar, salt, and 3 cups of water; bring to a boil. Reduce to a simmer; cover and cook for 25 minutes, or until the soup is richly flavored.

Makes 4 servings. Per serving: 282 calories, 8 g total fat (13% saturated), 9 g protein, 48 g carbohydrate, 13 g fiber, 0 mg cholesterol, 682 mg sodium

potato leek soup

This rich classic soup uses starchy potatoes to thicken and create a creamy consistency, so there's no need to add heavy cream. For a richer flavor, add the coconut milk.

2 TABLESPOONS OLIVE OIL

3 CELERY STALKS, COARSELY CHOPPED

2 MEDIUM ONIONS, CHOPPED

3 MEDIUM LEEKS (WHITE PORTION ONLY), COARSELY CHOPPED

1 MEDIUM GREEN BELL PEPPER, COARSELY CHOPPED

6 CLOVES GARLIC, MINCED

4 MEDIUM POTATOES, PEELED AND CUT INTO 1-INCH CHUNKS

2 CANS (14½-OUNCES EACH) REDUCED-SODIUM VEGETABLE BROTH

½ TEASPOON GROUND PEPPER

½ CUP COCONUT MILK, OPTIONAL

2 SCALLIONS, CHOPPED

1 In a large saucepan or Dutch oven, heat the oil over medium-high heat. Add the celery, onions, leeks, bell pepper, and garlic and cook, stirring frequently, for 5 minutes or until the vegetables are tender. Add the potatoes, broth, and ground pepper. Bring to a boil. Reduce to a simmer; cover and cook, stirring occasionally, for 15 minutes or until the potatoes are tender.

2 Puree the soup to the desired consistency using an immersion blender. Or, cool the soup slightly and puree in batches in a blender. Return to the pan. If desired, stir in the coconut milk and heat through. Sprinkle the soup with the scallions when serving.

Makes 4 servings. Per serving: 150 calories, 4 g total fat (25% saturated), 3 g protein, 27 g carbohydrate, 3 g fiber, 0 mg cholesterol, 263 mg sodium

lentil-tomato stew with browned onions

This hearty main course is rich in dietary fiber and phytonutrients, especially beta-carotene. If desired, serve the soup topped with some non-dairy, plant-based feta.

1   CUP DRIED SHIITAKE MUSHROOMS

1   CUP BOILING WATER

4   TEASPOONS OLIVE OIL

3   CARROTS, QUARTERED LENGTHWISE AND THINLY SLICED CROSSWISE

8   CLOVES GARLIC, THINLY SLICED

¾   CUP LENTILS, RINSED AND PICKED OVER

1   CUP CANNED CRUSHED TOMATOES

¾   TEASPOON SALT

¾   TEASPOON GROUND CUMIN

¾   TEASPOON GROUND GINGER

½   TEASPOON RUBBED SAGE

1   LARGE ONION, HALVED AND THINLY SLICED

2   TEASPOONS SUGAR

1   CUP FROZEN PEAS

1 In a small bowl, combine the shiitake mushrooms and boiling water. Let stand for 20 minutes, or until softened. With your fingers, remove the mushrooms from the soaking liquid, reserving the liquid. Trim any stems from the mushrooms and thinly slice the caps. Strain the reserved liquid through a fine-meshed sieve or coffee filter; set aside.

2 In a large saucepan, heat 3 teaspoons of the oil over medium heat. Add the carrots and garlic, and cook for 5 minutes, or until softened.

3 Stir in the lentils, tomatoes, salt, cumin, ginger, sage, mushrooms, and reserved liquid. Add 3 cups of water, and bring to a boil. Reduce to a simmer; cover and cook for 35 minutes, or until the lentils are tender.

4 Meanwhile, in a large skillet, heat the remaining 1 teaspoon oil over medium heat. Add the onion and sugar; cook, stirring frequently for 5 minutes, or until the onion is lightly browned.

5 Add the peas to the stew, and cook for 2 minutes to heat through. Serve the stew topped with the browned onions.

Makes 4 servings. Per serving: 290 calories, 5.5 g total fat (13% saturated), 15 g protein, 49 g carbohydrate, 10 g fiber, 0 mg cholesterol, 601 mg sodium

sweet potato stew

Okra and peanut butter contribute to the thickness and heartiness of this West African-inspired stew (these ingredients are common to West African cooking). In addition to huge amounts of beta-carotene supplied by the sweet potatoes, this dish is rich in fber and folate from the chickpeas.

1   TABLESPOON OLIVE OIL

1   MEDIUM ONION, FINELY CHOPPED

4   CLOVES GARLIC, MINCED

1   CUP CANNED CRUSHED TOMATOES

1   POUND SWEET POTATOES, PEELED AND CUT INTO ½-INCH CHUNKS

2   TABLESPOONS NATURAL CREAMY PEANUT BUTTER

½   TEASPOON SALT

½   TEASPOON CAYENNE PEPPER

10 OUNCES FROZEN CUT OR WHOLE OKRA, THAWED

1   CAN (15 OUNCES) LOW-SODIUM CHICKPEAS, RINSED AND DRAINED

1 Preheat the oven to 350°F. In a large nonstick Dutch oven or flameproof casserole, heat the oil over medium-high heat. Add the onion and garlic; cook for 2 minutes. Stir in ⅓ cup of water; cook until the onion is golden brown and tender.

2 Stir in the tomatoes, sweet potatoes, peanut butter, salt, cayenne, and 1½ cups of water; bring to a boil. Cover, transfer to the oven, and bake for 25 minutes.

3 Stir in the okra and chickpeas and return the pan to the oven; bake for 15 minutes, or until the okra is tender.

Makes 4 servings. Per serving: 333 calories, 10 g total fat (15% saturated), 13 g protein, 53 g carbohydrate, 13.5 g fiber, 0 mg cholesterol, 618 mg sodium

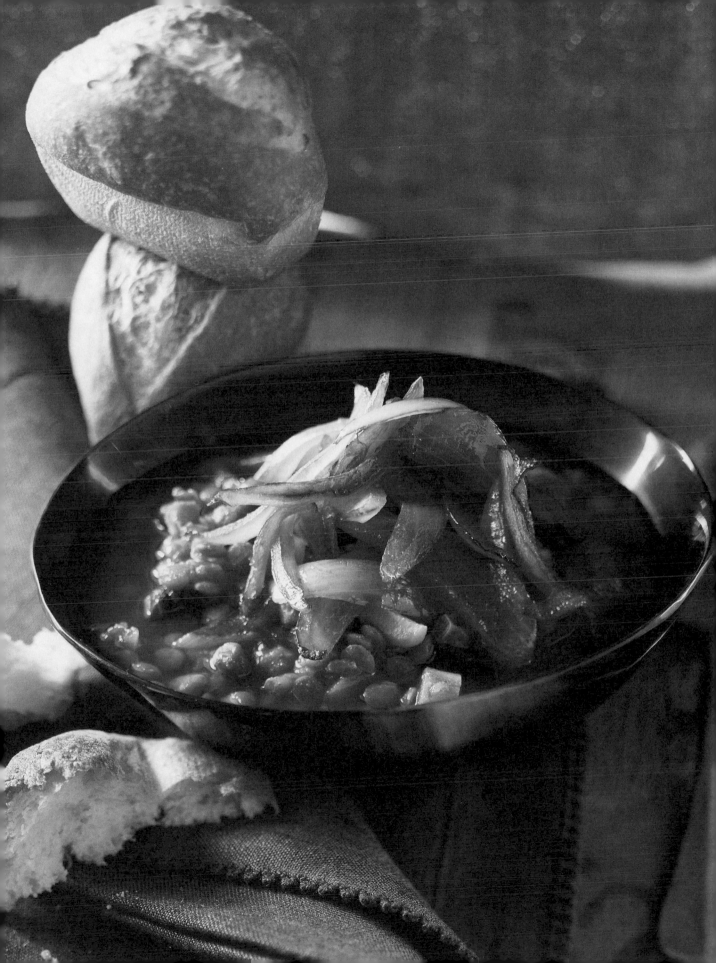

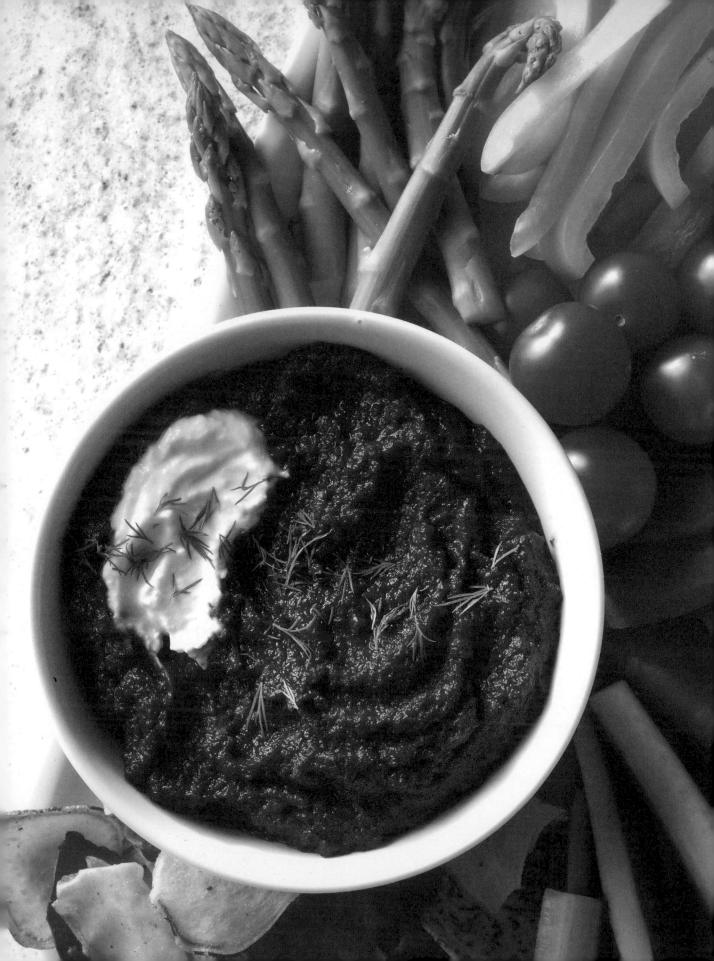

roasted beet & garlic hummus

Impress your guests with this bright pink beet hummus, surrounded with assorted vegetables and pita bread. It also makes a great sandwich spread in place of high-fat mayonnaise.

- 3 FRESH MEDIUM BEETS (ABOUT 1 POUND)
- 1 WHOLE GARLIC BULB
- ½ TEASPOON SALT
- ½ TEASPOON COARSELY GROUND PEPPER
- 1 TEASPOON PLUS ¼ CUP OLIVE OIL
- 1 CAN (15 OUNCES) CHICKPEAS, DRAINED AND RINSED
- 3 TABLESPOONS LEMON JUICE
- 2 TABLESPOONS TAHINI
- ½ TEASPOON GROUND CUMIN
- 4 TABLESPOONS DAIRY-FREE YOGURT
- MINCED FRESH DILL

1 Preheat the oven to 375°F. Pierce the beets and place in a microwave-safe bowl; cover loosely. Microwave on high for 4 minutes, turning halfway through. Cool slightly. Wrap the beets in individual foil packets.

2 Remove the papery outer skin from garlic bulb, but do not peel or separate the cloves. Cut in half crosswise. Sprinkle the halves with ¼ teaspoon salt and ¼ teaspoon pepper; drizzle with 1 teaspoon of oil. Wrap in individual foil packets. Roast the beets and garlic for about 45 minutes or until the beets are tender and the cloves are soft.

3 Remove from oven; unwrap. Rinse the beets with cold water; peel. Squeeze the garlic from skins into a food processor. Add the beets, chickpeas, lemon juice, tahini, cumin, the remaining ¼ cup olive oil, ¼ teaspoon salt, and ¼ teaspoon ground pepper. Process the mixture until smooth.

4 If desired, pulse 2 tablespoons of yogurt with the beet mixture. Dollop the remaining 2 tablespoons yogurt over the finished hummus and sprinkle with the dill when serving.

Makes 16 servings. Per serving: 87 calories, 5 g total fat (20% saturated), 2 g protein, 8 g carbohydrate, 2 g fiber, 0 mg cholesterol, 131 mg sodium

chili-lime roasted chickpeas

Here's a lighter snack than chips but just as enjoyable. Change up the flavors by substituting rosemary and thyme or lemon zest and freshly ground pepper for the spices in this recipe.

- 2 CANS (15 OUNCES EACH) CHICKPEAS, DRAINED, RINSED, AND PATTED DRY
- 2 TABLESPOONS EXTRA-VIRGIN OLIVE OIL
- 1 TABLESPOON CHILI POWDER
- 2 TEASPOONS GROUND CUMIN
- 1 TEASPOON GRATED LIME ZEST
- ¾ TEASPOON SEA SALT
- 1 TABLESPOON LIME JUICE

1 Preheat the oven to 400°F. Line a rimmed baking sheet with foil. Spread the chickpeas in a single layer over the foil, removing any loose skins. Bake for 40 minutes, stirring every 15 minutes or until very crunchy.

2 Meanwhile, in a small bowl, whisk together the oil, chili powder, cumin, zest, salt, and lime juice. Remove the chickpeas from oven and let cool for 5 minutes.

3 Drizzle the chickpeas with the oil mixture, shaking the pan to coat. Cool completely.

Makes 6 servings. Per serving: 178 calories, 8 g total fat (12% saturated), 6 g protein, 23 g carbohydrate, 6 g fiber, 23 mg cholesterol, 463 mg sodium

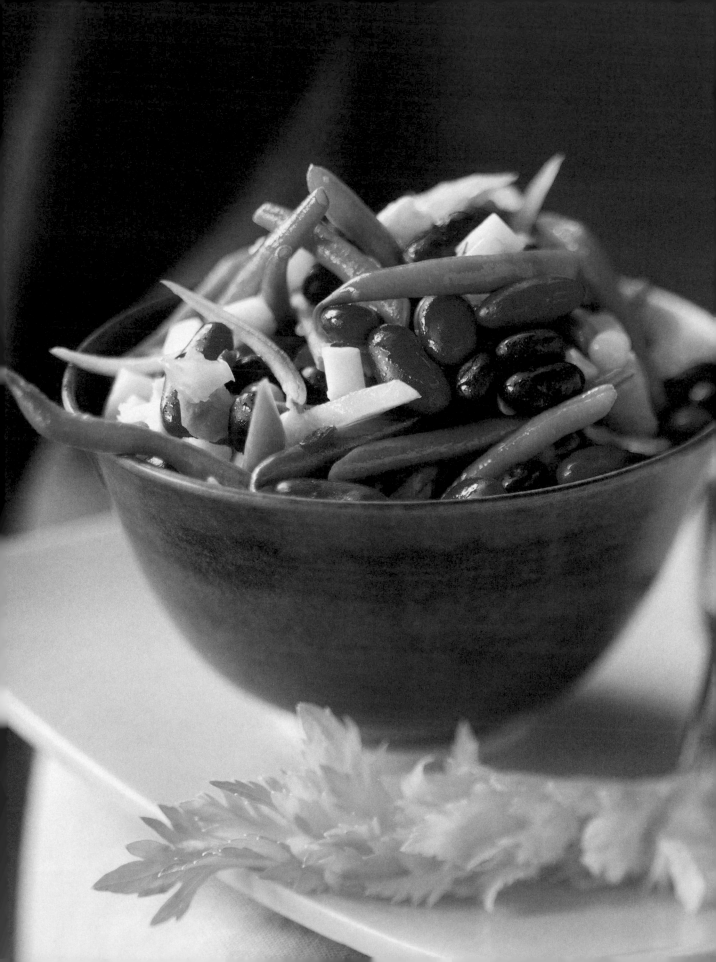

three-bean salad

Chipotle peppers, which are smoked jalapeños, are sold in cans, packed in adobo sauce (a spicy, chili- and vinegar-based sauce). Although the chipotles add depth of flavor and heat to the dish, you could make this dressing with 1 teaspoon of regular chili powder instead.

¼ CUP RED WINE VINEGAR

2 TABLESPOONS OLIVE OIL

1 TABLESPOON HONEY

1 CHIPOTLE PEPPER IN ADOBO, FINELY CHOPPED (2 TEASPOONS)

¼ TEASPOON SALT

12 OUNCES GREEN BEANS, HALVED

1 CUP FROZEN CORN KERNELS

1 CAN (15 OUNCES) BLACK BEANS, DRAINED AND RINSED

1 CAN (15 OUNCES) RED KIDNEY BEANS, DRAINED AND RINSED

1 CELERY STALK, DICED

1 CUP JULIENNE SLICED JICAMA

⅓ CUP FINELY CHOPPED RED ONION

1 In a large bowl, whisk together the vinegar, oil, honey, chipotle, and salt.

2 Meanwhile, in a large vegetable steamer, steam the green beans for 5 minutes, or until crisp-tender. Add the corn during the final minute of steaming. Transfer the hot vegetables to the bowl with the dressing, and toss to coat.

3 Add the black beans, kidney beans, celery, jicama, and onion; toss to combine.

Makes 4 servings. Per serving: 287 calories, 8 g total fat (11% saturated), 11 g protein, 45 g carbohydrate, 10 g fiber, 0 mg cholesterol, 536 mg sodium

roasted butternut panzanella

Butternut squash, pumpkin seeds, and maple syrup lend an autumnal feel to this bread salad. It's a good source of beta-carotene and lutein.

4 CUPS CUBED WHOLE-GRAIN BREAD

5 TABLESPOONS PLUS ¼ CUP OLIVE OIL

1 MEDIUM BUTTERNUT SQUASH (ABOUT 3 POUNDS), PEELED AND CUT INTO 1-INCH CUBES

½ TEASPOON GROUND GINGER

½ TEASPOON GROUND CUMIN

⅓ CUP RED WINE VINEGAR

¼ CUP MAPLE SYRUP

2 TABLESPOONS PREPARED HORSERADISH

½ TEASPOON SALT

½ TEASPOON PEPPER

¼ TEASPOON DRIED ROSEMARY, MINCED

1 CUP PUMPKIN SEEDS OR PEPITAS

1 CUP DRIED CRANBERRIES

4 SHALLOTS, FINELY CHOPPED (ABOUT ½ CUP)

1 Preheat the oven to 425°F. Place the bread cubes on a large rimmed baking sheet; toss with 2 table-spoons of oil. Bake for 10 minutes, stirring twice or until the bread is toasted. Transfer to a large bowl.

2 Place the squash in the same pan and toss with the ginger, cumin, and 3 tablespoons of the oil; toss to coat. Roast, stirring occasionally for 35 to 45 minutes or until the squash is tender and lightly browned.

3 Meanwhile, in a small saucepan over medium heat, combine the vinegar, syrup, horseradish, salt, pepper, and rosemary; cook, stirring frequently for 3 minutes or until heated through. Remove from heat; gradually whisk in the remaining ¼ cup of oil until blended.

4 To the bowl with the bread cubes, add the squash, pumpkin seeds, cranberries, and shallots. Drizzle the salad with ½ cup of dressing and toss to combine. (Save the remaining dressing for another use.)

Makes 8 servings. Per serving: 407 calories, 20 g total fat (15% saturated), 9 g protein, 54 g carbohydrate, 8 g fiber, 0 mg cholesterol, 387 mg sodium

◀ **three-bean salad**

spinach, sweet potato & shiitake salad

To save some time, instead of baking sliced sweet potatoes, you can microwave whole, unpeeled potatoes and then peel and slice them after cooking.

- 1 POUND SWEET POTATOES, PEELED, HALVED LENGTHWISE, AND CUT CROSSWISE INTO ½-INCH SLICES
- ⅓ CUP WALNUTS
- 1 TABLESPOON PLUS 4 TEASPOONS OLIVE OIL
- 2 CLOVES GARLIC, SLIVERED
- 12 OUNCES FRESH SHIITAKE MUSHROOMS, STEMS DISCARDED AND CAPS THICKLY SLICED
- ½ TEASPOON SALT
- 12 CUPS SPINACH LEAVES
- ½ CUP RED WINE VINEGAR
- 1 TABLESPOON DIJON MUSTARD

1 Preheat the oven to 400°F. Place the sweet potatoes on a lightly oiled baking sheet, and bake for 20 minutes, or until tender. Toast the walnuts in a separate pan in the oven for 5 minutes, or until crisp. When cool enough to handle, chop the nuts.

2 In a large skillet, heat 1 tablespoon of the oil over medium heat. Add the garlic, and cook for 30 seconds, or until fragrant.

3 Add half the mushrooms and ¼ teaspoon of the salt, and cook for 4 minutes, or until they begin to soften. Add the remaining mushrooms and ¼ teaspoon salt, and cook for 5 minutes, or until tender.

4 Place the spinach in a large bowl. Add the sweet potatoes and walnuts. Remove the mushrooms from the skillet with a slotted spoon, and add to the bowl with the spinach.

5 Add the vinegar, mustard, and remaining 4 teaspoons oil to the skillet, and whisk over high heat until warm. Pour the dressing over the salad, and toss to combine.

Makes 4 servings. *Per serving: 283 calories, 15 g total fat (12% saturated), 9 g protein, 32 g carbohydrate, 8.1 g fiber, 0 mg cholesterol, 524 mg sodium*

bulgur salad with tangerine-pomegranate dressing

Pomegranate molasses—a sweet-sour pomegranate concentrate—is available in Middle Eastern grocery stores, specialty food stores, and some supermarkets. If you can't find pomegranate molasses, substitute a mixture of currant jelly (2 tablespoons) and fresh lemon or lime juice (1 tablespoon).

- 1 CUP MEDIUM-GRAIN BULGUR
- 2½ CUPS BOILING WATER
- 1 TEASPOON GRATED TANGERINE OR ORANGE ZEST
- 1 CUP FRESH TANGERINE OR ORANGE JUICE
- 2 TABLESPOONS TOMATO PASTE
- 2 TABLESPOONS POMEGRANATE MOLASSES
- 2 TABLESPOONS OLIVE OIL
- ¾ TEASPOON SALT
- 1½ CUPS CORN KERNELS, THAWED IF FROZEN
- ⅔ CUP DRIED CHERRIES (3 OUNCES)
- ⅔ CUP THINLY SLICED SCALLIONS
- ⅓ CUP ROASTED PEANUTS, COARSELY CHOPPED

1 In a large bowl, combine the bulgur and the boiling water. Let stand for 30 minutes at room temperature. Drain well.

2 While the bulgur soaks, in a large bowl, whisk together the tangerine zest, tangerine juice, tomato paste, pomegranate molasses, oil, and salt.

3 Add the drained bulgur to the dressing, and fluff with a fork. Add the corn, cherries, scallions, and peanuts, tossing to combine. Serve at room temperature or chilled.

Makes 4 servings. *Per serving: 414 calories, 14 g total fat (14% saturated), 10 g protein, 69 g carbohydrate, 10 g fiber, 0 mg cholesterol, 520 mg sodium*

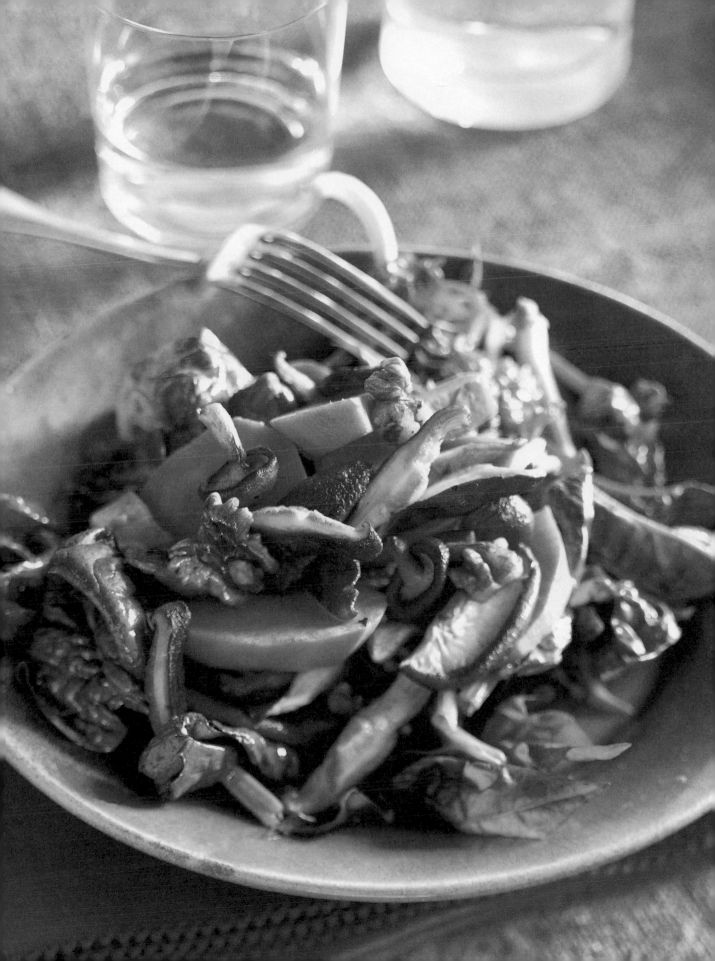

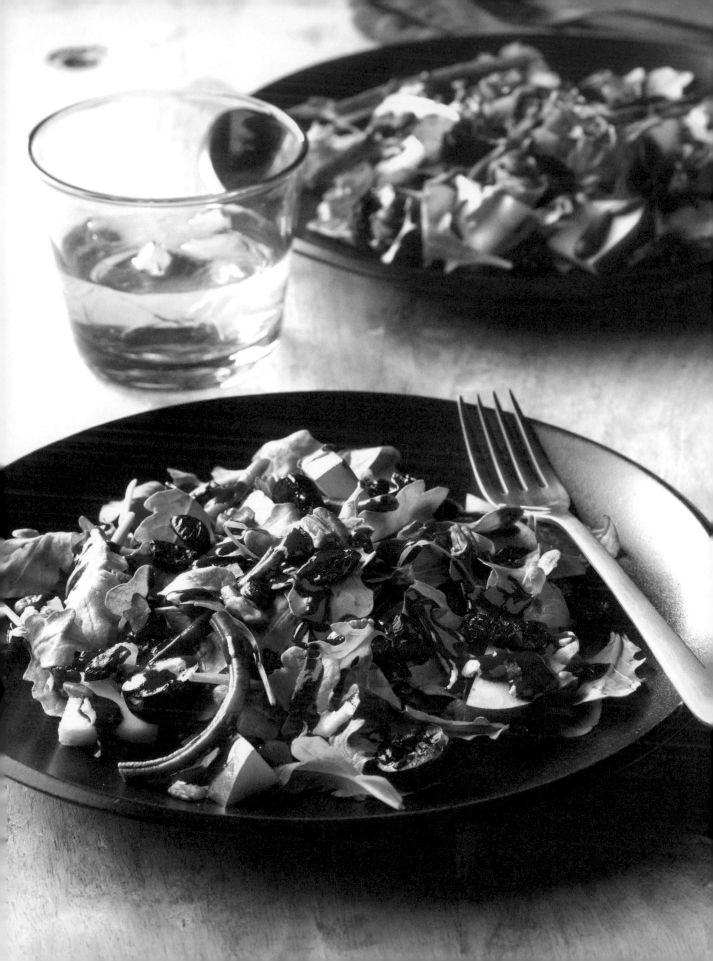

chocolate, pear & cherry salad

Unexpected dark chocolate blends with vinegar and oil for a delicious dressing that complements the bitter arugula and sweet fruits.

- ¾ CUP CUT FRENCH GREEN BEANS (HARICOTS VERTS)
- ⅛ TEASPOON SALT
- ⅛ TEASPOON PEPPER
- 3 TABLESPOONS OLIVE OIL
- ¼ CUP BALSAMIC VINEGAR
- 1 OUNCE DARK CHOCOLATE, CHOPPED
- 1 TABLESPOON RED WINE VINEGAR
- 4 CUPS FRESH ARUGULA
- 1 MEDIUM PEAR, PEELED AND CUT INTO ½-INCH CHUNKS
- ½ CUP FROZEN PITTED SWEET CHERRIES, THAWED AND HALVED
- ¼ CUP DRIED CRANBERRIES
- 3 TABLESPOONS CHOPPED PECANS
- 1 TABLESPOON MINCED DRIED APRICOTS

1 Preheat the oven to 350°F. In an 8-inch square baking dish, toss the beans with the salt, pepper, and 1 tablespoon of olive oil. Roast for 15 minutes or until the beans are tender. Remove from the oven. Toss the beans with the balsamic vinegar; cover, and refrigerate for 2 hours.

2 Meanwhile, in a small glass bowl, microwave the chocolate for 30 seconds, stirring, or until smooth. Whisk in the red wine vinegar and the remaining 2 tablespoons of oil.

3 Divide the arugula between 2 salad bowls. Drizzle with the chocolate mixture. Top with the pear, cherries, cranberries, and green beans. Sprinkle with the pecans and apricots.

Makes 2 servings. *Per serving: 511 calories, 33 g total fat (18% saturated), 4 g protein, 62 g carbohydrate, 8 g fiber, 2 mg cholesterol, 166 mg sodium*

pomegranate persimmon salad

Fall fruits and kale combine beautifully in this maple-glazed salad. If planning on leftovers, keep the salad and fruits separate from the dressing until just before serving.

- ½ CUP OLIVE OIL
- ½ CUP MAPLE SYRUP
- ¼ CUP RICE VINEGAR
- 2 TABLESPOONS DIJON MUSTARD
- ¼ TEASPOON SALT
- ¼ TEASPOON PEPPER
- 2 PACKAGES (10 OUNCES EACH) BABY KALE SALAD BLEND
- 3 RIPE FUYU PERSIMMONS OR 3 PLUMS, SLICED
- 1 CUP POMEGRANATE SEEDS

1 In a large bowl, whisk together the oil, maple syrup, vinegar, mustard, salt, and pepper.

2 To serve, add the salad blend and persimmons to the bowl and toss to coat. Sprinkle with the pomegranate seeds.

Makes 12 servings. *Per serving: 175 calories, 9 g total fat (22% saturated), 2 g protein, 23 g carbohydrate, 0 mg cholesterol, 220 mg sodium*

◄ chocolate, pear & cherry salad

colorful quinoa salad

Vitamin C-rich lime juice and bell peppers enhance the absorption of iron from the quinoa.

1 CUP QUINOA, RINSED

2 CUPS FRESH BABY SPINACH, THINLY SLICED

1 CUP GRAPE TOMATOES, HALVED

1 MEDIUM CUCUMBER, SEEDED AND FINELY CHOPPED

2 MEDIUM BELL PEPPERS SUCH AS RED AND ORANGE, FINELY CHOPPED

2 SCALLIONS, FINELY CHOPPED

3 TABLESPOONS LIME JUICE

2 TABLESPOONS OLIVE OIL

4 TEASPOONS HONEY

1 TABLESPOON GRATED LIME ZEST

2 TEASPOONS MINCED FRESH GINGER

¼ TEASPOON SALT

1 In a large saucepan, bring 2 cups of water to a boil. Add the quinoa and return to a boil. Reduce to a simmer; cover and cook for 12 minutes or until tender. Drain. Transfer to a large bowl; cool completely.

2 Stir the spinach, tomatoes, cucumber, peppers, and scallions into the quinoa. In a small bowl, whisk together lime juice, oil, honey, lime zest, ginger, and salt. Drizzle over the quinoa mixture; toss to coat. Refrigerate until serving.

Makes 8 servings. Per serving: 143 calories, 5 g total fat (20% saturated), 4 g protein, 23 g carbohydrate, 3 g fiber, 0 mg cholesterol, 88 mg sodium

bean & barley salad

Canned beans are packed in a salt brine as a preservative and rinsing the beans removes almost one-third of the salt from the beans. Opting, instead, for low-sodium beans cuts the sodium content by 40%.

¾ CUP QUICK-COOKING BARLEY

1 CAN (16 OUNCES) LOW-SODIUM KIDNEY BEANS, DRAINED AND RINSED

1 CAN (15 OUNCES) LOW-SODIUM BLACK BEANS, DRAINED AND RINSED

1 CAN (11 OUNCES) WHOLE KERNEL CORN, DRAINED

1 LARGE RED BELL PEPPER, FINELY CHOPPED

6 SCALLIONS, SLICED

⅓ CUP MINCED FRESH CILANTRO

½ CUP OLIVE OIL

⅓ CUP RED WINE VINEGAR

2 CLOVES GARLIC, MINCED

1½ TEASPOONS CHILI POWDER

¾ TEASPOON GROUND CUMIN

½ TEASPOON SALT

¼ TEASPOON CRUSHED RED PEPPER FLAKES

1 Prepare the barley according to package directions. Transfer to a large bowl; stir in the beans, corn, bell pepper, scallions, and cilantro.

2 In a small bowl, whisk together the oil, vinegar, garlic, chili powder, cumin, salt, and pepper flakes. Pour over salad; toss to coat. Refrigerate until serving.

Makes 6 servings. Per serving: 286 calories, 18 g total fat (14% saturated), 12 g protein, 48 g carbohydrate, 12 g fiber, 0 mg cholesterol, 348 mg sodium

great grain salad

Chewy whole grains marry well with crunchy nuts and seeds and tender, sweet dried fruits in this salad. Serve over greens for a phytonutrient-rich meal.

- ½ CUP MEDIUM PEARL BARLEY
- ½ CUP UNCOOKED WILD RICE
- ⅔ CUP UNCOOKED BROWN BASMATI RICE
- ⅔ CUP WALNUT OR OLIVE OIL
- ⅔ CUP RASPBERRY VINEGAR
- 2 TEASPOONS ORANGE JUICE
- 1 TEASPOON SALT
- 1 TEASPOON PEPPER
- ½ CUP SLIVERED ALMONDS
- ½ CUP SUNFLOWER SEEDS
- ½ CUP HULLED PUMPKIN SEEDS OR PEPITAS
- ½ CUP GOLDEN RAISINS
- ½ CUP CHOPPED DRIED APRICOTS
- ½ CUP DRIED CRANBERRIES
- ⅓ CUP MINCED FRESH PARSLEY
- 4 TEASPOONS GRATED ORANGE ZEST

1 In a large saucepan, bring 4 cups of water to a boil. Add the barley and wild rice and return to a boil. Reduce to simmer; cover and cook for 55 to 65 minutes or until tender.

2 Meanwhile, cook the basmati rice according to package directions. Cool the barley, wild rice, and basmati rice to room temperature.

3 In a large bowl, whisk together the oil, vinegar, orange juice, salt, and pepper. Add the barley and wild rice, basmati rice, almonds, sunflower seeds, pumpkin seeds, raisins, apricots, cranberries, parsley, and orange zest; toss to coat well. Cover and refrigerate for at least 2 hours before serving.

Makes 12 servings. *Per serving: 368 calories, 22 g total fat (14% saturated), 8 g protein, 39 g carbohydrate, 4 g fiber, 0 mg cholesterol, 281 mg sodium*

asian grains & veggies

Great for a last-minute supper, this one-dish meal is ready in under 30 minutes.

- ⅔ CUP UNCOOKED LONG-GRAIN RICE
- ⅔ CUP QUICK-COOKING BARLEY
- ½ TEASPOON SALT
- 2 TABLESPOONS OLIVE OIL
- 1 LARGE ONION, COARSELY CHOPPED
- 2 CARROTS, COARSELY CHOPPED
- 1 RED BELL PEPPER, COARSELY CHOPPED
- 1 SMALL TURNIP, COARSELY CHOPPED
- ½ CUP CHOPPED CELERY OR CELERY ROOT
- 1 TABLESPOON MINCED FRESH GINGER
- 1 PACKAGE (10 OUNCES) FRESH SPINACH, TORN
- 1 CUP CANNED PINTO BEANS, DRAINED AND RINSED
- 2 TABLESPOONS REDUCED-SODIUM SOY SAUCE

1 In a small saucepan, bring 2⅔ cups of water to a boil. Stir in the rice, barley, and salt and return to a boil. Reduce to simmer; cover and cook for 15 minutes or until tender. Remove from the heat; let stand for 5 minutes.

2 Meanwhile, in a large saucepan or Dutch oven, heat the oil over medium-high heat. Add the onion, carrots, bell pepper, turnip, celery, and ginger; cook for 5 minutes, stirring frequently, until crisp-tender.

3 Stir in the spinach, beans, soy sauce, and the rice mixture; cook, stirring for 3 minutes or until heated through.

Makes 6 servings. *Per serving: 264 calories, 6 g total fat (25% saturated), 8 g protein, 47 g carbohydrate, 8 g fiber, 0 mg cholesterol, 516 mg sodium*

brown rice & chickpea pilaf

Although intended as a main course, this fiber- and folate-rich pilaf could just as easily serve 6 to 8 people as a side dish.

- 1 TABLESPOON OLIVE OIL
- 1 LARGE RED ONION, FINELY CHOPPED
- 5 CLOVES GARLIC, THINLY SLICED
- 12 OUNCES GREEN CABBAGE, CUT INTO 1-INCH CHUNKS (ABOUT 6 CUPS)
- ¾ CUP LONG-GRAIN BROWN RICE
- ½ TEASPOON SALT
- 1 CAN (15 OUNCES) CHICKPEAS, DRAINED AND RINSED
- 1 CUP CANNED TOMATOES, CHOPPED WITH THEIR JUICE
- ¾ CUP RAISINS

1 In a large saucepan, heat the oil over medium heat. Add the onion and garlic; cook, stirring frequently for 7 minutes, or until the onion is tender.

2 Stir in the cabbage; cover and cook for 5 minutes, or until the cabbage begins to wilt.

3 Stir in the brown rice, 2 cups of water, and the salt; bring to a boil. Reduce to a simmer; cover and cook for 25 minutes, or until the rice is almost done.

4 Stir in the chickpeas, tomatoes, and raisins; bring to a boil. Reduce to a simmer; cover and cook for 10 minutes, or until the rice is tender.

Makes 4 servings. Per serving: 392 calories, 7 g total fat (12% saturated), 11 g protein, 75 g carbohydrate, 9.8 g fiber, 0 mg cholesterol, 565 mg sodium

toasted buckwheat pilaf with dried fruit

Toasting brings out the flavors of many ingredients, especially nuts and grains. This pilaf calls for whole grains of buckwheat (called groats) that have been preroasted. This form of buckwheat is sold in most supermarkets as "kasha" and comes in both whole-grain and cracked versions.

- ½ CUP WALNUTS
- 1 TABLESPOON OLIVE OIL
- 1 RED BELL PEPPER, DICED
- 4 CLOVES GARLIC, MINCED
- 1 CUP WHOLE-GRAIN ROASTED BUCKWHEAT GROATS (KASHA)
- ½ CUP RED LENTILS
- 3 CUPS BOILING WATER
- ¾ TEASPOON DRIED ROSEMARY, MINCED
- ¾ TEASPOON SALT
- ½ TEASPOON BLACK PEPPER
- ⅔ CUP DRIED APRICOTS, DICED
- ⅔ CUP DRIED FIGS, DICED
- ¼ CUP CHOPPED PARSLEY

1 Preheat the oven to 350°F. Place the walnuts on a rimmed baking sheet and toast in the oven for 5 to 7 minutes, or until crisp and fragrant. When cool enough to handle, coarsely chop.

2 In a large skillet, heat the oil over medium heat. Add the bell pepper and garlic, and cook for 4 minutes, or until the pepper is tender.

3 Stir in the buckwheat and red lentils, and cook for 3 minutes, or until the buckwheat is well coated.

4 Add the boiling water, rosemary, salt, and black pepper; bring to a boil. Reduce to a simmer; cover and cook for 15 minutes, or until the buckwheat is tender. Stir in the walnuts, apricots, figs, and parsley.

Makes 4 servings. Per serving: 482 calories, 13 g total fat (12% saturated), 16 g protein, 85 g carbohydrate, 13 g fiber, 0 mg cholesterol, 453 mg sodium

toasted buckwheat pilaf with dried fruit ▶

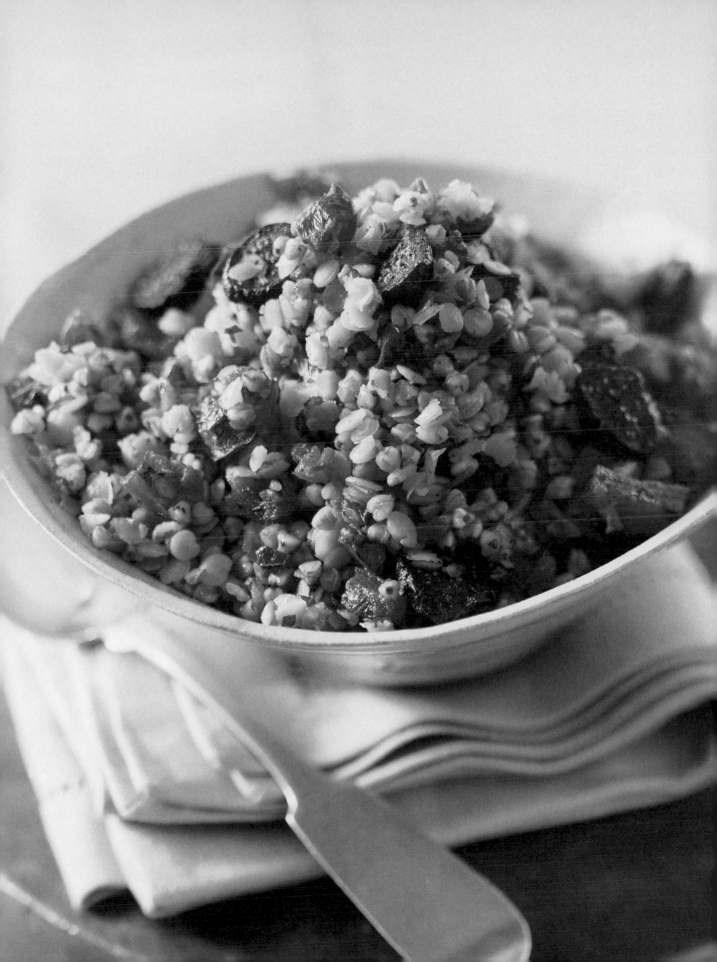

corn & tortilla strata

A strata—a layered casserole with an exotic Italian name but humble North American roots—is most commonly made with bread. We've given it a twist by using corn tortillas instead. Corn tortillas have no fat and considerably less sodium than bread.

1 TABLESPOON OLIVE OIL

3 CLOVES GARLIC, MINCED

8 OUNCES FRESH SHIITAKE MUSHROOMS, STEMS REMOVED AND CAPS THINLY SLICED

10 OUNCES FROZEN CHOPPED COLLARD GREENS, THAWED AND SQUEEZED DRY

3 CUPS UNSWEETENED SOY MILK

¼ TEASPOON SALT

¼ TEASPOON CAYENNE PEPPER

3 TABLESPOONS FLOUR

1½ CUPS FROZEN CORN KERNELS

½ CUP DAIRY-FREE CHEDDAR SHREDS

5 CORN TORTILLAS (6-INCH DIAMETER), HALVED

1 Preheat the oven to 375°F. In a large saucepan, heat the oil over medium heat. Add the garlic, and cook for 10 seconds. Stir in the mushrooms, and cook, stirring frequently for 3 minutes, or until firm-tender. Stir in the collards, and cook, stirring for 5 minutes, or until the collards are tender.

2 In a small bowl, whisk the milk, salt, and cayenne into the flour until smooth.

3 Whisk the milk mixture into the collards; cook, stirring frequently for 3 to 5 minutes, or until the sauce is creamy and lightly thickened. Stir in the corn. Remove from the heat, and stir in the shreds until melted.

4 Arrange 5 tortilla halves over the bottom of a 9 x 9-inch glass baking dish. Top with half of the collard mixture. Place the remaining tortillas on top and spoon the remaining collard mixture over the tortillas. Bake for 25 minutes, or until the strata is bubbling hot.

Makes 4 servings. Per serving: 366 calories, 15.5 g total fat (45% saturated), 11 g protein, 51 g carbohydrate, 7 g fiber, 0 mg cholesterol, 563 mg sodium

southwestern pizza

The secret ingredient in this pizza crust is carrot juice. It imparts a lovely golden color to the dough. Look for dairy-free or vegan cheese alternatives in the refrigerated section of your supermarket.

1 TABLESPOON ACTIVE DRY YEAST

¼ CUP WARM (105°F TO 115°F) WATER

3½ CUPS WHOLE-WHEAT PASTRY FLOUR

½ CUP YELLOW CORNMEAL

2 TABLESPOONS CHILI POWDER

1 TABLESPOON GROUND CUMIN

1½ TEASPOONS SALT

1 CUP CARROT JUICE

3 TABLESPOONS OLIVE OIL

1 LARGE RED BELL PEPPER, THINLY SLICED

1 LARGE GREEN BELL PEPPER, THINLY SLICED

1 LARGE ONION, HALVED AND THINLY SLICED

1 CUP CORN KERNELS

2 TEASPOONS DRIED OREGANO

8 OUNCES DAIRY-FREE MOZZARELLA SHREDS

1 In a measuring cup, sprinkle the yeast over the warm water. Let stand for 5 minutes to dissolve.

2 In a large bowl, combine the flour, cornmeal, chili powder, cumin, and salt. Stir in the yeast mixture, carrot juice, and 2 tablespoons of the oil. Transfer to a lightly floured surface, and knead for 7 to 10 minutes, or until the dough is smooth and elastic.

3 Transfer the dough to a large oiled bowl, cover with a dampened cloth, and let stand for 1½ hours in a warm draft-free spot, or until doubled in volume. Punch the dough down and divide in half. Cover and let rest for 15 minutes.

4 In a medium bowl, toss the peppers, onion, corn, and oregano with the remaining 1 tablespoon oil.

5 Roll each portion of the dough to a 10-inch round; place each on a parchment-lined baking sheet. Top each with the vegetables and shreds; let stand for 20 minutes. Meanwhile, preheat the oven to 450°F.

6 Bake for 20 to 25 minutes, reversing the top and bottom pizzas midway, until the crust is crisp.

Makes 8 servings. Per serving: 440 calories, 15 g total fat (38% saturated), 16 g protein, 61 g carbohydrate, 5 g fiber, 30 mg cholesterol, 625 mg sodium

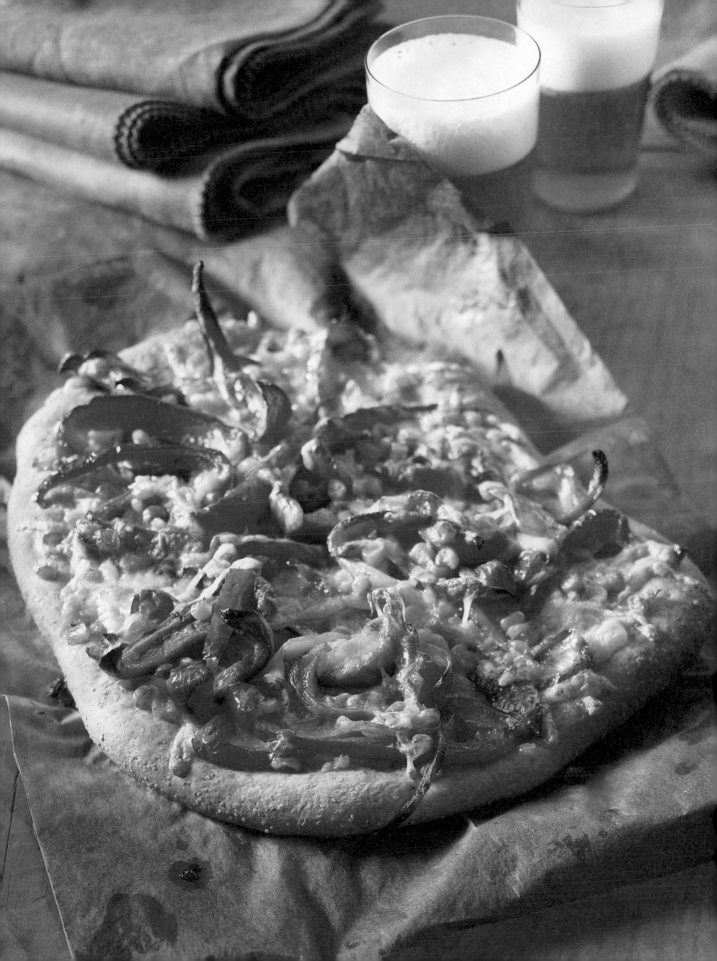

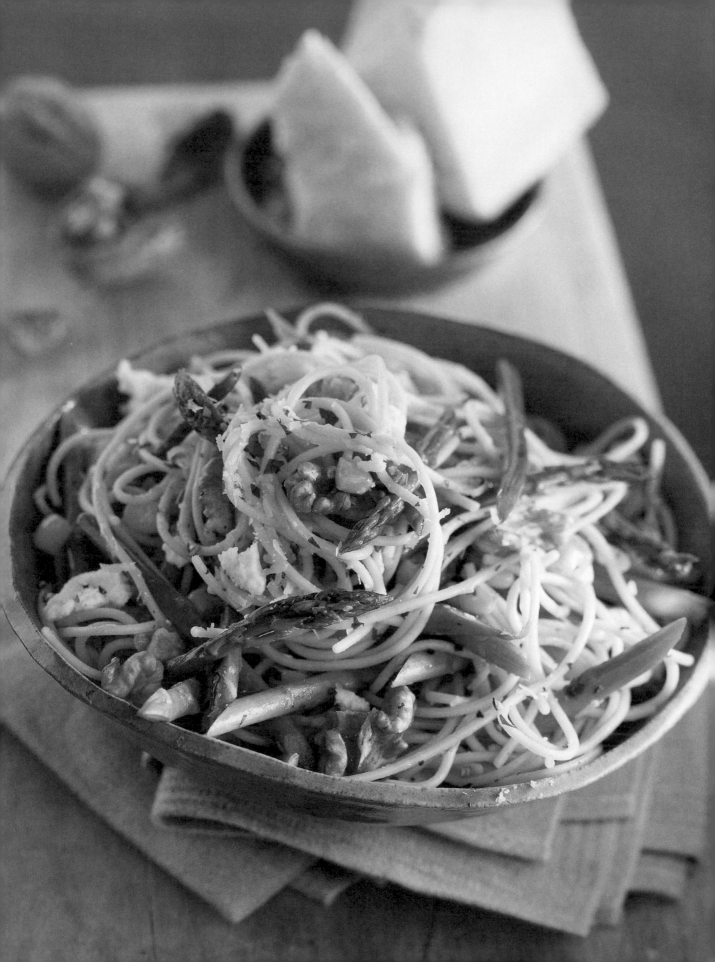

gluten-free pasta with roasted asparagus

There are many delicious gluten-free pasta alternatives to wheat-based pastas. Look for corn, brown rice, quinoa, or a combination of several flours. Or give the lentil or bean versions a try.

¼ CUP WALNUTS

1½ POUNDS ASPARAGUS, CUT INTO 1-INCH LENGTHS

1½ CUPS FROZEN CORN KERNELS

1 TABLESPOON OLIVE OIL

8 OUNCES GLUTEN-FREE SPAGHETTI

2 OUNCES DAIRY-FREE FETA, CRUMBLED

2 TABLESPOONS CHOPPED PARSLEY

½ TEASPOON SALT

¼ TEASPOON PEPPER

1 Preheat the oven to 350°F. Place the walnuts on a rimmed baking sheet and toast in the oven for 5 to 7 minutes, or until crisp and fragrant. Increase the oven temperature to 450°F. When the walnuts are cool enough to handle, coarsely chop them.

2 In a 13 x 9-inch baking dish, toss the asparagus with the corn and oil. Bake for 10 minutes or until the asparagus is tender and lightly browned.

3 Meanwhile, in a large pot of boiling water, cook the pasta according to package directions. Drain, reserving ¾ cup of the pasta cooking water. Transfer the pasta to a large bowl.

4 To the pasta in the bowl, add the asparagus and corn, the reserved cooking liquid, feta, parsley, salt, and pepper; toss well to combine. Serve the pasta sprinkled with the walnuts.

Makes 4 servings. Per serving: 424 calories, 15 g total fat (33% saturated), 9 g protein, 64 g carbohydrate, 9.6 g fiber, 11 mg cholesterol, 404 mg sodium

pasta with cabbage, apples & leeks

For a calcium boost, add a cup of plain dairy-free yogurt to the cabbage mixture before tossing it with the pasta.

2 TABLESPOONS OLIVE OIL

2 LEEKS, HALVED LENGTHWISE, THINLY SLICED CROSSWISE, AND WELL WASHED

3 CUPS PACKED SHREDDED GREEN CABBAGE (ABOUT 12 OUNCES)

3 CLOVES GARLIC, MINCED

2 LARGE RED APPLES (UNPEELED), CUT INTO ½-INCH CHUNKS

½ TEASPOON SALT

½ TEASPOON PEPPER

2 TABLESPOONS CIDER VINEGAR

1 TABLESPOON DIJON MUSTARD

8 OUNCES FARFALLE (BOW-TIE) PASTA

1 In a large skillet, heat the oil over medium heat. Add the leeks, and cook, stirring frequently for 5 minutes or until tender. Add the cabbage and garlic, and increase the heat to high; cook, stirring frequently for 5 minutes, or until the cabbage is golden brown.

2 Add the apples, salt, and pepper; cook for 2 minutes or until the apple is crisp-tender. Stir in the vinegar and mustard, and cook for 30 seconds to blend the flavors.

3 In a large pot of boiling water, cook the pasta according to package directions. Drain, reserving ½ cup of the pasta cooking water. Transfer the drained pasta to a large bowl. Add the cabbage-apple mixture and the reserved pasta cooking water; toss to combine.

Makes 4 servings. Per serving: 385 calories, 8.3 g total fat (14% saturated), 9 g protein, 70 g carbohydrate, 6.1 g fiber, 0 mg cholesterol, 411 mg sodium

◀ **gluten-free pasta with roasted asparagus**

pasta with broccoli-basil sauce

It's a common kitchen trick to use some of the pasta cooking water to help blend pasta sauce ingredients. For this sauce, the heat of the cooking water is also helpful in melting the Parmesan.

10 OUNCES WHOLE-GRAIN PASTA SHELLS

1 TABLESPOON OLIVE OIL

1 LARGE RED ONION, FINELY CHOPPED

6 CLOVES GARLIC, MINCED

2 CUPS CANNED CRUSHED TOMATOES

2 TABLESPOONS TOMATO PASTE

½ TEASPOON CRUSHED RED PEPPER FLAKES

¼ TEASPOON SALT

4 CUPS SMALL BROCCOLI FLORETS

1 CUP CHOPPED FRESH BASIL

¼ OUNCE DAIRY-FREE SHREDDED PARMESAN

1 In a large pot of boiling water, cook the pasta according to package directions. Drain, reserving ½ cup of the pasta cooking water.

2 Meanwhile, in a large skillet, heat the oil over medium heat. Add the onion and garlic, and cook, stirring frequently for 7 minutes, or until the onion is tender.

3 Add the crushed tomatoes, tomato paste, red pepper flakes, and salt; bring to a boil. Reduce to a simmer; cover and cook for 5 minutes.

4 Stir in the broccoli; cook, uncovered, for 5 minutes, or until the broccoli is crisp-tender. Transfer the sauce to a large bowl. Add the basil, drained pasta, reserved liquid, and the Parmesan. Toss to combine well.

Makes 4 servings. Per serving: 444 calories, 1 g total fat (6% saturated), 26 g protein, 73 g carbohydrate, 8.2 g fiber, 18 mg cholesterol, 853 mg sodium

farfalle with winter squash sauce

Creamy, sweet butternut squash puree, enriched with dairy-free Parmesan and flecked with red bell pepper and raisins, makes a delicious and unusual pasta sauce. This dish provides ample amounts of beta-carotene, and also vitamin C, folate, selenium, and several B vitamins.

⅓ CUP RAISINS

1 CUP BOILING WATER

8 OUNCES FARFALLE (BOW-TIE) PASTA

1 TABLESPOON OLIVE OIL

1 LARGE RED BELL PEPPER, DICED

4 CLOVES GARLIC, MINCED

16 OUNCES FROZEN BUTTERNUT SQUASH PUREE, THAWED

1 TEASPOON RUBBED SAGE

1 TEASPOON SALT

½ TEASPOON BLACK PEPPER

3 TABLESPOONS DAIRY-FREE CREAM CHEESE

¼ CUP DAIRY-FREE SHREDDED PARMESAN

1 In a small bowl, soak the raisins in boiling water for 5 minutes, or until plump. In a large pot of boiling water, cook the pasta according to package directions. Drain, reserving ⅓ cup of the pasta cooking water.

2 While the pasta cooks, in a large skillet, heat the oil over medium heat. Add the bell pepper and garlic; cook, stirring frequently for 5 minutes, or until the pepper is tender. Add the squash puree, sage, salt, and black pepper; cook until heated through.

3 Stir in the raisins and their soaking liquid and the cream cheese, and cook until the cream cheese has melted. Transfer to a large bowl. Add the pasta, the reserved cooking liquid, and the Parmesan; toss to combine.

Makes 4 servings. Per serving: 418 calories, 8.7 g total fat (39% saturated), 14 g protein, 73 g carbohydrate, 7.4 g fiber, 13 mg cholesterol, 760 mg sodium

farfalle with winter squash sauce ▶

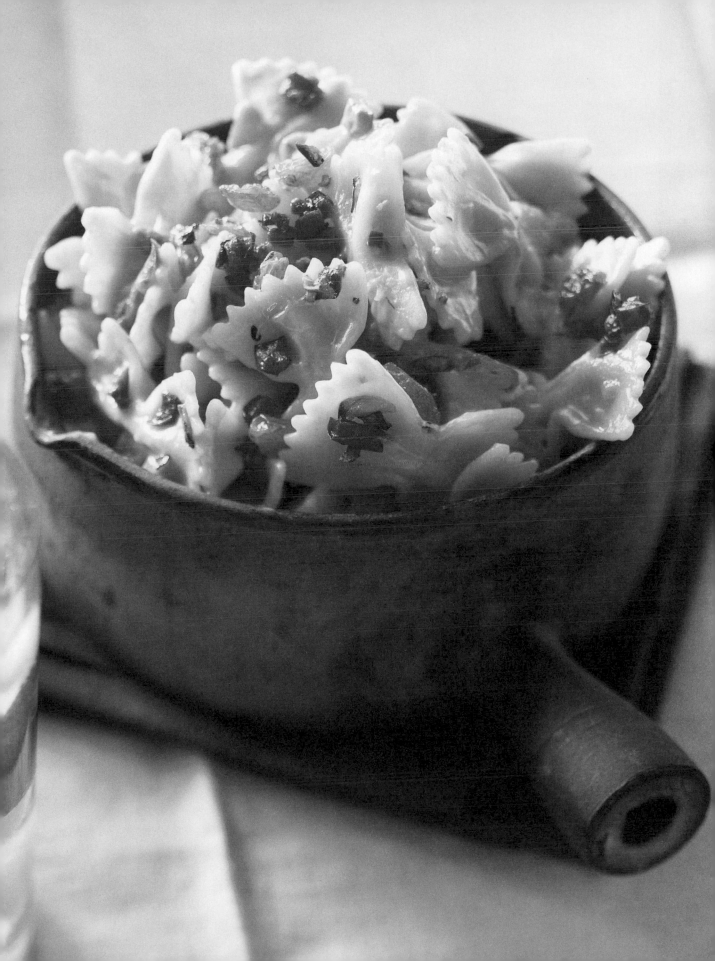

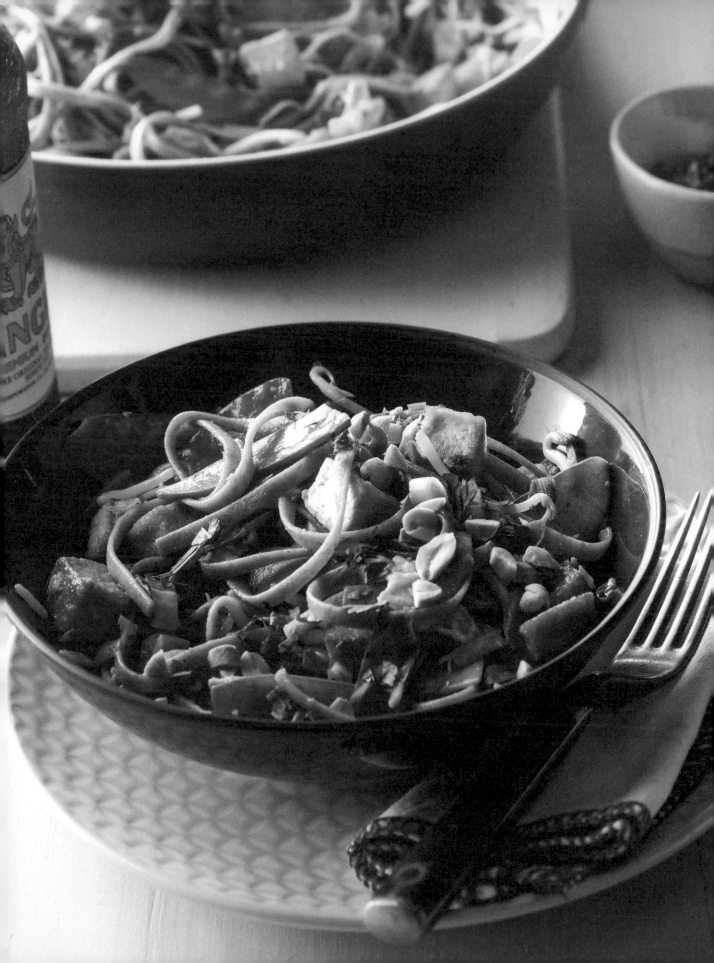

vegetable pad thai

Classic flavors of Thailand abound in this fragrant and flavorful dish featuring stir-fried vegetables, tofu, and whole-wheat noodles. New to tofu? This recipe gives the entree its satisfying protein, for a delicious way to introduce it to your diet.

- 1 PACKAGE (12 OUNCES) WHOLE-WHEAT FETTUCCINE
- ⅓ CUP REDUCED-SODIUM SOY SAUCE
- ¼ CUP RICE VINEGAR
- 2 TABLESPOONS BROWN SUGAR
- 1 TABLESPOON LIME JUICE
- 3 TEASPOONS CANOLA OIL
- 1 PACKAGE (12 OUNCES) EXTRA-FIRM TOFU, DRAINED AND CUT INTO ½-INCH CUBES
- 2 MEDIUM CARROTS, SHREDDED
- 2 CUPS FRESH SNOW PEAS, HALVED
- 3 CLOVES GARLIC, MINCED
- 2 CUPS BEAN SPROUTS
- 3 SCALLIONS, CHOPPED
- ½ CUP MINCED FRESH CILANTRO
- ¼ CUP UNSALTED PEANUTS, CHOPPED

1 In a large pot of boiling water, cook the fettuccine according to package directions.

2 While the pasta cooks, in a small bowl, whisk together the soy sauce, vinegar, brown sugar, and lime juice until smooth.

3 In a nonstick large skillet or wok, heat 2 teaspoons of oil over medium-high heat. Stir-fry the tofu for 5 minutes or until golden brown. Remove to a plate and keep warm. Stir-fry the carrots and snow peas in the remaining 1 teaspoon of oil for 2 minutes. Add the garlic and cook 1 minute or until the vegetables are crisp-tender.

4 Drain the pasta; add to the vegetable mixture. Stir in the vinegar mixture and add to the skillet. Bring to a boil. Add the tofu, bean sprouts, and scallions; heat through. Sprinkle with the cilantro and peanuts.

Makes 4 servings. Per serving: 501 calories, 12.3 g total fat (21% saturated), 48 g protein, 50 g carbohydrate, 5.9 g fiber, 172 mg cholesterol, 792 mg sodium

soba noodles with ginger-sesame dressing

Bright green edamame are whole, immature soybeans and a great way to sneak more soy into your diet. Look for them in the frozen vegetable section of the supermarket.

- ⅓ CUP REDUCED-SODIUM SOY SAUCE
- ¼ CUP PACKED BROWN SUGAR
- 2 TABLESPOONS RICE VINEGAR
- 2 TABLESPOONS CANOLA OIL
- 2 TABLESPOONS ORANGE JUICE
- 1 TABLESPOON MINCED FRESH GINGER
- 1 TEASPOON SESAME OIL
- 1 CLOVE GARLIC, MINCED
- 1 TEASPOON SRIRACHA CHILI SAUCE OR ½ TEASPOON HOT PEPPER SAUCE
- ½ POUND UNCOOKED JAPANESE SOBA NOODLES OR WHOLE-WHEAT LINGUINI
- 2 CUPS FROZEN SHELLED EDAMAME, THAWED
- 1 PACKAGE (14 OUNCES) COLESLAW MIX
- 1 CUP SHREDDED CARROTS
- 1 CUP THINLY SLICED SCALLIONS
- 3 TABLESPOONS SESAME SEEDS, TOASTED

1 In a small bowl, whisk together the soy sauce, sugar, vinegar, canola oil, orange juice, ginger, sesame oil, garlic, and Sriracha.

2 In a large pot of boiling water, cook the noodles according to package directions, adding the edamame during the last 5 minutes of cooking. Drain. Rinse the noodles and edamame in cold water; drain again.

3 To serve, in a large bowl, combine the coleslaw mix, carrots, scallions, noodles, and edamame. Add the soy mixture; toss to coat. Top with the sesame seeds.

Makes 4 servings. Per serving: 349 calories, 11 g total fat (9% saturated), 14 g protein, 54 g carbohydrate, 5 g fiber, 0 mg cholesterol, 816 mg sodium

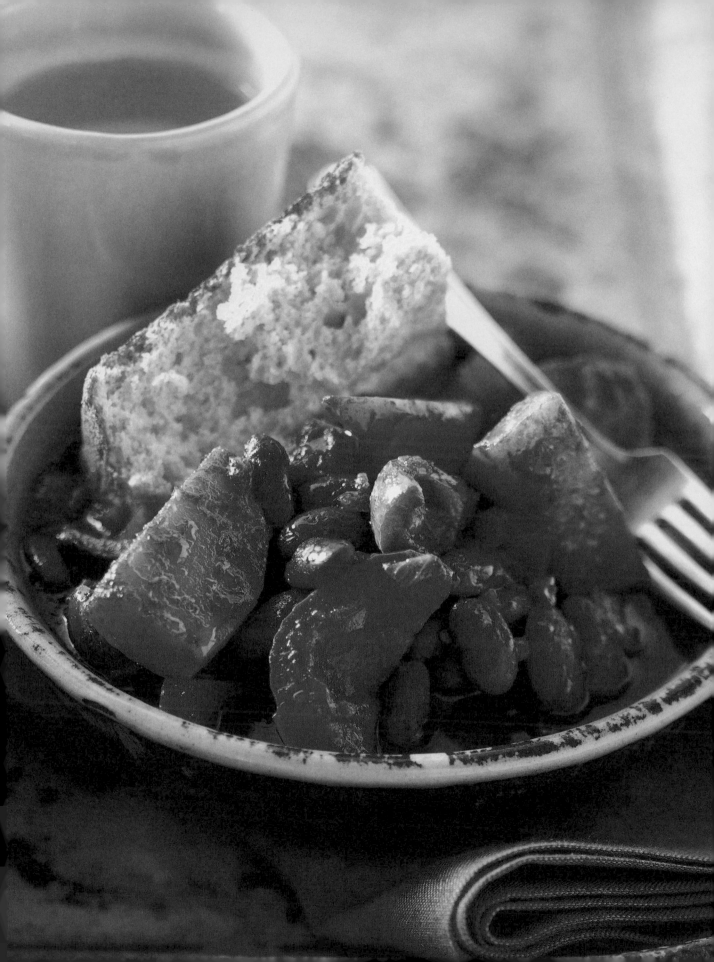

chunky chili

If you don't have the time to soak and cook dried beans, substitute 2½ cups of rinsed and drained canned beans. If you can't find chipotle peppers in adobo sauce (they're sold in cans and can be found in the international section of many supermarkets), substitute 1 teaspoon of hot chili powder.

1	CUP DRIED RED KIDNEY BEANS
1	TABLESPOON OLIVE OIL
1	LARGE ONION, FINELY CHOPPED
3	CLOVES GARLIC, MINCED
1	LARGE RED BELL PEPPER, CUT INTO ½-INCH CHUNKS
1	LARGE GREEN BELL PEPPER, CUT INTO ½-INCH CHUNKS
2	CUPS BUTTERNUT SQUASH (1-INCH) CUBES
2	TABLESPOONS UNSWEETENED COCOA POWDER
1	TABLESPOON LIGHT BROWN SUGAR
1	TEASPOON DRIED MARJORAM
½	TEASPOON SALT
1½	CUPS CANNED CRUSHED TOMATOES
1	CHIPOTLE PEPPER IN ADOBO, MINCED (2 TEASPOONS)

1 In a large saucepan, combine the kidney beans with water to cover by 3 inches; bring to a boil. Reduce to a simmer; cover and cook for 2¼ to 2½ hours, or until the beans are tender. Drain, reserving 1 cup of the liquid.

2 In a Dutch oven or flameproof casserole, heat the oil over medium heat. Add the onion and garlic, and cook for 7 minutes, or until tender. Stir in the bell peppers and butternut squash, and cook for 4 minutes, or until the peppers are crisp-tender. Add the cocoa powder, brown sugar, marjoram, and salt, stirring to coat.

3 Stir in the drained beans, the reserved liquid, the tomatoes, and chipotle pepper; bring to a boil. Reduce to a simmer; cover and cook for 30 minutes to blend the flavors.

Makes 4 servings. Per serving: 293 calories, 4.7 g total fat (16% saturated), 14 g protein, 54 g carbohydrate, 9.4 g fiber, 0 mg cholesterol, 477 mg sodium

stir-fried broccoli, shiitakes & new potatoes

Broccoli stalks are full of flavor (and nutrients). To use them, first separate them from the florets. Then trim the tough end of the stalks and peel off the tough outer layer. Thinly slice the peeled stalks crosswise and cook them along with the florets.

2	TABLESPOONS OLIVE OIL
12	OUNCES SMALL RED-SKINNED POTATOES, CUT INTO ½-INCH CHUNKS
¾	TEASPOON SALT
8	OUNCES FRESH SHIITAKE MUSHROOMS, STEMS DISCARDED AND CAPS QUARTERED
4	CUPS BROCCOLI FLORETS AND SLICED STALKS
3	SCALLIONS, THINLY SLICED
4	CLOVES GARLIC, MINCED

1 In a large skillet, heat the oil over medium heat. Add the potatoes and ¼ teaspoon of the salt; cook, stirring frequently for 10 minutes, or until the potatoes are golden brown.

2 Add the mushrooms. Reduce the heat to low; cover and cook for 4 minutes, or until the mushrooms have softened.

3 Add the broccoli, scallions, and garlic; cook, stirring frequently for 2 minutes, or until the scallions are tender. Add ¾ cup of water and the remaining ½ teaspoon salt, and cook, uncovered, for 5 minutes, or until the broccoli is crisp-tender.

Makes 4 servings. Per serving: 170 calories, 7.2 g total fat (13% saturated), 6 g protein, 24 g carbohydrate, 4.6 g fiber, 0 mg cholesterol, 467 mg sodium

artichokes with lentils & lima beans

A wonderful combination of textures and flavors, this vegetarian dish is also a nutritional powerhouse: One serving provides a very healthy dose of fiber, potassium, and beta-carotene.

 4 LARGE ARTICHOKES
 3 TABLESPOONS FRESH LEMON JUICE
 1 TABLESPOON OLIVE OIL
 1 SMALL ONION, FINELY CHOPPED
 3 CLOVES GARLIC, MINCED
 1 LARGE CARROT, DICED
 ¾ CUP LENTILS, PICKED OVER AND RINSED
 1½ CUPS CARROT JUICE
 ¾ TEASPOON SALT
 ½ TEASPOON DRIED THYME
 10 OUNCES LIMA BEANS

1 To trim the artichokes: Remove the tough outer leaves. Trim the tough end of the stem; then, with a paring knife, peel the tough skin off the remaining stem. Cut off the top of the artichoke to just about 1 inch above the base. Halve the artichokes lengthwise, then scoop out and discard the chokes. Halve the artichokes again. Place the cleaned artichokes in a bowl with cold water to cover. Add 1 tablespoon of the lemon juice; set aside.

2 In a Dutch oven, heat the oil over medium heat. Add the onion and garlic; cook, stirring frequently for 5 minutes, or until the onion is golden brown. Stir in the carrot, and cook for 4 minutes.

3 Remove the artichokes from the water and place in the Dutch oven. Stir in the lentils, the remaining 2 tablespoons lemon juice, the carrot juice, salt, thyme, and 1 cup of water; bring to a boil. Reduce to a simmer; cover and cook for 25 minutes.

4 Stir in the lima beans, and cook for 10 minutes, or until the artichokes, lima beans, and lentils are tender.

Makes 4 servings. Per serving: 367 calories, 4 g total fat (25% saturated), 22 g protein, 67 g carbohydrate, 18 g fiber, 0 mg cholesterol, 907 mg sodium

bok choy, tofu & mushroom stir-fry

In addition to the phytoestrogens from the tofu, this stir-fry is also rich in calcium, selenium, beta-carotene, and vitamin C.

 15 OUNCES EXTRA-FIRM TOFU
 3 TABLESPOONS REDUCED-SODIUM SOY SAUCE
 4 TEASPOONS DARK BROWN SUGAR
 1½ TEASPOONS CORNSTARCH
 4 TEASPOONS OLIVE OIL
 4 SCALLIONS, THINLY SLICED
 2 TABLESPOONS MINCED FRESH GINGER
 3 CLOVES GARLIC, MINCED
 8 OUNCES FRESH SHIITAKE MUSHROOMS, STEMS REMOVED AND CAPS QUARTERED
 8 OUNCES BUTTON MUSHROOMS, HALVED
 1 LARGE HEAD BOK CHOY, SLICED CROSSWISE INTO 1-INCH STRIPS

1 Halve the block of tofu horizontally, then cut each piece into 12 squares or triangles; set aside. In a small bowl, whisk together the soy sauce, brown sugar, cornstarch, and ½ cup of water; set aside.

2 In a large nonstick skillet, heat 2 teaspoons of the oil over medium heat. Add the scallions, ginger, and garlic; cook for 1 minute, or until tender.

3 Stir in the shiitake and button mushrooms. Add ½ cup of water; cover and cook, stirring occasionally for 5 minutes, or until the mushrooms are tender. Transfer to a bowl.

4 Add the remaining 2 teaspoons oil and the bok choy to the pan; cook, stirring frequently for 5 minutes, or until the bok choy is tender.

5 Return the mushroom-scallion mixture to the pan and add the tofu. Stir the soy sauce mixture to recombine, and add it to the pan. Cook for 2 minutes, or until the tofu is heated through and the vegetables are coated with the sauce.

Makes 4 servings. Per serving: 240 calories, 11 g total fat (11% saturated), 20 g protein, 20 g carbohydrate, 4 g fiber, 0 mg cholesterol, 615 mg sodium

bok choy, tofu & mushroom stir-fry ▶

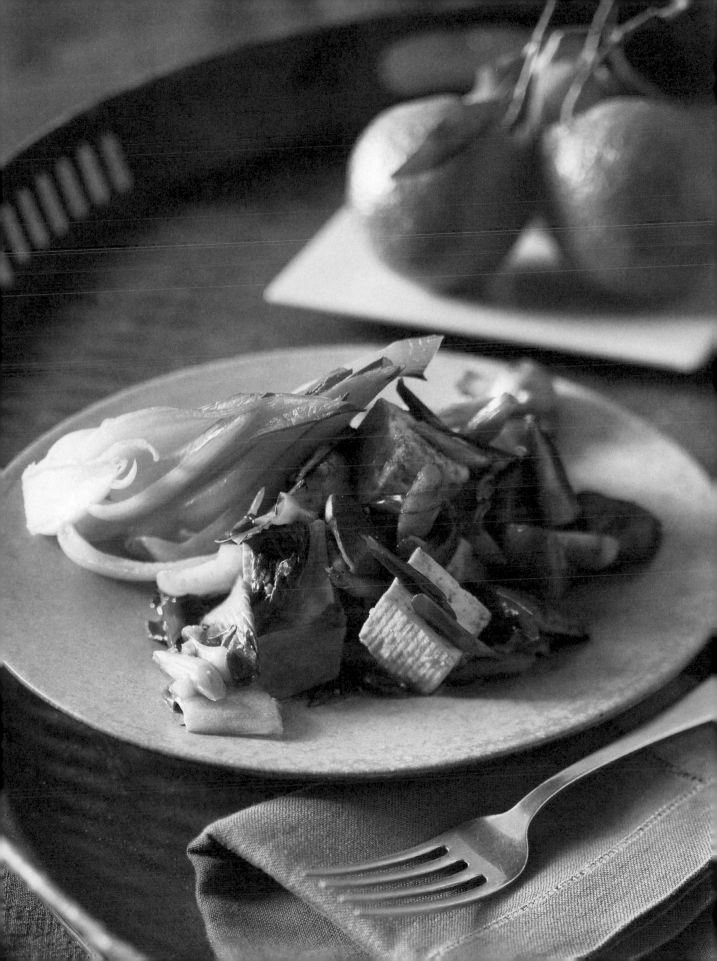

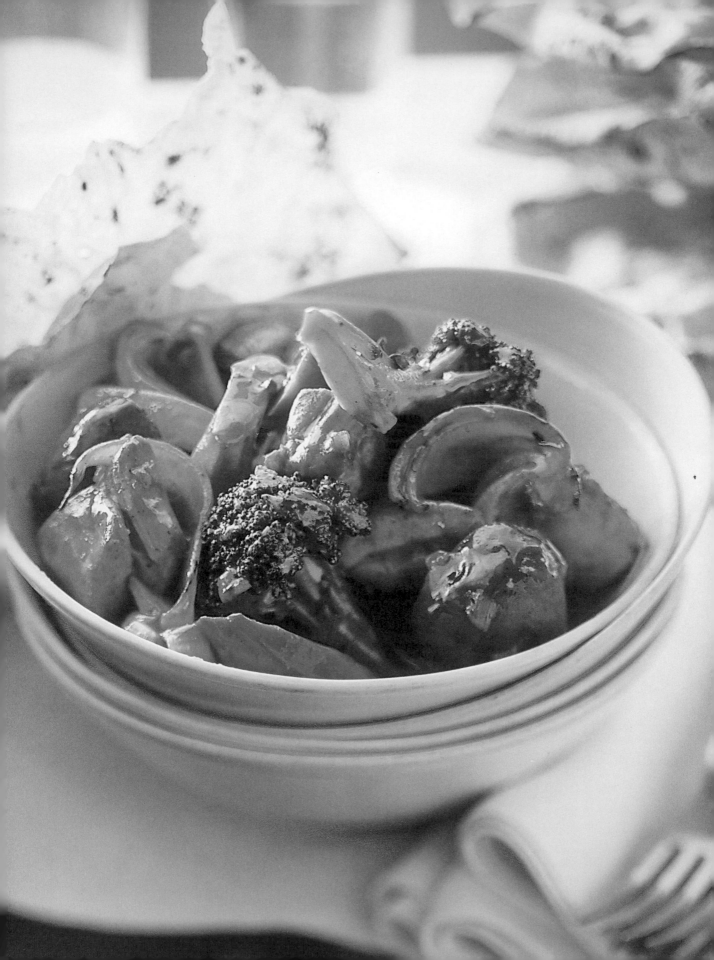

rich curried vegetables

The homemade curry powder for this vegetable dish has an especially high proportion of phytonutrient-rich turmeric and ginger.

- 1 TABLESPOON TURMERIC
- 1½ TEASPOONS GROUND GINGER
- 1 TEASPOON SALT
- ½ TEASPOON CINNAMON
- ½ TEASPOON SUGAR
- ½ TEASPOON PEPPER
- 2 TEASPOONS OLIVE OIL
- 1 MEDIUM ONION, HALVED AND THICKLY SLICED
- 4 CLOVES GARLIC, MINCED
- 3 CARROTS, THICKLY SLICED
- 1½ CUPS BUTTERNUT SQUASH (1-INCH) CUBES
- 1 POUND SMALL RED-SKINNED POTATOES, QUARTERED
- 2 TEASPOONS CREAMY PEANUT BUTTER
- 4 CUPS BROCCOLI FLORETS

1 In a medium bowl, stir together the turmeric, ginger, salt, cinnamon, sugar, and pepper.

2 In a nonstick Dutch oven, heat the oil over medium heat. Add the onion and garlic, and cook, stirring frequently for 7 minutes, or until the onion is tender. Stir in the spice mixture and cook for 1 minute.

3 Add 2½ cups of water, the carrots, butternut squash, potatoes, and peanut butter and bring to a boil. Reduce to a simmer; cover and cook for 20 minutes, or until the potatoes and squash are tender.

4 Add the broccoli; cover and cook for 5 minutes, or until the broccoli is tender.

Makes 4 servings. *Per serving: 234 calories, 7 g total fat (13% saturated), 18 g protein, 38 g carbohydrate, 8 g fiber, 0 mg cholesterol, 414 mg sodium*

penne with kale and onion

Kale, garlic, and onion bring an array of phytonutrients, including plant-based calcium, to this quick pasta dish. Add a can of low-sodium beans for a hearty dinner ready in less than 20 minutes.

- 2 TABLESPOONS OLIVE OIL
- 1 MEDIUM ONION, SLICED
- 8 CLOVES GARLIC, THINLY SLICED
- 3 CUPS WHOLE-GRAIN PENNE PASTA
- 6 CUPS CHOPPED FRESH KALE
- ½ TEASPOON SALT

1 In a large skillet, heat 1 tablespoon oil over medium heat. Add the onion and cook, stirring frequently for 15 minutes or until the onion is golden brown. Add the garlic and cook for 1 minute.

2 While the onion cooks, in a large pot, cook the penne according to package directions, adding the kale to the boiling water after 5 minutes. Drain; reserve ½ cup of the pasta cooking water.

3 To serve, place the pasta in a large bowl. Drizzle with the remaining 1 tablespoon of oil, the salt, onion mixture, and some of the pasta water until of the desired consistency.

Makes 4 servings. *Per serving: 287 calories, 7.5 g total fat (20% saturated), 9 g protein, 46 g carbohydrate, 3 g fiber, 0 mg cholesterol, 309 mg sodium*

coconut-ginger chickpeas & tomatoes

Warming ginger and jalapeño add zest to chickpeas and tomatoes in a broth of cooling coconut milk. Delicious as is, adding steamed greens such as bok choy or spinach will enhance the flavor and boost the phytonutrients of this dish.

- 2 TABLESPOONS CANOLA OIL
- 2 MEDIUM ONIONS, CHOPPED
- 3 LARGE TOMATOES, SEEDED AND CHOPPED
- 1 JALAPEÑO PEPPER, SEEDED AND CHOPPED
- 1 TABLESPOON MINCED FRESH GINGER
- 2 CANS (15 OUNCES EACH) CHICKPEAS, DRAINED AND RINSED
- ½ TEASPOON SALT
- 1 CUP LIGHT COCONUT MILK
- 3 TABLESPOONS MINCED FRESH CILANTRO
- 4½ CUPS HOT COOKED BROWN RICE

1 In a large skillet, heat the oil over medium-high heat. Add the onions; cook, stirring frequently for 5 minutes or until browned. Add the tomatoes, jalapeño, and ginger; cook, stirring for 3 minutes or until the vegetables are tender.

2 Stir in the chickpeas, ¼ cup of water, and salt; bring to a boil. Reduce to a simmer, and cook, uncovered for 5 minutes or until the liquid is almost evaporated. Remove from the heat; stir in the coconut milk and cilantro. Serve over the rice.

Makes 6 servings. Per serving: 402 calories, 12 g total fat (25% saturated), 11 g protein, 65 g carbohydrate, 10 g fiber, 0 mg cholesterol, 397 mg sodium

broiled marinated tofu

These marinated tofu "steaks" can be served hot, cold, or at room temperature. Serve 4 tofu triangles as a main course (perhaps on a bed of shredded spinach), or serve 2 to 3 as a first course or as part of a buffet. If you can find pressed tofu, skip step 1.

- 2 BLOCKS (16 OUNCES EACH) FIRM TOFU
- ¼ CUP REDUCED-SODIUM SOY SAUCE
- 2 TABLESPOONS FRESH LEMON JUICE
- 4 TEASPOONS DARK BROWN SUGAR
- 2 TEASPOONS DARK SESAME OIL
- 4 TEASPOONS SESAME SEEDS
- 4 SCALLIONS, THINLY SLICED

1 Slice each block of tofu in half horizontally. Lay the 4 pieces of tofu on a cutting board and place a can or small bowl under one end of the board to tilt it slightly. Set the board so that the low end hangs over the sink. Cover the tofu with paper towels, place another cutting board on top and weight it with a heavy pan or a couple of cans. Let drain for 2 hours.

2 In a shallow container large enough to hold the tofu in a single layer, whisk together the soy sauce, lemon juice, sugar, and sesame oil. Place the pressed tofu in the pan and let stand for 3 hours, or until the marinade has been absorbed about halfway up the tofu, turning once (there should still be some marinade in the container).

3 Preheat the broiler. Remove the tofu from the marinade, reserving any leftover. Place the tofu on a broiler pan, and broil 6 inches from the heat for 5 minutes per side, or until richly browned.

4 Meanwhile, in a small skillet, toast the sesame seeds over low heat for 3 minutes, or until golden.

5 To serve, cut each piece of tofu into 4 triangles and sprinkle with the scallions, sesame seeds, and any leftover marinade.

Makes 4 servings. Per serving: 461 calories, 27 g total fat (14% saturated), 44 g protein, 20 g carbohydrate, 0.7 g fiber, 0 mg cholesterol, 642 mg sodium

broiled marinated tofu ▶

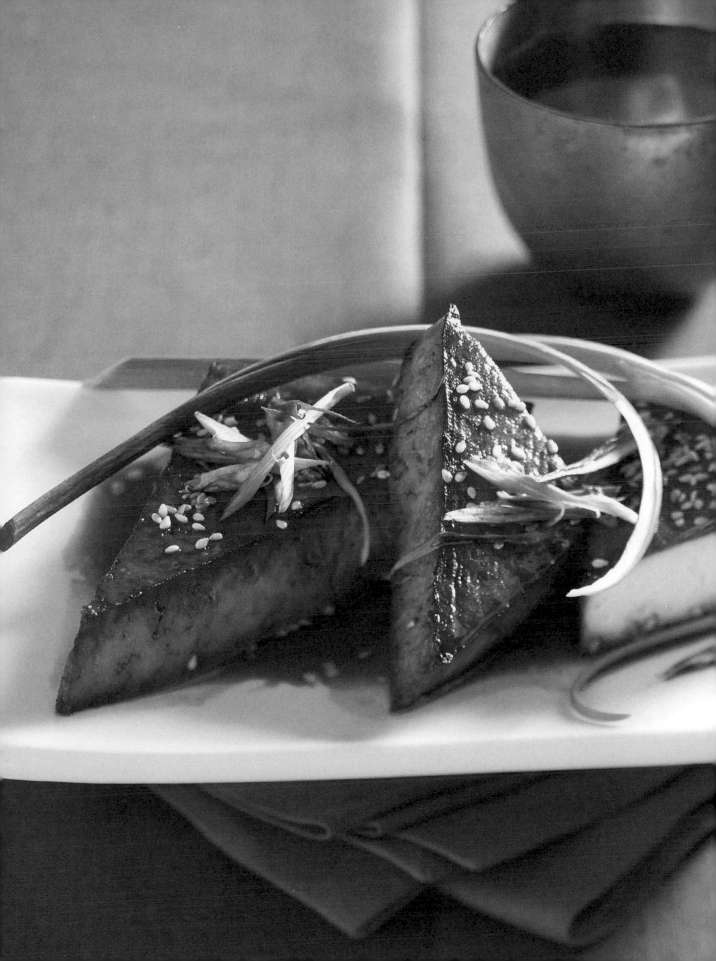

roasted harvest vegetables

Fall and winter vegetables stand up well to roasting, and you can easily mix and match. You could make this with parsnips or carrots instead of brussels sprouts, or throw in some small onions. This particular combination is rich in fiber, potassium, beta-carotene, and calcium (most of which comes from the squash and brussels sprouts, not the Parmesan!).

- 3 TABLESPOONS OLIVE OIL
- 6 CLOVES GARLIC, SLICED
- 3 CUPS BUTTERNUT SQUASH (1-INCH) CUBES
- 10 OUNCES BRUSSELS SPROUTS, TRIMMED AND HALVED LENGTHWISE
- 8 OUNCES FRESH SHIITAKE MUSHROOMS, STEMS DISCARDED AND CAPS THICKLY SLICED
- 2 LARGE RED APPLES (UNPEELED), CUT INTO 1-INCH CHUNKS
- ¼ CUP OIL-PACKED SUN-DRIED TOMATOES, DRAINED AND THINLY SLICED
- 1 TEASPOON DRIED ROSEMARY, MINCED
- ½ TEASPOON SALT
- ¼ CUP DAIRY-FREE PARMESAN

1 Preheat the oven to 400°F. In a large roasting pan, combine the olive oil and garlic. Heat for 3 minutes in the oven. Add the squash, brussels sprouts, mushrooms, apples, sun-dried tomatoes, rosemary, and salt; toss to combine.

2 Roast for 35 minutes, or until the vegetables are tender; toss the vegetables every 10 minutes. Sprinkle the Parmesan over the vegetables, and roast for 5 minutes.

Makes 4 servings. Per serving: 237 calories, 10 g total fat (0% saturated), 3 g protein, 39 g carbohydrate, 9.3 g fiber, 0 mg cholesterol, 269 mg sodium

braised artichokes, potatoes & peas

In order to preserve the most fiber and phyto-nutrients in the artichokes, they are not trimmed all the way down to their hearts: A good 1 inch of the leaves is left on.

- 4 LARGE ARTICHOKES
- 4 TABLESPOONS FRESH LEMON JUICE
- 2 TABLESPOONS OLIVE OIL
- 1 SMALL RED ONION, FINELY CHOPPED
- 3 CLOVES GARLIC, MINCED
- ¾ TEASPOON DRIED MARJORAM
- ¾ TEASPOON SALT
- 1 POUND SMALL RED-SKINNED POTATOES, CUT INTO ½-INCH CUBES
- 1½ CUPS FROZEN PEAS
- ½ CUP CHOPPED PARSLEY

1 To trim the artichokes: Remove the tough outer leaves. Trim the tough end of the stem; then, with a paring knife, peel off the tough skin of the remaining stem. Cut off the top of the artichoke to just about 1 inch above the base. Halve the artichokes; scoop out and discard the chokes. Halve the artichokes again. Place the cleaned artichokes in a bowl with cold water to cover. Add 1 tablespoon of the lemon juice and set aside.

2 In a large skillet, heat the oil over medium heat. Add the onion and garlic, and cook, stirring frequently for 5 minutes, or until the onion is light golden.

3 Lift the artichokes from the water and add them to the skillet, stirring to coat. Add 1½ cups of water, the remaining 3 tablespoons lemon juice, the marjoram, and ¼ teaspoon of the salt; bring to a boil. Reduce to a simmer; cover and cook for 10 minutes.

4 Stir in the potatoes and the remaining ½ teaspoon of salt; cover and cook for 15 to 20 minutes, or until the potatoes and artichokes are tender.

5 Stir in the peas and parsley; cover and cook for 5 minutes, or until the peas are heated through.

Makes 4 servings. Per serving: 289 calories, 7.5 g total fat (13% saturated), 11 g protein, 50 g carbohydrate, 13 g fiber, 0 mg cholesterol, 662 mg sodium

roasted harvest vegetables ▶

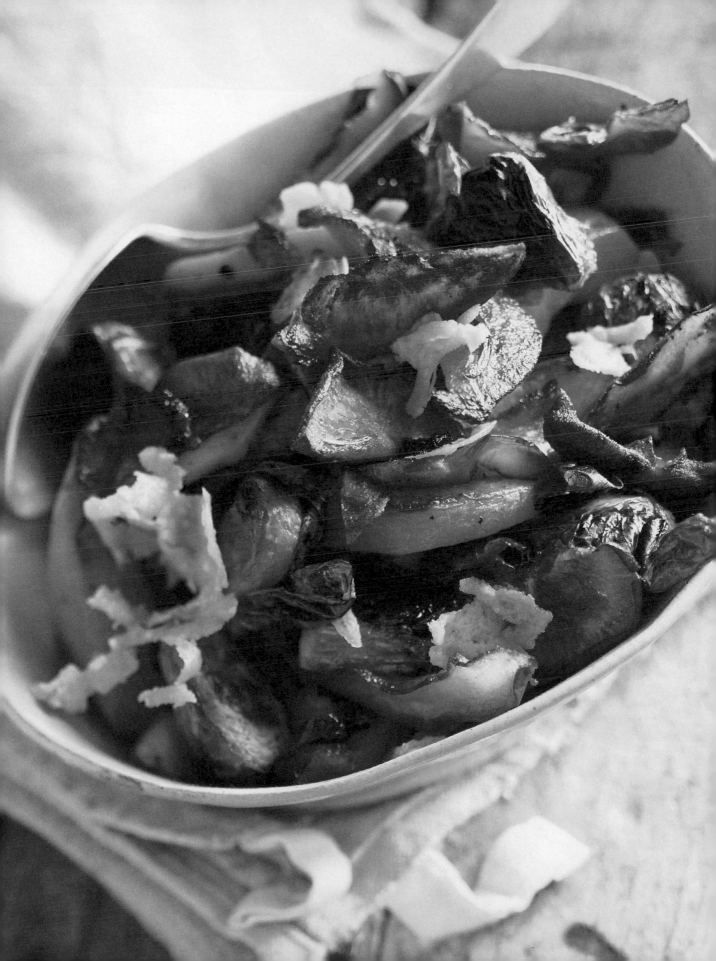

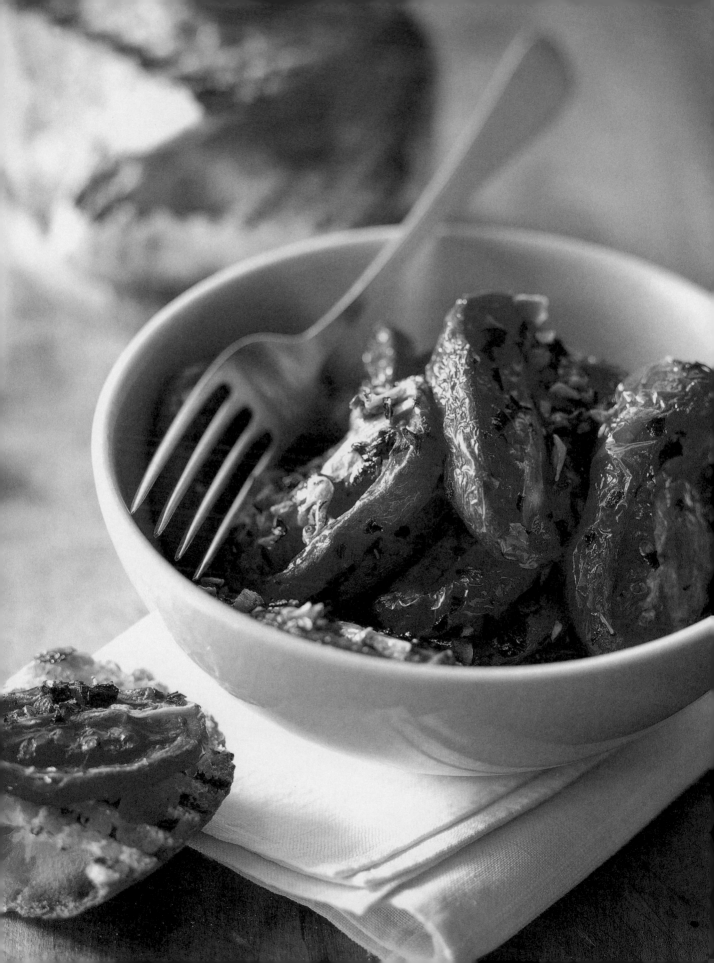

roasted tomatoes with garlic & herbs

Even in the winter months, when plum tomatoes are not at their best, these taste like a burst of summer. Although they do bake a long time, they require very little attention. Once baked, they'll keep for several days in the refrigerator. Eat them as is or use them in pasta sauces and salads.

- 3 POUNDS PLUM TOMATOES, HALVED LENGTHWISE
- 2 TABLESPOONS OLIVE OIL
- 5 CLOVES GARLIC, MINCED
- ½ CUP FINELY CHOPPED FRESH BASIL
- 2 TABLESPOONS MINCED FRESH ROSEMARY
- 1 TEASPOON SUGAR
- ¾ TEASPOON SALT

1 Preheat the oven to 250°F. Line a large rimmed baking sheet with foil.

2 In a large bowl, toss the tomatoes with the oil, garlic, basil, rosemary, sugar, and salt. Place the tomatoes cut-side up in the prepared pan, and bake for 3 hours, or until the tomatoes have collapsed and their skins have wrinkled.

3 Serve at room temperature or chilled.

Makes 4 servings. *Per serving: 148 calories, 8 g total fat (13% saturated), 4 g protein, 19 g carbohydrate, 5.4 g fiber, 0 mg cholesterol, 468 mg sodium*

roasted jerusalem artichokes & garlic

Also known as sunchokes, Jerusalem artichokes have a creamy consistency and nutty flavor when roasted. They are a rich source of inulin, which may prove helpful in maintaining the balance between good and bad bacteria in the intestines.

- 2 TABLESPOONS OLIVE OIL
- 12 CLOVES GARLIC, UNPEELED
- 1 TABLESPOON DRIED ROSEMARY, MINCED
- 2 POUNDS JERUSALEM ARTICHOKES, WELL SCRUBBED AND SLICED ½ INCH THICK
- ½ TEASPOON SALT

1 Preheat the oven to 400°F. In a roasting pan large enough to hold the Jerusalem artichokes in a single layer, combine the oil, garlic, and rosemary. Heat the pan in the oven for 3 to 5 minutes, or until the oil begins to sizzle.

2 Add the Jerusalem artichokes, and toss well to coat with the oil. Roast the artichokes, shaking the pan occasionally, for 35 to 40 minutes, or until the artichokes are tender. Sprinkle the salt over the artichokes and serve.

Makes 4 servings. *Per serving: 248 calories, 6.9 g total fat (14% saturated), 5 g protein, 43 g carbohydrate, 4.2 g fiber, 0 mg cholesterol, 301 mg sodium*

colorful stuffed peppers with feta

The bean mixture used to stuff these peppers has seasonings (cocoa, cinnamon, oregano, and raisins) that are reminiscent of a Latin American meat dish called picadillo.

- 1 LARGE RED BELL PEPPER, HALVED LENGTHWISE AND SEEDED
- 1 LARGE GREEN BELL PEPPER, HALVED LENGTHWISE AND SEEDED
- 1 TABLESPOON OLIVE OIL
- 1 LARGE RED ONION, FINELY CHOPPED
- 5 CLOVES GARLIC, MINCED
- 1 CAN (15 OUNCES) CANNELLINI BEANS, DRAINED AND RINSED
- 2 TABLESPOONS TOMATO PASTE
- 2 TEASPOONS SESAME SEEDS
- 1½ TEASPOONS UNSWEETENED COCOA POWDER
- ½ TEASPOON DRIED OREGANO
- ½ TEASPOON GROUND CINNAMON
- ¼ TEASPOON SALT
- 1½ CUPS CANNED CRUSHED TOMATOES
- ½ CUP RAISINS
- 2 OUNCES DAIRY-FREE FETA

1 In a vegetable steamer, cook the pepper halves, cut-side down, for 10 minutes, or until crisp-tender.

2 Meanwhile, in a medium nonstick skillet, heat the oil over low heat. Add the onion and garlic, and cook for 5 minutes, or until the onion is golden brown. Measure out ¼ cup of the onion mixture and transfer to a bowl. Add the beans and tomato paste to the bowl, and mash with a potato masher or a spoon.

3 To the onion mixture remaining in the skillet, add the sesame seeds, cocoa powder, oregano, cinnamon, and salt; cook for 1 minute. Stir in the crushed tomatoes and raisins; bring to a boil. Reduce to a simmer; cover and cook for 5 minutes to blend the flavors. Transfer to a food processor or blender and puree.

4 Return the puree to the skillet and stir in ⅓ cup of water. Add the steamed peppers, cut-side up. Spoon the bean mixture into the peppers; cover and cook for 5 minutes, or until the bean mixture is heated through. Spoon a little of the sauce over the beans and sprinkle with the feta; cover and cook for 2 minutes to melt the feta.

5 To serve, spoon some of the sauce onto each plate; top with a pepper half and a little more sauce.

Makes 4 servings. Per serving: 288 calories, 10 g total fat (37% saturated), 8 g protein, 42 g carbohydrate, 9.2 g fiber, 0 mg cholesterol, 527 mg sodium

garlic mashed potatoes & peas

Here's comfort food at its best. Plant-based sour cream adds a slight tang to these mashed potatoes, while tarragon underscores the sweetness of the peas. Lots of garlic and sautéed scallions round out the flavors.

- 1½ POUNDS BAKING POTATOES, PEELED AND CUT INTO LARGE CHUNKS
- 8 CLOVES GARLIC, PEELED AND CRUSHED
- 1 TEASPOON SALT
- 1½ CUPS FROZEN PEAS
- ½ CUP DAIRY-FREE SOUR CREAM
- 1 TEASPOON DRIED TARRAGON
- 1 TABLESPOON OLIVE OIL
- 8 SCALLIONS, THINLY SLICED

1 In a large saucepan, combine the potatoes, garlic, ¼ teaspoon of the salt, and water to cover by 1 inch; bring to a boil. Reduce to a simmer and cook for 20 minutes, or until the potatoes are tender. Add the peas, and cook for 1 minute. Drain.

2 Return the potatoes, peas, and garlic to the saucepan. Add the remaining ¾ teaspoon salt, sour cream, and tarragon. With a potato masher, mash the potatoes until creamy.

3 In a small skillet, heat the oil over medium heat. Add the scallions, and cook for 3 minutes, or until very soft. Stir the scallions into the mashed potato mixture, and cook over low heat until the potatoes are heated through.

Makes 4 servings. Per serving: 205 calories, 4 g total fat (17% saturated), 8 g protein, 36 g carbohydrate, 4.9 g fiber, 0 mg cholesterol, 689 mg sodium

grilled veggie tortillas

Similar to a pizza, these grilled tortillas are loaded with antioxidant-rich vegetables. Best with fresh herbs, you can substitute 1 teaspoon dried Italian seasoning if desired.

- 2 TABLESPOONS PLANT-BASED MAYONNAISE
- 1 TABLESPOON PREPARED PESTO
- 1½ TEASPOONS MINCED FRESH BASIL
- 1½ TEASPOONS MINCED FRESH OREGANO
- 1 SMALL ZUCCHINI, CUT LENGTHWISE INTO ½-INCH SLICES
- 1 SMALL YELLOW SUMMER SQUASH, CUT LENGTHWISE INTO ½-INCH SLICES
- ½ SMALL RED BELL PEPPER, CUT IN HALF
- 1 TABLESPOON OLIVE OIL
- ¼ TEASPOON SALT
- 1 SMALL TOMATO, CHOPPED
- 2 WHOLE-WHEAT TORTILLAS (8 INCHES)
- ½ CUP DAIRY-FREE MOZZARELLA SHREDS

1 Preheat the grill to medium heat. In a small bowl, combine the mayonnaise, pesto, basil, and oregano.

2 Brush the zucchini, summer squash, and pepper with 2½ teaspoons of oil. Sprinkle with the salt. Grill the vegetables over medium heat for 4 minutes on each side or until tender. Cut the vegetables into ½-inch chunks and place in a small bowl; stir in the tomato.

3 Brush both sides of the tortillas with the remaining ½ teaspoon of oil. Grill 1 side for 3 minutes or until puffed. Transfer to a cutting board.

4 Spread the grilled sides of the tortillas with the mayonnaise mixture. Top with the vegetable mixture and sprinkle with the shreds. Grill, covered, for 3 minutes or until the shreds are melted.

Makes 4 servings. Per serving: 420 calories, 26 g total fat (42% saturated), 9 g protein, 36 g carbohydrate, 5 g fiber, 0 mg cholesterol, 795 mg sodium

eggplant-portobello sandwich loaf

Grilled eggplant and portobello mushrooms fill this hearty sandwich with a touch of marinara and basil. This recipe works well in the oven too; just broil the vegetables and sandwich, adding 3 to 5 more minutes to the cook times.

- 1 LOAF (1 POUND) WHOLE-GRAIN ITALIAN BREAD
- ½ CUP OLIVE OIL
- 2 TEASPOONS MINCED GARLIC
- 1 TEASPOON ITALIAN SEASONING
- ½ TEASPOON SALT
- ¼ TEASPOON PEPPER
- 1 LARGE EGGPLANT (1 POUND), CUT INTO 1/2-INCH SLICES
- 1 PACKAGE (6 OUNCES) SLICED PORTOBELLO MUSHROOMS
- 1 CUP MARINARA SAUCE
- 2 TABLESPOONS MINCED FRESH BASIL
- ½ CUP DAIRY-FREE MOZZARELLA SHREDS

1 Cut the bread lengthwise in half. Carefully hollow out the top and bottom, leaving a ½-inch shell; set aside. In a small bowl, combine the oil, garlic, Italian seasoning, salt, and pepper. Brush over the eggplant and mushrooms.

2 Grill the eggplant and mushrooms, covered, over medium heat for 5 minutes on each side, or until the vegetables are tender.

3 Spread half of the marinara sauce over the bottom piece of bread. Top with the eggplant and mushrooms. Spread with the remaining sauce; top with the basil and mozzarella. Cover with the bread top.

4 Wrap the loaf in a large piece of heavy-duty foil (about 28 inches x 18 inches); seal tightly. Grill, covered, over medium heat for 4 minutes on each side.

Makes 4 servings. Per serving: 522 calories, 30 g total fat (13% saturated fat), 10 g protein, 60 g carbohydrate, 7 g fiber, 2 mg cholesterol, 795 mg sodium

lentil sloppy joes

Enjoy these finger-licking sandwiches bursting with antioxidant-rich vegetables and lentils. So tasty, no one will ever notice the protein is from lentils. Store leftover sloppy joe mixture in the refrigerator for up to 4 days or freeze for up to 3 months.

- 2 TABLESPOONS OLIVE OIL
- 1 LARGE SWEET ONION, COARSELY CHOPPED
- 1 MEDIUM GREEN BELL PEPPER, COARSELY CHOPPED
- 1 MEDIUM RED BELL PEPPER, COARSELY CHOPPED
- 1 MEDIUM CARROT, SHREDDED
- 6 CLOVES GARLIC, MINCED
- 2½ CUPS REDUCED-SODIUM VEGETABLE BROTH
- 1 CUP DRIED RED LENTILS, RINSED
- 5 PLUM TOMATOES, CHOPPED
- 1 CAN (8 OUNCES) TOMATO SAUCE
- 2 TABLESPOONS CHILI POWDER
- 2 TABLESPOONS YELLOW MUSTARD
- 4½ TEASPOONS CIDER VINEGAR
- 2 TEASPOONS VEGAN WORCESTERSHIRE SAUCE
- 2 TEASPOONS HONEY
- 1½ TEASPOONS TOMATO PASTE
- ¼ TEASPOON SALT
- ⅛ TEASPOON PEPPER
- 14 WHOLE-WHEAT HAMBURGER BUNS, SPLIT AND TOASTED

1 In a large skillet, heat the oil over medium-high heat. Add the onion, peppers, and carrot and cook, stirring frequently for 7 minutes or until the vegetables are tender. Add the garlic and cook for 1 minute.

2 Stir in the broth and lentils and bring to a boil. Reduce to a simmer; cook, uncovered, stirring occasionally, for about 15 minutes or until the lentils are tender.

3 Stir in the chopped tomatoes, tomato sauce, chili powder, mustard, vinegar, Worcestershire sauce, honey, tomato paste, salt, and pepper. Bring to a boil. Reduce to a simmer; cook, uncovered, for 10 minutes or until thickened. Serve on the buns.

Makes 14 servings. Per serving: 522 calories, 30 g total fat (13% saturated fat), 10 g protein, 60 g carbohydrate, 7 g fiber, 2 mg cholesterol, 795 mg sodium

grilled bean burgers

These juicy veggie patties have major flavor from cumin, garlic, and a little chili powder. They hold their own against any veggie burger available at the supermarket.

- 1 TABLESPOON OLIVE OIL
- 1 LARGE ONION, FINELY CHOPPED
- 4 CLOVES GARLIC, MINCED
- 1 MEDIUM CARROT, SHREDDED
- 1½ TEASPOONS CHILI POWDER
- 1 TEASPOON GROUND CUMIN
- ¼ TEASPOON PEPPER
- 1 CAN (15 OUNCES) PINTO BEANS, RINSED AND DRAINED
- 1 CAN (15 OUNCES) BLACK BEANS, RINSED AND DRAINED
- 2 TABLESPOONS DIJON MUSTARD
- 2 TABLESPOONS REDUCED-SODIUM SOY SAUCE
- 1 TABLESPOON KETCHUP
- 1½ CUPS QUICK-COOKING OATS
- 8 WHOLE-WHEAT HAMBURGER BUNS, SPLIT
- 8 LETTUCE LEAVES
- ½ CUP SALSA

1 In a large nonstick skillet, heat the oil over medium-high heat; cook the onion for 2 minutes. Add the garlic and cook, stirring frequently for 1 minute. Stir in the carrot, chili powder, cumin, and pepper; cook, stirring frequently for 3 minutes or until the carrot is tender. Remove from heat.

2 In a large bowl, mash the pinto and black beans using a potato masher. Stir in the mustard, soy sauce, ketchup, and carrot mixture. Add the oats, mixing well. Shape into eight 3½-inch patties.

3 Place the burgers on an oiled grill rack over medium heat or on a greased rack of a broiler pan. Grill, covered, or broil 4 inches from the heat until lightly browned and heated through, 4 to 5 minutes per side. Serve on buns with the lettuce and salsa.

Makes 8 servings. Per serving: 305 calories, 5 g total fat (1 g saturated), 12 g protein, 54 g carbohydrate, 10 g fiber, 0 mg cholesterol, 736 mg sodium

lentil sloppy joes ▶

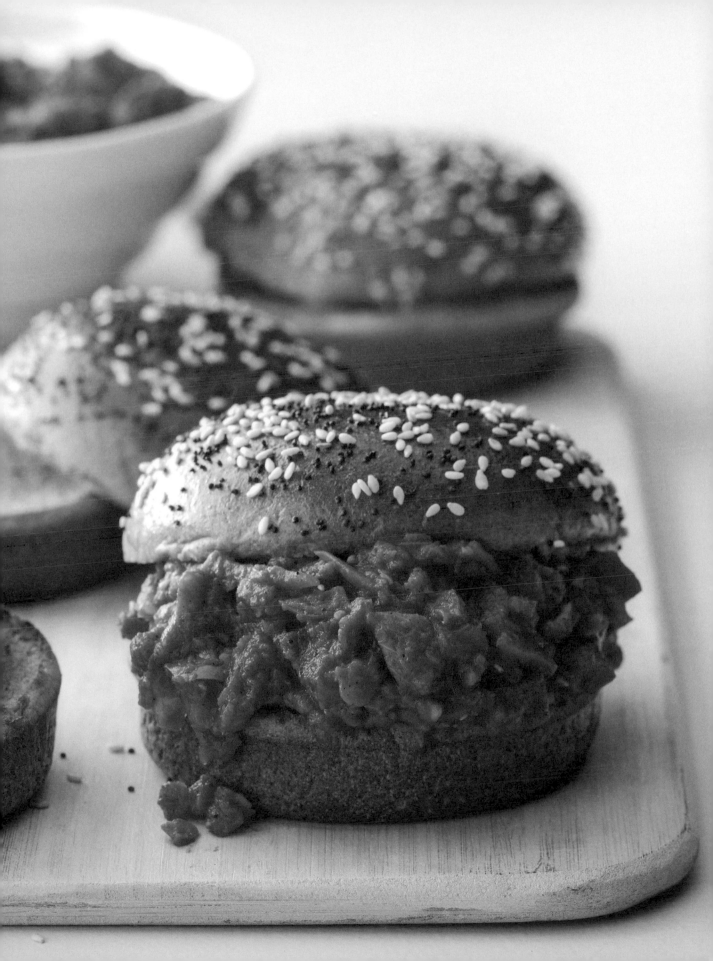

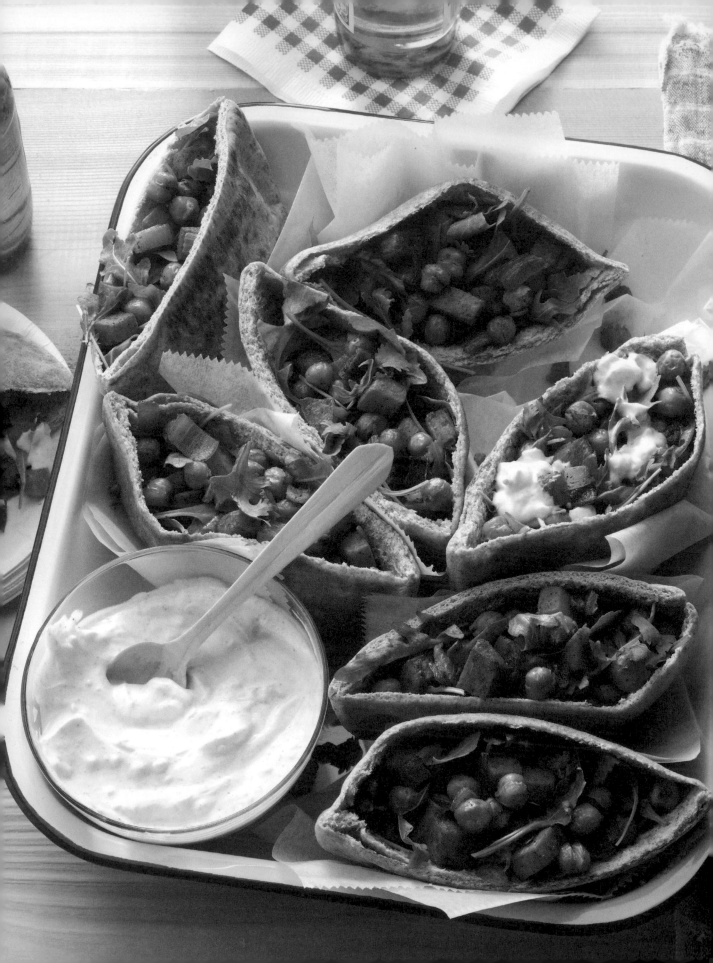

roasted sweet potato & chickpea pitas

Here's a hearty take on Mediterranean food, this time with sweet potatoes tucked inside. These unique pockets are delicious for lunch or dinner.

2   MEDIUM SWEET POTATOES (ABOUT 1¼ POUNDS), PEELED AND CUBED

2   CANS (15 OUNCES EACH) CHICKPEAS, RINSED AND DRAINED

1   MEDIUM RED ONION, FINELY CHOPPED

2   TEASPOONS GARAM MASALA

3   TABLESPOONS OLIVE OIL

½   TEASPOON SALT

1   CUP PLAIN DAIRY-FREE YOGURT

2   CLOVES GARLIC, MINCED

1   TABLESPOON LEMON JUICE

1   TEASPOON GROUND CUMIN

2   CUPS ARUGULA OR BABY SPINACH

12   WHOLE-WHEAT PITA POCKET HALVES, WARMED

¼   CUP MINCED FRESH CILANTRO

1 Preheat the oven to 400°F. Place the potatoes in a large microwave-safe bowl; microwave, covered, on high for 5 minutes. Stir in the chickpeas, onion, garam masala, 2 tablespoons of oil, and ¼ teaspoon of salt.

2 Spread onto a large rimmed baking sheet. Roast for 15 minutes or until the potatoes are tender. Cool slightly.

3 In a small bowl, stir together the yogurt, garlic, lemon juice, and cumin.

4 To serve, toss the potato mixture with the arugula and spoon into the pitas. Top the pitas with the yogurt sauce and the cilantro.

Makes 6 servings. Per serving: 462 calories, 15 g total fat (20% saturated), 14 g protein, 72 g carbohydrate, 12 g fiber, 0 mg cholesterol, 662 mg sodium

tasty lentil tacos

Chili powder, cumin, and oregano add zesty Tex-Mex flavors to these lentils. Cooking the lentils in the broth that becomes the base of the sauce protects the B vitamins from being washed away as they would be if the cooking liquid were drained.

1   TEASPOON CANOLA OIL

1   MEDIUM ONION, FINELY CHOPPED

1   CLOVE GARLIC, MINCED

1   CUP DRIED LENTILS, RINSED

1   TABLESPOON CHILI POWDER

2   TEASPOONS GROUND CUMIN

1   TEASPOON DRIED OREGANO

2½   CUPS VEGETABLE BROTH

1   CUP SALSA

12   TACO SHELLS

1   CUP DAIRY-FREE CHEDDAR SHREDS

1½   CUPS SHREDDED LETTUCE

1   CUP CHOPPED FRESH TOMATOES

1 In a large nonstick skillet, heat the oil over medium heat. Add the onion and garlic and cook for 5 minutes or until the onion is tender. Add the lentils, chili powder, cumin, and oregano; cook, stirring frequently for 1 minute. Stir in the broth; bring to a boil. Reduce to a simmer; cook, covered, for 25 minutes or until the lentils are tender.

2 Cook, uncovered, stirring occasionally for 8 minutes or until the mixture is thickened. With a fork, mash the lentils slightly then stir in the salsa and cook to heat through.

3 To serve, divide the lentil mixture among the taco shells. Top with the shreds, lettuce, and tomatoes.

Makes 6 servings. Per serving: 319 calories, 13 g total fat (31% saturated), 10 g protein, 46 g carbohydrate, 6 g fiber, 0 mg cholesterol, 642 mg sodium,

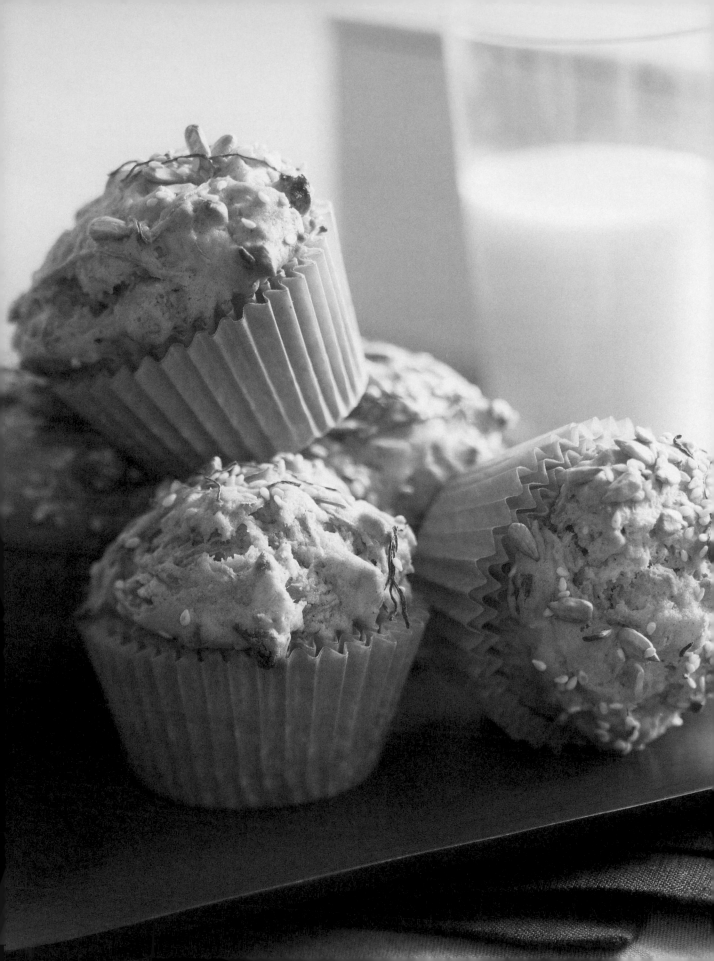

carrot-apricot muffins

Bursting with good-for-you ingredients—carrots, sunflower seeds, and apricots—these muffins make a substantial breakfast or afternoon snack.

- 1 CUP OAT, SOY, OR ALMOND MILK
- 1 TABLESPOON CIDER VINEGAR
- 1 TABLESPOON GROUND FLAXSEEDS
- 1¾ CUPS WHOLE-WHEAT PASTRY FLOUR
- 2 TEASPOONS BAKING POWDER
- ¾ TEASPOON CINNAMON
- ¾ TEASPOON GROUND CARDAMOM
- ¾ TEASPOON GROUND GINGER
- ½ TEASPOON BAKING SODA
- ½ TEASPOON SALT
- ½ CUP FIRMLY PACKED LIGHT BROWN SUGAR
- ¼ CUP LIGHT OLIVE OIL
- ⅔ CUP SUNFLOWER SEEDS
- 3 TABLESPOONS SESAME SEEDS
- 3 LARGE CARROTS, SHREDDED (1½ CUPS)
- ½ CUP DRIED APRICOTS, FINELY CHOPPED

1 Preheat the oven to 350°F. Grease 12 muffin cups or fill with foil-lined muffin liners. In a measuring cup, combine the milk and vinegar. In a small bowl, whisk together the flaxseeds and 3 tablespoons water. Set both aside for 5 minutes.

2 In a large bowl, combine the flour, baking powder, cinnamon, cardamom, ginger, baking soda, and salt.

3 In a separate bowl, whisk together the brown sugar, oil, milk mixture, and flaxseed mixture until well combined. Make a well in the center of the dry ingredients, pour in the milk mixture, and stir until just combined.

4 Fold in the sunflower seeds, sesame seeds, carrots, and apricots.

5 Spoon the batter into the prepared muffin cups, and bake for 30 minutes, or until a toothpick inserted in the center of a muffin comes out clean. Remove the muffins from the pan and cool on a wire rack.

Makes 12 muffins. Per muffin: 233 calories, 9 g total fat (6% saturated), 5 g protein, 32 g carbohydrate, 1.6 g fiber, 0 mg cholesterol, 222 mg sodium

chocolate banana muffins

When bananas are overripe, peel them, place in an airtight container, and freeze for up to 4 months. When preparing these muffins, remove the bananas to a bowl to thaw. Don't worry if they are brown. They will still taste great.

- 1½ CUPS WHOLE-WHEAT PASTRY FLOUR
- ⅔ CUP SUGAR
- ½ CUP BAKING COCOA
- 1 TEASPOON BAKING POWDER
- ½ TEASPOON BAKING SODA
- 1⅓ CUPS MASHED RIPE BANANAS (ABOUT 2 TO 3 MEDIUM)
- ½ CUP DAIRY-FREE PLAIN YOGURT
- ⅓ CUP CANOLA OIL
- 1½ TEASPOONS VANILLA EXTRACT

1 Preheat the oven to 350°F. Grease 12 muffin cups or fill with foil-lined muffin liners.

2 In a large bowl, whisk together the flour, sugar, cocoa, baking powder, and baking soda.

3 In a separate bowl, whisk together the bananas, yogurt, oil, and vanilla until blended. Add to flour mixture; stir just until moistened.

4 Fill the muffin cups three-fourths full with the batter. Bake for 15 minutes or until a toothpick inserted in the center of a muffin comes out clean. Cool for 5 minutes before removing the muffins to a wire rack. Serve warm.

Makes 12 muffins. Per muffin: 196 calories, 7 g fat (27% saturated fat), 3 g protein, 38 g carbohydrate, 2 g fiber, 0 mg cholesterol, 99 mg sodium

chewy honey granola bars

Sure to become a favorite, these bars have sweetness from the honey, chewiness from the raisins, hints of chocolate and cinnamon, and a bit of crunch. Freeze in an airtight container for up to 3 months.

- 3 CUPS OLD-FASHIONED OATS
- 2 CUPS UNSWEETENED PUFFED WHEAT CEREAL
- 1 CUP WHOLE-GRAIN FLOUR
- ⅓ CUP CHOPPED WALNUTS
- ⅓ CUP RAISINS
- ⅓ CUP MINIATURE DAIRY-FREE CHOCOLATE CHIPS
- 1 TEASPOON BAKING SODA
- 1 TEASPOON GROUND CINNAMON
- 1 CUP HONEY
- ¼ CUP DAIRY-FREE BUTTER OR MARGARINE, MELTED
- 1 TEASPOON VANILLA EXTRACT

1 Preheat the oven to 350°F. Coat a 13 x 9-inch baking dish with cooking spray.

2 In a large bowl, combine the oats, wheat cereal, flour, walnuts, raisins, chips, baking soda, and cinnamon. In a small bowl, combine the honey, butter, and vanilla; pour over the oat mixture and mix well. (Mixture will be sticky.)

3 Press the mixture into the pan. Bake for 14 to 18 minutes or until set and the edges are lightly browned. Cool on a wire rack. Cut into 8 bars.

Makes 8 servings. Per serving: 319 calories, 13 g total fat (13% saturated), 3 g protein, 50 g carbohydrate, 3.4 g fiber, 0 mg cholesterol, 177 mg sodium

cranberry-peanut cereal bars

Flaxseeds, rich in antioxidants called lignans, are also a good source of fiber and omega-3 fatty acids. Flaxseeds add a slightly nutty flavor and some good-for-you fat to these bars.

- 3 CUPS PUFFED WHOLE-GRAIN CEREAL, LIKE KASHI
- ½ CUP CHOPPED DRY-ROASTED UNSALTED PEANUTS
- ¼ CUP CHOPPED UNSWEETENED DRIED CRANBERRIES
- 3 TABLESPOONS GROUND FLAXSEEDS
- ⅓ CUP CREAMY PEANUT BUTTER
- ½ CUP AGAVE SYRUP OR HONEY

1 Preheat the oven to 350°F. Coat an 8 x 8-inch metal baking pan with cooking spray.

2 In a large bowl, combine the cereal, peanuts, cranberries, and flaxseeds.

3 In a small saucepan over low heat, combine the peanut butter and agave. Cook, stirring constantly for 1 minute or until the mixture boils. Stir into the cereal mixture until well blended. Scrape into the prepared pan and press down firmly to compact.

4 Bake for 15 minutes, or until the edges are golden. Cool completely on a rack. Cut into 24 squares.

Makes 24 servings. Per serving: 112 calories, 4 g total fat (25% saturated), 3 g protein, 19 g carbohydrate, 2 g fiber, 0 mg cholesterol, 78 mg sodium

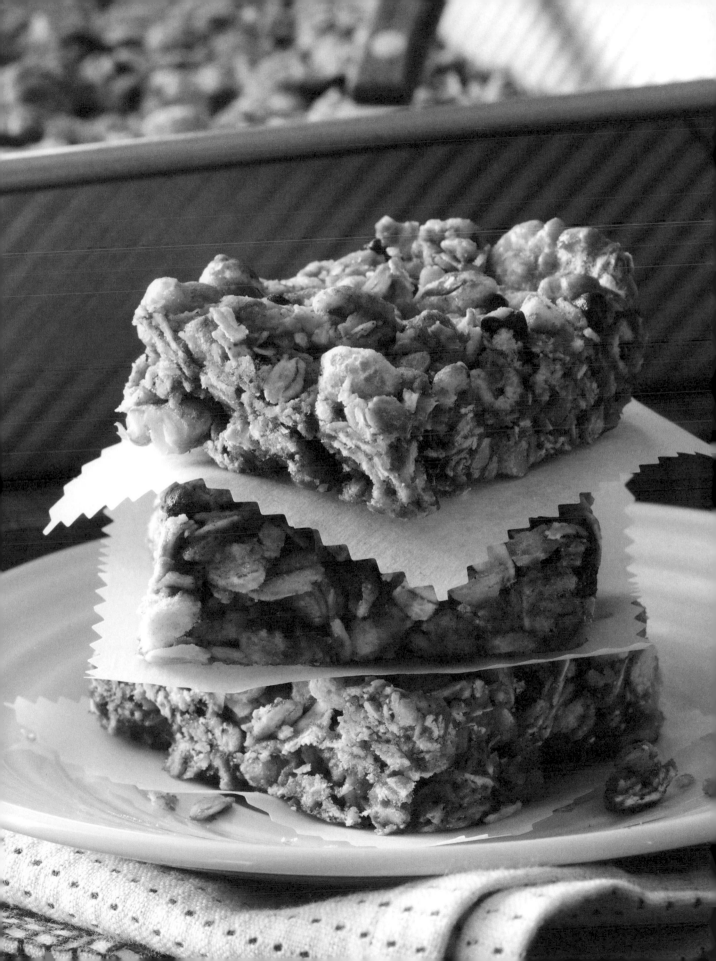

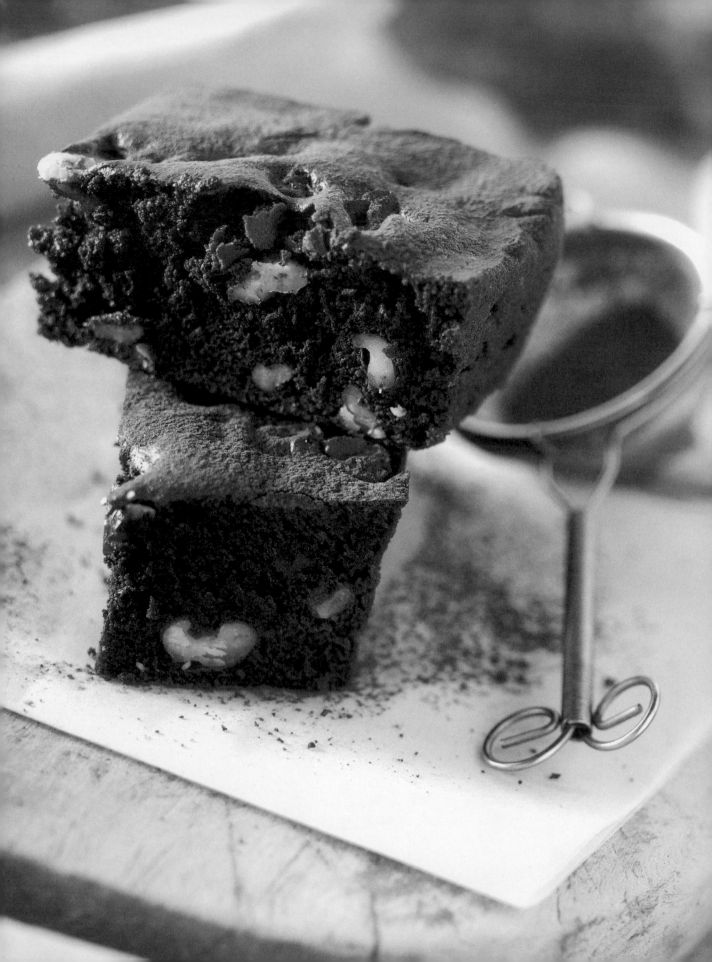

fig bars with sesame crust

Carrots, rich in beta-carotene, are added to the filling of these bar cookies to lighten and sweeten the mixture.

- ½ CUP NATURAL ALMONDS
- 1 TABLESPOON SESAME SEEDS
- 1 CUP WHOLE-WHEAT PASTRY FLOUR
- ⅓ CUP CONFECTIONERS' SUGAR
- ½ TEASPOON SALT
- ⅓ CUP DARK SESAME OIL
- 1½ TEASPOONS GRATED ORANGE ZEST
- 1 CUP DRIED FIGS, COARSELY CHOPPED
- 2 CARROTS, VERY THINLY SLICED
- ¾ CUP ORANGE JUICE
- 2 TABLESPOONS FRESH LEMON JUICE
- ¾ TEASPOON GROUND CARDAMOM
- 1 TEASPOON VANILLA EXTRACT

1 Preheat the oven to 350°F. Place the almonds and sesame seeds on a rimmed baking sheet and toast in the oven for 5 to 7 minutes, or until the almonds are fragrant and the seeds golden.

2 Transfer the almonds and sesame seeds to a food processor. Add the flour, confectioners' sugar, and salt; process until powdery. Add the sesame oil and orange zest, and process until evenly moistened.

3 Press the crust mixture into a 9 x 9-inch metal baking pan. With the tines of a fork, prick the dough all over and bake for 20 minutes. Cool on a wire rack.

4 While the crust bakes, in a medium saucepan, combine the figs, carrots, orange juice, lemon juice, and cardamom; bring to a boil over medium heat. Reduce to a simmer; cover and cook 20 minutes, or until the figs and carrots are soft and most of the liquid has been absorbed. Cool to room temperature.

5 Transfer the fig-carrot mixture to a food processor. Add the vanilla, and process to a coarse puree. Spread the mixture over the crust, and bake for 20 minutes. Cool in the pan on a wire rack before slicing into 32 pieces.

Makes 32 cookies. Per cookie: 75 calories, 3.6 g total fat (0% saturated), 1 g protein, 10 g carbohydrate, 1.1 g fiber, 0 mg cholesterol, 39 mg sodium

peanut butter brownies with walnuts & cranberries

Peanut butter and olive oil replace the butter in these brownies, and walnuts and cranberries add some healthful phytochemicals.

- 1 TABLESPOON GROUND FLAXSEEDS
- ⅔ CUP WHOLE-WHEAT PASTRY FLOUR
- ½ CUP UNSWEETENED COCOA POWDER
- 1 TEASPOON BAKING POWDER
- ¼ TEASPOON BAKING SODA
- ¼ TEASPOON SALT
- ¾ CUP FIRMLY PACKED LIGHT BROWN SUGAR
- ¼ CUP CREAMY PEANUT BUTTER
- 3 TABLESPOONS LIGHT OLIVE OIL
- 2 TEASPOONS VANILLA EXTRACT
- ½ CUP CHOPPED WALNUTS
- ⅓ CUP DRIED CRANBERRIES OR CHERRIES
- 1 OUNCE 60% DARK CHOCOLATE, CHOPPED

1 Preheat the oven to 350°F. Lightly grease an 8 x 8-inch metal baking pan. In a small bowl, whisk together the flaxseeds and 3 tablespoons water. Set aside for 5 minutes. On a sheet of wax paper, combine the flour, cocoa powder, baking powder, baking soda, and salt.

2 In a medium bowl, with an electric mixer, beat together the brown sugar, peanut butter, oil, and flaxseed mixture until well combined. Beat in the vanilla. On low speed, add the flour mixture. Fold in the walnuts, cranberries, and chocolate. Spread into the prepared pan.

3 Bake for 25 to 30 minutes, or until a toothpick inserted in the center comes out clean, but with some crumbs clinging to it. Cool in the pan on a wire rack before cutting into 8 brownies.

Makes 8 brownies. Per brownie: 309 calories, 16 g total fat (19% saturated), 6 g protein, 40 g carbohydrate, 3.2 g fiber, 12 mg cholesterol, 228 mg sodium

panforte cluster cookies

A true panforte is a dense, nearly flourless nut cake from Siena, Italy. Here is a cookie-size adaptation made with nutrient-rich dried fruits and crystallized ginger in place of some of the nuts.

- 1 CUP NATURAL ALMONDS
- ½ CUP DICED DRIED PINEAPPLE (3½ OUNCES)
- ½ CUP DICED DRIED MANGO (3 OUNCES)
- ⅓ CUP DRIED CRANBERRIES, FINELY CHOPPED
- ¼ CUP CHOPPED CRYSTALLIZED GINGER (1½ OUNCES)
- ½ CUP WHOLE-WHEAT PASTRY FLOUR
- ¾ TEASPOON CINNAMON
- ¼ TEASPOON GROUND CORIANDER
- ¼ TEASPOON ALLSPICE
- ¼ TEASPOON NUTMEG
- ¼ TEASPOON SALT
- ⅓ CUP HONEY
- ⅓ CUP SUGAR

1 Preheat the oven to 350°F. Place the almonds on a rimmed baking sheet and toast in the oven for 5 to 7 minutes, or until crisp and fragrant. Leave the oven on. When the almonds are cool enough to handle, finely chop them.

2 Line a large baking sheet with parchment paper or a silicone baking sheet.

3 In a large bowl, combine the pineapple, mango, cranberries, ginger, and almonds. On a sheet of wax paper, stir together the flour, cinnamon, coriander, allspice, nutmeg, and salt.

4 In a small saucepan, stir together the honey and sugar; bring to a boil over medium heat. Boil for 2 minutes. Pour the hot honey mixture over the fruit mixture, and stir to combine. Add the flour mixture and stir until combined.

5 With dampened hands, shape the dough into walnut-size pieces. Place 1 inch apart on the prepared baking sheet, then flatten each to ¼-inch thickness. Bake for 10 minutes, or until just set. Cool on the pan for 5 minutes before transferring to a wire rack to cool completely.

Makes 32 cookies. Per cookie: 75 calories, 2.2 g total fat (0% saturated), 1 g protein, 14 g carbohydrate, 0.8 g fiber, 0 mg cholesterol, 23 mg sodium

chocolate chip cookies

Using whole-wheat pastry flour instead of all-purpose flour adds fiber to recipes without a noticeable difference. Because the bran of the wheat kernel is removed in all-purpose white flour, so too are many of the nutrients—B vitamins, iron, calcium, and protein—present in whole-wheat flours. Because whole-wheat pastry flour is more finely ground than regular whole-wheat flour, it easily mimics nutrient-deficient white flour in baked goods.

- 1 CUP PACKED DARK BROWN SUGAR
- ½ CUP CANOLA OIL
- 6 TABLESPOONS VANILLA SOY MILK
- ¼ CUP UNSWEETENED APPLESAUCE
- 2 TEASPOONS VANILLA EXTRACT
- 1 TEASPOON BAKING SODA
- ¾ TEASPOON SALT
- 2¼ CUPS WHOLE-WHEAT PASTRY FLOUR
- 1 CUP DAIRY-FREE SEMISWEET CHOCOLATE CHIPS
- ½ CUP FINELY CHOPPED WALNUTS

1 In a large bowl, whisk together the brown sugar, oil, milk, applesauce, and vanilla until well blended. Stir in the baking soda and salt until blended. Add the flour; mix until combined. Stir in chocolate chips and nuts. Cover and refrigerate for 1 hour.

2 Preheat the oven to 375°F. Line 2 baking sheets with parchment paper or silicone baking sheets.

3 Drop the dough by rounded tablespoonfuls 2 inches apart onto the baking sheets. Bake for 10 to 12 minutes or until the edges are lightly browned. Cool on the pan for 1 minutes before transferring to a wire rack to cool completely.

Makes 42 cookies. Per cookie: 111 calories, 5 g total fat (20% saturated fat), 1g protein, 16 g carbohydrate, 1g fiber, 0 mg cholesterol, 76 mg sodium

kiwi-mango salad

While the avocado may come as a surprise in this dessert salad, its smooth, silky texture and rich flavor are a nice counterpoint to the other fruits. Prepare this shortly before serving, or the fruit—especially the banana—will become mushy as the acid in the lime juice starts to break it down.

¼ CUP FRESH LIME JUICE

2 TABLESPOONS SUGAR

2 TABLESPOONS MINCED FRESH MINT LEAVES

6 KIWIFRUIT, PEELED, QUARTERED LENGTHWISE, AND CUT CROSSWISE INTO THIRDS

2 BANANAS, HALVED LENGTHWISE AND THICKLY SLICED

1 MANGO, PEELED AND CUT INTO 1-INCH CHUNKS

1 AVOCADO, PEELED AND CUT INTO 1-INCH CHUNKS

In a large bowl, whisk together the lime juice, sugar, and mint. Add the kiwifruit, bananas, mango, and avocado; toss well. Refrigerate for up to 1 hour before serving.

Makes 4 servings. Per serving: 267 calories, 8.6 g total fat (16% saturated), 3 g protein, 51 g carbohydrate, 6.7 g fiber, 0 mg cholesterol, 14 mg sodium

blushing applesauce

Making your own applesauce is a cinch, and when the apples are combined with grape juice, cinnamon, and a hint of black pepper, the sauce is much more interesting than the store-bought variety. In addition to adding some sweetness and the "blush" color, the purple grape juice provides the heart-healthy phytochemical resveratrol.

4 LARGE GRANNY SMITH APPLES, PEELED, CORED, AND HALVED

2 CUPS UNSWEETENED CONCORD GRAPE JUICE

2 TABLESPOONS HONEY

½ TEASPOON CINNAMON

¼ TEASPOON BLACK PEPPER

1 TEASPOON VANILLA EXTRACT

1 In a medium saucepan, combine the apples, grape juice, honey, cinnamon, and pepper; bring to a boil over medium heat. Reduce to a gentle boil and cook for 30 minutes, or until the apples are slightly chunky and the mixture has become thick.

2 Remove from the heat and stir in the vanilla. If you prefer a smoother applesauce, mash with a potato masher or immersion blender. Serve the applesauce chilled or at room temperature.

Makes 4 servings. Per serving: 200 calories, 0.5 g total fat (15% saturated), 0 g protein, 51 g carbohydrate, 2.8 g fiber, 0 mg cholesterol, 1 mg sodium

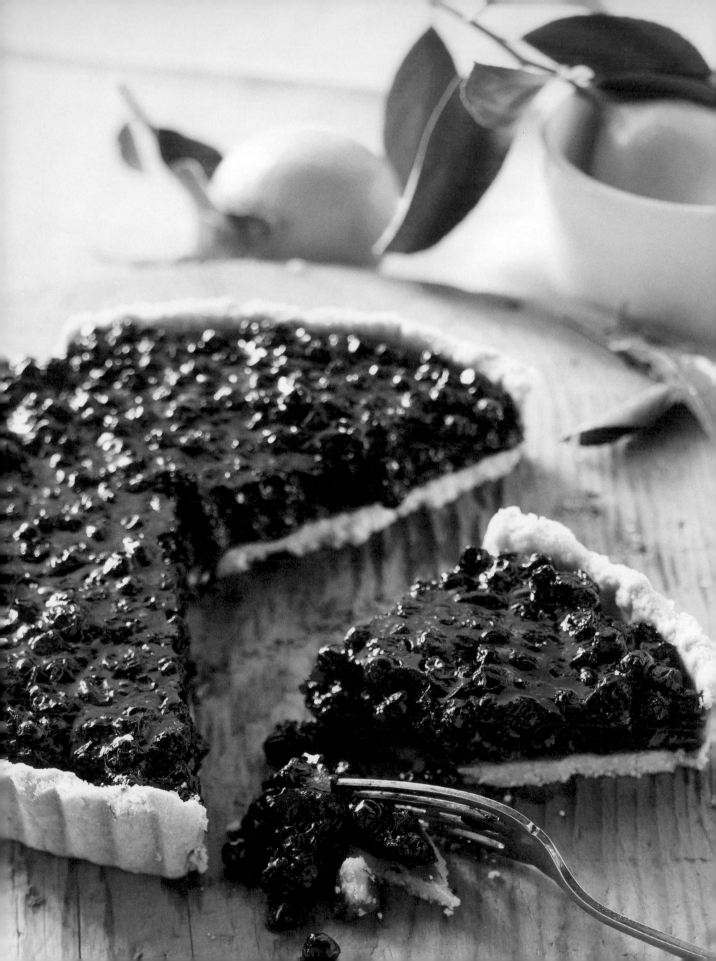

blueberry-orange tart

Don't be surprised by the small amount of pepper in the filling—it heightens the blueberry flavor. The dough for the tart shell is made with monounsaturated olive oil instead of butter.

1½ CUPS WHOLE-WHEAT PASTRY FLOUR

⅓ CUP CONFECTIONERS' SUGAR

2 TEASPOONS GRATED ORANGE ZEST

½ TEASPOON BAKING POWDER

½ TEASPOON SALT

¼ CUP PLUS 3 TABLESPOONS OLIVE OIL

2 TABLESPOONS PLUS ¼ CUP ORANGE JUICE

2 BAGS (12 OUNCES EACH) FROZEN UNSWEETENED BLUEBERRIES

8 TABLESPOONS GRANULATED SUGAR

½ TEASPOON PEPPER

⅛ TEASPOON NUTMEG

3 TABLESPOONS CORNSTARCH

1 In a large bowl, stir together the flour, confectioners' sugar, orange zest, baking powder, and salt. Add the oil and 2 tablespoons of the orange juice, and stir until the mixture comes together. Transfer the dough to a lightly floured work surface and knead 10 times, or until the dough forms a ball. Flatten into a disk, wrap in plastic wrap, and let stand for 30 minutes at room temperature.

2 Preheat the oven to 350°F. With your fingertips, gently press the dough onto the bottom and sides of a 9-inch tart pan with a removable bottom. Prick the bottom of the shell with a fork and line the pan with foil. Fill the foil with pie weights or dried beans, and bake the shell for 15 minutes. Remove the foil and weights, and bake the shell for 10 minutes, or until golden brown. Cool on a wire rack.

3 Meanwhile, in a saucepan, combine the blueberries, the remaining ¼ cup orange juice, 6 tablespoons of the granulated sugar, the pepper, and nutmeg; bring to a boil. Reduce to a simmer and cook for 5 minutes.

4 In a small bowl, stir together the remaining 2 tablespoons granulated sugar and the cornstarch. Stir the cornstarch mixture into the berries, and cook for 2 minutes, or until the berry mixture is thick.

5 Cool the blueberry mixture to room temperature, then spoon into the baked shell. Chill the tart for 1 hour before serving.

Makes 8 servings. Per serving: 319 calories, 13 g total fat (13% saturated), 3 g protein, 50 g carbohydrate, 4 g fiber, 0 mg cholesterol, 177 mg sodium

banana bread pudding

Made with rice milk instead of cow's milk, and thickend with cornstarch instead of whole eggs, this sweet, mildly spiced banana bread pudding is rich tasting without being high in fat. Soothing to both the body and spirit, the pudding is a good source of B vitamins, potassium, folate, and selenium.

16 OUNCES WHOLE-GRAIN ITALIAN BREAD, CUT INTO 1-INCH PIECES (ABOUT 6 CUPS)

1 POUND VERY RIPE BANANAS

2½ CUPS RICE MILK

¼ CUP FIRMLY PACKED DARK BROWN SUGAR

3 TABLESPOONS CORNSTARCH OR ARROWROOT POWDER

½ TEASPOON VANILLA EXTRACT

¼ TEASPOON GRATED NUTMEG

¼ TEASPOON SALT

1 Preheat the oven to 400°F. Toast the bread cubes for 7 to 10 minutes, or until crisp. Remove from the oven and reduce the oven temperature to 350°F. In a large bowl, mash the bananas with a potato masher or a fork.

2 In a medium saucepan, whisk together the milk, brown sugar, and cornstarch until combined and no lumps remain. Cook over medium heat for 5 minutes, whisking frequently, until the mixture starts to boil and thickens. Whisk into the bananas along with the vanilla, nutmeg, and salt.

3 Place the toasted bread cubes in a 9 x 9-inch glass baking dish. Pour the banana mixture over the bread.

4 Bake for 35 minutes, or until the pudding is set. Cool to room temperature before serving.

Makes 4 servings. Per serving: 341 calories, 4.6 g total fat (3% saturated), 8 g protein, 69 g carbohydrate, 4 g fiber, 0 mg cholesterol, 477 mg sodium

◀ **blueberry-orange tart**

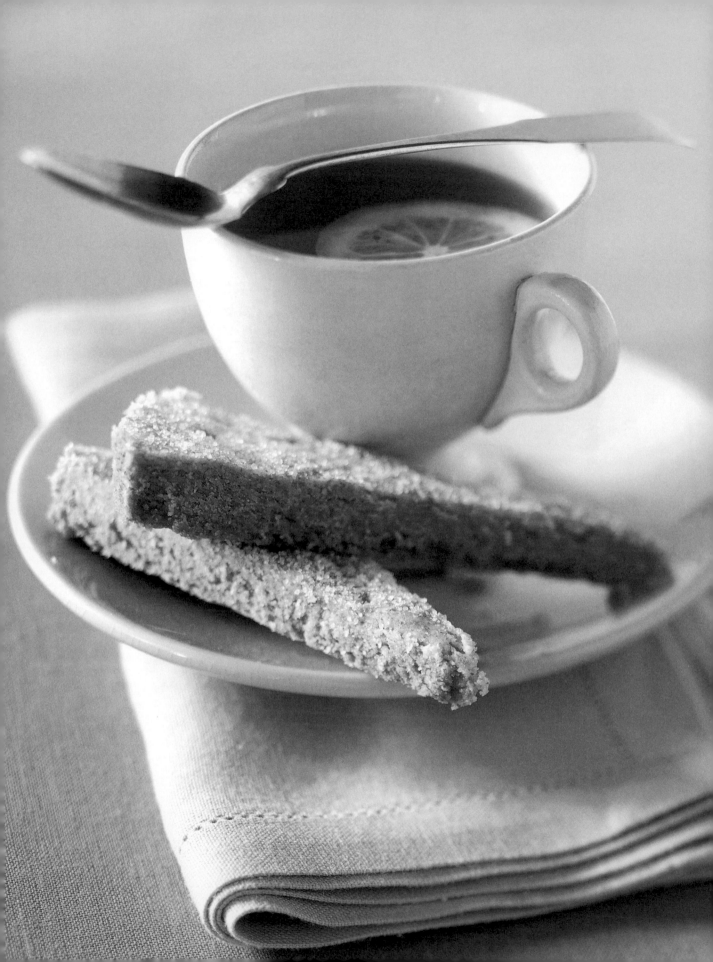

walnut shortbread

Although shortbread is usually made with butter, we've found that replacing it with ground walnuts, olive oil, and walnut oil works beautifully. The result is a rich-tasting cookie with no cholesterol and healthful monounsaturated fats instead of saturated fats. Walnuts and walnut oil also have ellagic acid, a potent antioxidant.

⅔ CUP WALNUTS

1¼ CUPS WHOLE-WHEAT PASTRY FLOUR

½ CUP CONFECTIONERS' SUGAR

¼ TEASPOON SALT

¼ CUP WALNUT OR LIGHT OLIVE OIL

¼ CUP LIGHT OLIVE OIL

1½ TEASPOONS GRATED LEMON ZEST

1 TEASPOON VANILLA EXTRACT

1 Preheat the oven to 325°F. Place the walnuts on a rimmed baking sheet and toast in the oven for 5 to 7 minutes, or until crisp and fragrant. Leave on the oven. Cool the walnuts, then transfer to a food processor with the flour, and process until the nuts are finely ground.

2 Transfer the flour-walnut mixture to a large bowl. Stir in the confectioners' sugar and salt. Add the walnut oil, olive oil, lemon zest, and vanilla, and stir until well combined.

3 Press the dough onto the bottom of a 9-inch tart pan with a removable bottom. With the tines of a fork, prick the dough. With a sharp knife, score the dough into 16 wedges, cutting almost, but not quite through, to the bottom.

4 Bake for 30 minutes, or until crisp and light golden. Check the shortbread after 20 minutes; if it is overbrowning, decrease the oven temperature to 300°F. Remove from the oven and, while the shortbread is still warm, cut the wedges through to the bottom. Cool in the pan on a wire rack.

Makes 8 servings. Per serving: 273 calories, 19 g total fat (11% saturated), 3 g protein, 24 g carbohydrate, 1.7 g fiber, 0 mg cholesterol, 73 mg sodium

creamy citrus & vanilla rice pudding

Rice milk is used here instead of cow's milk for a creamy, lactose-free pudding. Soy, oat, or almond millk will work as well. The basmati rice is used for extra flavor, but long-grain rice would be fine.

4 CUPS RICE MILK

3 STRIPS (3 x ½ INCH EACH) ORANGE ZEST

3 STRIPS (3 x ½ INCH EACH) LIME ZEST

1 CINNAMON STICK, SPLIT LENGTHWISE

½ TEASPOON SALT

½ CUP BASMATI OR JASMINE RICE

⅓ CUP CORNSTARCH OR ARROWROOT POWDER

¼ CUP SUGAR

½ TEASPOON VANILLA EXTRACT

1 In a large saucepan, stir together 3½ cups of the rice milk, orange and lime zests, cinnamon, and salt. Add the rice, and bring to a simmer over medium-low heat. Cover and cook for 15 minutes, stirring occasionally.

2 Meanwhile, in a medium bowl, whisk together the cornstarch and sugar. Whisk in the remaining ½ cup rice milk until smooth.

3 Uncover the rice and cook, stirring frequently for 15 minutes, or until the rice is very tender. Whisk the cornstarch mixture into the saucepan. Cook, stirring constantly, for 1 minute, or until the pudding is thickened.

4 Transfer the pudding to a bowl and stir in the vanilla. When cool, remove the orange zest, lime zest, and cinnamon stick. Cool to room temperature, then cover and refrigerate until serving time.

Makes 4 servings. Per serving: 251 calories, 2.75 g total fat (0% saturated), 4 g protein, 56 g carbohydrate, 0.3 g fiber, 0 mg cholesterol, 394 mg sodium

cherry crisp

For an even better-tasting crisp, use fresh cherries. To get the amount of pitted cherries you need here, buy 2 pounds of fresh cherries and pit them; this should yield the same quantity as the 24 ounces of frozen pitted cherries. Sour cherries (pie cherries)—fresh or frozen—can be substituted for the sweet cherries, but increase the granulated sugar in the cherry mixture to ⅓ or ½ cup, to taste.

- ¼ CUP GRANULATED SUGAR
- 2 TABLESPOONS CORNSTARCH
- 1 TEASPOON CINNAMON
- ½ TEASPOON SALT
- ⅛ TEASPOON ALLSPICE
- 2 TEASPOONS GRATED LIME ZEST
- 2 BAGS (12 OUNCES EACH) FROZEN PITTED SWEET CHERRIES, THAWED
- 1 TABLESPOON FRESH LIME JUICE
- ¾ CUP OLD-FASHIONED ROLLED OATS
- ⅓ CUP WHOLE-WHEAT PASTRY FLOUR
- ⅓ CUP FIRMLY PACKED LIGHT BROWN SUGAR
- 3 TABLESPOONS COLD DAIRY-FREE BUTTER OR MARGARINE, CUT UP

1 Preheat the oven to 400°F. In a large bowl, stir together the granulated sugar, cornstarch, cinnamon, ¼ teaspoon of the salt, the allspice, and lime zest. Add the cherries and lime juice, tossing to coat. Transfer to a 9 x 9-inch glass baking dish; set aside.

2 In a medium bowl, stir together the remaining ¼ teaspoon salt, the oats, flour, and brown sugar. With a pastry blender or two knives, cut in the butter until the mixture resembles coarse crumbs. Sprinkle the mixture over the fruit.

3 Bake for 25 minutes, or until the fruit is bubbly and piping hot and the topping is golden brown and crisp.

Makes 6 servings. Per serving: 257 calories, 6.9 g total fat (55% saturated), 4 g protein, 48 g carbohydrate, 1.4 g fiber, 16 mg cholesterol, 201 mg sodium

fruit & nut-studded amaranth pudding

Cultivated since ancient times, amaranth is rich in magnesium, iron, fiber, and the amino acid lysine (which is rare in plant sources). You'll find amaranth in health-food stores. In this homey pudding, the amaranth remains somewhat crunchy and has a nutty flavor, which is emphasized by the addition of pine nuts.

- 2 TABLESPOONS PINE NUTS
- 3 CUPS UNSWEETENED SOY MILK
- 1 CUP WHOLE-GRAIN AMARANTH
- ¼ CUP MAPLE SUGAR
- 2 TEASPOONS GRATED ORANGE ZEST
- 2 TEASPOONS GRATED LEMON ZEST
- ¼ TEASPOON GROUND CARDAMOM
- ¼ TEASPOON SALT
- ⅓ CUP RAISINS
- ½ TEASPOON VANILLA EXTRACT

1 Preheat the oven to 350°F. Place the pine nuts on a rimmed baking sheet and toast in the oven for 3 minutes, or until golden brown.

2 In a large saucepan, combine the milk, amaranth, maple sugar, orange zest, lemon zest, cardamom, and salt; bring to a boil. Reduce to a simmer; cover and cook, stirring occasionally for 35 minutes, or until the amaranth is tender.

3 Remove from the heat and stir in the pine nuts, raisins, and vanilla. Serve the pudding at room temperature or chilled.

Makes 4 servings. Per serving: 354 calories, 7.4 g total fat (32% saturated), 15 g protein, 60 g carbohydrate, 8.6 g fiber, 7 mg cholesterol, 248 mg sodium

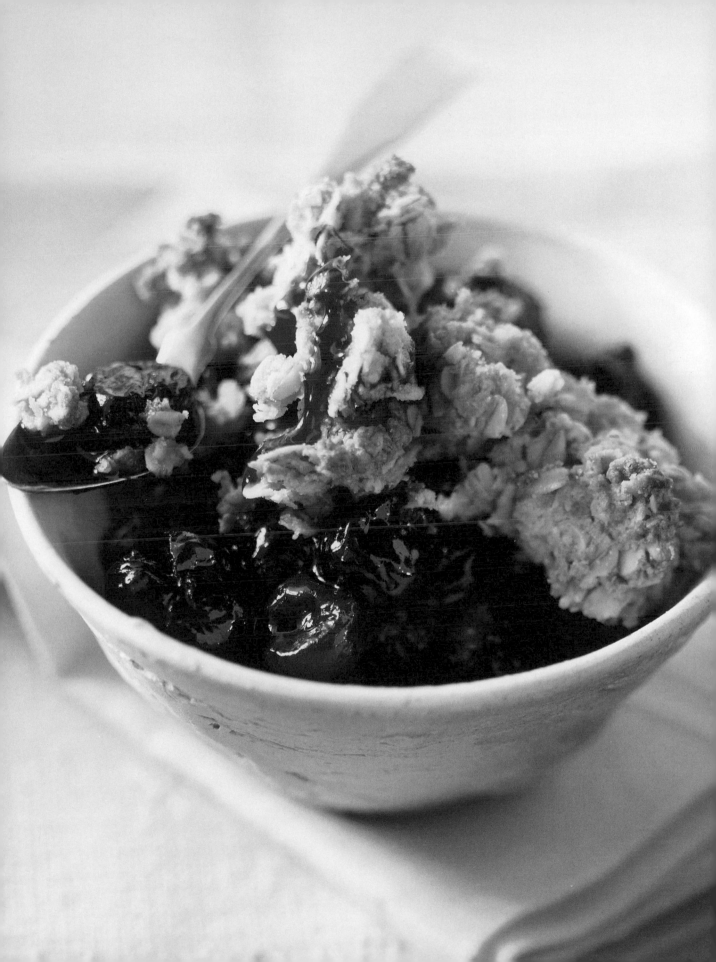

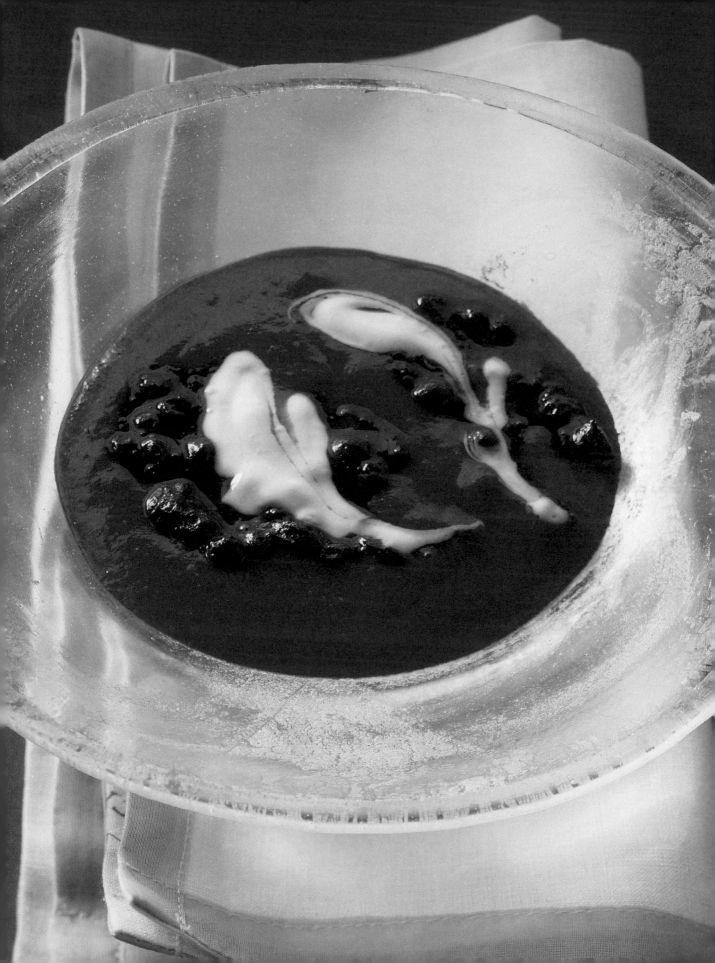

three-berry fool

Although many recipes call for straining out the seeds from raspberry purees and sauces, we have purposely left them in, because the seeds account for a goodly amount of the dietary fiber. When purchasing the yogurt, opt for one that's a Greek-style if possible.

- 1 QUART PLAIN DAIRY-FREE YOGURT
- 1 PACKAGE (12 OUNCES) FROZEN UNSWEETENED RASPBERRIES, THAWED
- 2 CUPS FROZEN UNSWEETENED STRAWBERRIES, THAWED
- ½ CUP SUGAR
- 1½ TEASPOONS VANILLA EXTRACT
- 3 TEASPOONS CORNSTARCH BLENDED WITH 2 TABLESPOONS WATER
- 1 PACKAGE (12 OUNCES) FROZEN UNSWEETENED BLUEBERRIES
- 2 TABLESPOONS ORANGE JUICE
- ¼ TEASPOON PEPPER
- ¼ TEASPOON ALLSPICE
- 1 TABLESPOON FRESH LEMON JUICE

1 Spoon the yogurt into a fine-mesh strainer or a coffee filter set over a bowl to catch the drips. Let the yogurt stand for 4 hours at room temperature.

2 In a food processor, combine the raspberries, strawberries, ¼ cup of the sugar, and ½ teaspoon of the vanilla; puree. Transfer the puree to a small saucepan and bring to a boil over medium heat. Stir in half of the cornstarch mixture and bring to a boil. Boil, stirring constantly for 1 minute, until lightly thickened. Cool to room temperature, transfer to a bowl, cover, and refrigerate.

3 In a small saucepan, combine 2 tablespoons of the sugar, the blueberries, orange juice, pepper, and allspice; bring to a simmer over low heat. Cook, stirring frequently for 5 minutes, or until the blueberries are tender. Stir in the remaining cornstarch mixture and bring to a boil; cook, stirring constantly, for 1 minute, or until thickened. Transfer to a bowl and stir in the lemon juice; cover and refrigerate.

4 In a medium bowl, combine the drained yogurt, the remaining 2 tablespoons sugar, and the remaining 1 teaspoon vanilla.

5 To serve, spoon the raspberry-strawberry mixture into 4 bowls. Spoon the blueberry mixture into the center and top with the yogurt. Gently swirl the mixture to lightly marble the yogurt with fruit puree.

Makes 4 servings. Per serving: 331 calories, 4.5 g total fat (0% saturated), 13 g protein, 63 g carbohydrate, 2.8 g fiber, 6 mg cholesterol, 75 mg sodium

mint-chocolate chip pudding

The soy milk used in this recipe is unsweetened but if you'd prefer to use flavored soy milk such as vanilla, which is sweetened, reduce the brown sugar by ⅓ cup.

- ⅔ CUP FIRMLY PACKED DARK BROWN SUGAR
- ⅓ CUP CORNSTARCH
- 3 TABLESPOONS UNSWEETENED COCOA POWDER
- ½ TEASPOON SALT
- 3 CUPS UNSWEETENED SOY MILK
- ½ TEASPOON PURE MINT EXTRACT
- ½ TEASPOON VANILLA EXTRACT
- ¼ CUP DAIRY-FREE MINI CHOCOLATE CHIPS (1 OUNCE)

1 In a large saucepan, stir together the brown sugar, cornstarch, cocoa powder, and salt. Gradually whisk in the soy milk until smooth.

2 Bring to a boil over medium heat, stirring constantly. Boil for 1 minute, or until the pudding is thick. Remove from the heat and stir in the mint and vanilla extracts. Cool to room temperature and stir in the chocolate chips.

3 Spoon into 4 dessert dishes. Cover and refrigerate for 2 hours, or until chilled.

Makes 4 servings. Per serving: 291 calories, 5.3 g total fat (27% saturated), 8 g protein, 53 g carbohydrate, 1.3 g fiber, 0 mg cholesterol, 387 mg sodium

◄ **three-berry fool**

strawberry citrus ice

Daiquiri fans will love this ice! The combination of strawberries, lime juice, and orange juice becomes a health version of the cocktail and a source of vitamin C.

¾ CUP SUGAR

3 CUPS FRESH STRAWBERRIES, HULLED

¼ CUP LIME JUICE

¼ CUP ORANGE JUICE

1 In a small saucepan, bring the sugar and ½ cup water to a boil; cook, stirring constantly 4 minutes or until the sugar is dissolved. Remove to a bowl; cool slightly. Refrigerate the syrup, covered, for 2 hours or until cold.

2 In a blender, process the strawberries, lime juice, and orange juice until smooth. Add the sugar syrup; pulse to blend.

3 Pour the strawberry mixture into the cylinder of an ice cream maker; freeze according to manufacturer's directions. Serve immediately or store in a freezer container, allowing about 1-inch headspace for expansion.

Makes 7 servings. Per serving: 128 calories, 0 g total fat (0% saturated fat), 1 g protein, 33 g carbohydrate, 1 g fiber, 0 mg cholesterol, 1 mg sodium

sonoran sunset watermelon ice

If you didn't think watermelon and cilantro could go together in a dessert, this recipe will give you a pleasant surprise! Sprinkle pomegranate seeds and a sprig of cilantro on top for extra flair.

½ CUP SUGAR

4 CUPS CUBED SEEDLESS WATERMELON

3 TABLESPOONS LIME JUICE

2 TABLESPOONS POMEGRANATE JUICE

1 TABLESPOON MINCED FRESH CILANTRO

DASH SALT

1 In a small saucepan, bring the sugar and ¼ cup water to a boil; cook, stirring constantly 4 minutes or until the sugar is dissolved. Remove to a bowl; cool slightly. Refrigerate the syrup, covered, for 2 hours or until cold.

2 Puree the watermelon in a blender. Transfer to a large bowl; stir in the sugar syrup, lime juice, pomegranate juice, cilantro, and salt. Refrigerate until cold.

3 Pour the watermelon mixture into the cylinder of an ice cream maker; freeze according to manufacturer's directions. Serve immediately or store in a freezer container, allowing about 1-inch headspace for expansion.

Makes 4 servings. Per serving: 100 calories, 0 g total fat (0% saturated), 1 g protein, 26 g carbohydrate, 0 g fiber, 0 mg cholesterol, 246 mg sodium

almond butter swirl cream

This ice cream substitute is bursting with almond flavor and a creamy chocolate finish.

- 2 CUPS LITE CANNED COCONUT MILK
- 1 CUP UNSWEETENED ALMOND MILK
- ½ CUP ALMOND BUTTER (OR OTHER NUT BUTTER)
- ½ CUP SUGAR
- ½ TEASPOON SEA SALT
- ½ CUP DAIRY-FREE CHOCOLATE CHIPS, MELTED

1 In a large bowl, whisk together the coconut milk, almond milk, almond butter, sugar, and salt until well blended.

2 Pour the mixture into the cylinder of an ice cream maker no more than two-thirds full. Freeze according to manufacturer's directions, slowly adding the melted chocolate during the last 2 minutes of processing.

3 Serve immediately, or transfer to a freezer container, allowing about 1-inch headspace for expansion.

Makes 8 servings. Per serving: 271 calories, 18 g fat (38% saturated), 4.8 g protein, 26 g carbohydrate, 3 mg fiber, 0 mg cholesterol, 146 mg sodium

strawberry-citrus freezer pops

Keep a batch of these pops in the freezer for when you're craving a sweet snack. Feel free to substitute blueberries or peeled peaches for the strawberries and oranges or tangerines for the clementine.

- 2 CUPS FRESH STRAWBERRIES, SLICED
- 1 TABLESPOON SUGAR
- 10 FREEZER-POP MOLDS OR 10 PAPER CUPS (3-OUNCE SIZE) AND 10 WOODEN POP STICKS
- 2 CUPS CLEMENTINE SEGMENTS (ABOUT 10), SEEDED IF NECESSARY
- 6 TABLESPOONS ORANGE JUICE

1 Place the strawberries, sugar, and 6 tablespoons water in a food processor; pulse until combined.

Divide the strawberry mixture among the freezer-pop molds or paper cups.

2 Top the molds with their lids or holders; if using cups, top the cups with foil and insert popsicle sticks through foil. Freeze until firm, about 2 hours.

3 Wipe the food processor clean. Add the clementine and orange juice; pulse the mixture until well combined. Spoon the clementine mixture over the strawberry layer. Freeze for 2 to 4 hours, covered, or until firm.

Makes 10 servings. Per serving: 82 calories, 0 g total fat (0% saturated fat), 1 g protein, 20 g carbohydrate, 3 g fiber, 0 mg cholesterol, 3 mg sodium

quick mango sorbet

This refreshing dessert comes together in minutes. Keep frozen mango and passion fruit juice on hand for last-minute guests. To make it a bit creamy, substitute canned coconut milk for the juice.

- 1 PACKAGE (16 OUNCES) FROZEN MANGO CHUNKS, SLIGHTLY THAWED
- ½ CUP PASSION FRUIT JUICE
- 2 TABLESPOONS SUGAR

1 Place the mango, passion fruit juice, and sugar in a blender; cover and process until smooth.

2 Serve immediately, or transfer to a freezer container, allowing about 1-inch headspace for expansion. Freeze for 2 to 4 hours or until firm.

Makes 4 servings. Per serving: 91 calories, 0 g total fat (0% saturated fat), 1 g protein, 24 g carbohydrate, 2 g fiber, 0 mg cholesterol, 2 mg sodium

gluten-free chocolate cupcakes

Dusting these cupcakes with confectioners' sugar instead of topping with frosting keeps the calories and fat to a minimum while offering a sweet treat. Try sprinkling with cinnamon or cocoa powder for a change of pace.

- 2 CUPS GLUTEN-FREE OAT FLOUR
- 1 CUP SUGAR
- ¼ CUP UNSWEETENED COCOA POWDER
- 1 TEASPOON BAKING SODA
- ½ TEASPOON SALT
- ⅓ CUP CANOLA OIL
- 1 TEASPOON CIDER VINEGAR
- ½ TEASPOON VANILLA EXTRACT
- 2 TEASPOONS CONFECTIONERS' SUGAR

1 Preheat the oven to 350°F. Line a 12-cup muffin pan with paper cupcake liners.

2 In a large bowl, whisk together the flour, sugar, cocoa powder, baking soda, and salt. In a separate bowl, combine the oil, vinegar, vanilla, and 1 cup water. Stir the oil mixture into the flour mixture just until moistened.

3 Fill the prepared cupcake liners with the batter three-quarters full. Bake for 20 to 25 minutes or until a toothpick inserted in the center comes out clean. Cool the pan on a wire rack for 10 minutes. Remove the cupcakes to the rack to cool completely.

4 To serve, dust the cupcakes with the confectioners' sugar.

Makes 12 cupcakes. Per cupcake: 187 calories, 8 g total fat (12% saturated), 2 g protein, 29 g carbohydrate, 2 g fiber, 0 mg cholesterol, 203 mg sodium

vanilla cupcakes

An occasional dessert treat makes life enjoyable and while these cupcakes are plant-based, they still should be saved for special occasions and holidays. You can change up the flavors by adding grated orange or lemon zest, chopped pecans, or spices like pumpkin pie spice to the batter.

- 2½ CUPS WHOLE-WHEAT PASTRY FLOUR
- 2 TEASPOONS BAKING POWDER
- ½ TEASPOON BAKING SODA
- ¼ TEASPOON SALT
- 1¾ CUPS REFRIGERATED UNSWEETENED COCONUT MILK
- 1½ CUPS SUGAR
- ⅓ CUP CANOLA OIL
- 2 TABLESPOONS CIDER VINEGAR
- 1 TEASPOON VANILLA EXTRACT
- 1 CUP DAIRY-FREE BUTTER OR MARGARINE, SOFTENED
- 3 CUPS CONFECTIONERS' SUGAR
- 2 TEASPOONS VANILLA EXTRACT

1 Preheat the oven to 350°F. Line two 12-cup muffin pans with paper cupcake liners.

2 In a large bowl, whisk together the flour, baking powder, baking soda, and salt. In a small bowl, whisk together the coconut milk, sugar, oil, vinegar, and vanilla. Stir the milk mixture into the flour mixture just until moistened.

3 Fill the prepared cupcake liners with the batter half full. Bake for 15 to 20 minutes or until a toothpick inserted in the center comes out clean. Cool the pans on wire racks for 10 minutes. Remove the cupcakes to the racks to cool completely.

4 For the frosting, in a large bowl, with an electric mixer, beat the butter until light and fluffy. Beat in confectioners' sugar and vanilla. Frost the cupcakes.

Makes 24 cupcakes. Per cupcake: 255 calories, 11 g total fat (18% saturated), 1 g protein, 38 g carbohydrate, 1.6 g fiber, 0 mg cholesterol, 180 mg sodium

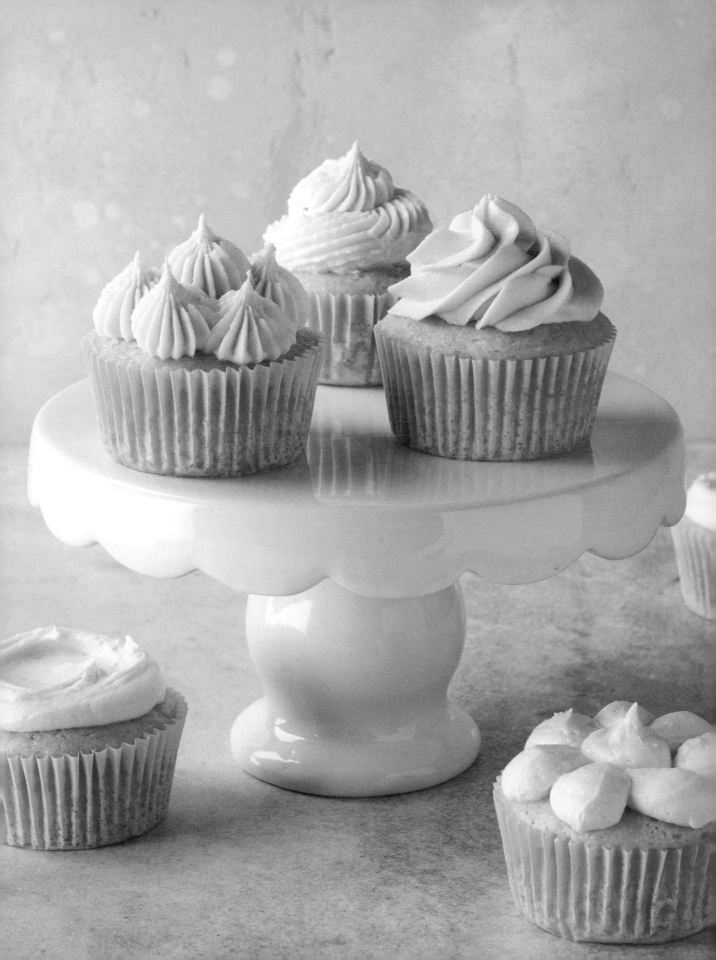

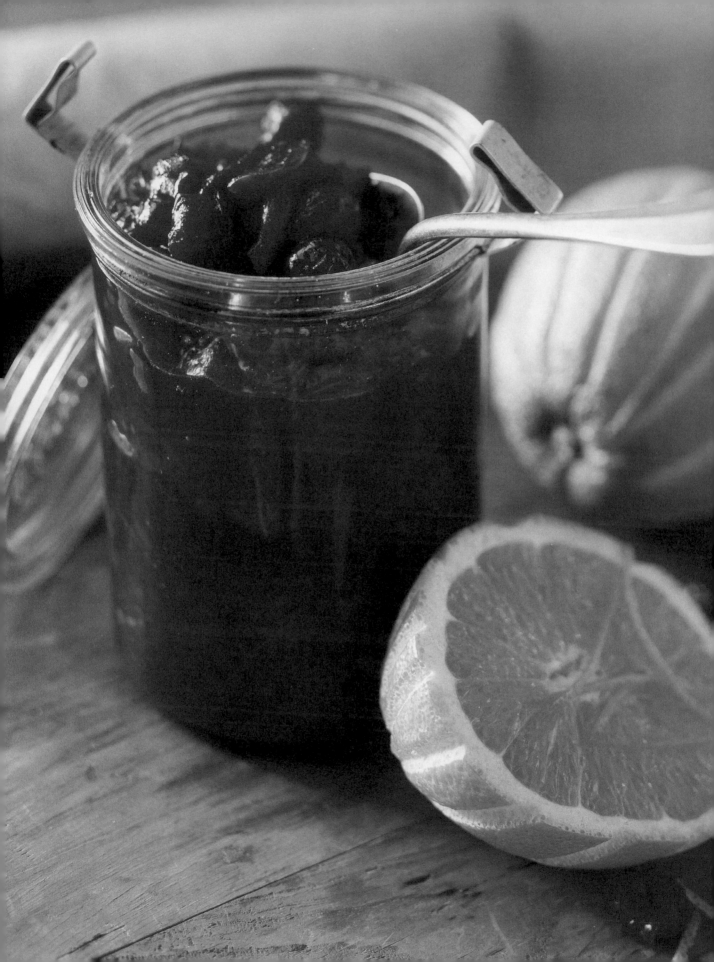

wasabi-miso dressing

Wasabi, a type of horseradish, can be found in paste form or as a powder in Asian food markets and in the international section of supermarkets. Once opened, store the wasabi in the refrigerator—it will keep for several months. Serve this spicy dressing on mixed greens, sliced cucumbers, or in a edamame salad.

- 2 TABLESPOONS WASABI POWDER
- 2 TABLESPOONS YELLOW SHIRO MISO PASTE
- ¼ CUP FRESH LIME JUICE
- 1 TABLESPOON DARK SESAME OIL
- 1 TABLESPOON HONEY
- ½ TEASPOON SALT
- ½ TEASPOON GROUND GINGER

1 In a medium bowl, stir together the wasabi powder and 2 tablespoons of water to form a paste. Stir in the miso.

2 Whisk in the lime juice, sesame oil, honey, salt, and ginger until smooth.

Makes 4 servings. Per serving: 74 calories, 4 g total fat (14% saturated), 2 g protein, 10 g carbohydrate, 0.5 g fiber, 0 mg cholesterol, 603 mg sodium

savory cranberry chutney

It's getting easier to make cranberry dishes year-round now that many supermarkets have figured out that cranberries freeze well. If you're fond of cranberries, you can buy several bags of fresh cranberries when they're available in the late fall, and simply throw them into the freezer for later use.

- 2 TEASPOONS OLIVE OIL
- 1 LARGE RED ONION, FINELY CHOPPED
- 3 CLOVES GARLIC, MINCED
- 1 PACKAGE (16 OUNCES) FRESH OR FROZEN CRANBERRIES
- ½ CUP FIRMLY PACKED LIGHT BROWN SUGAR
- ½ CUP DRIED CHERRIES
- 2 TEASPOONS GRATED ORANGE ZEST
- ½ CUP ORANGE JUICE
- ½ TEASPOON PEPPER
- ¼ TEASPOON SALT
- ⅛ TEASPOON ALLSPICE

1 In a large saucepan, heat the oil over medium-low heat. Add the onion and garlic; cook, stirring frequently for 7 minutes, or until the onion is tender.

2 Stir in the cranberries, brown sugar, dried cherries, orange zest, orange juice, pepper, salt, and allspice. Cook, stirring occasionally for 10 minutes, or until the berries have popped. Cool to room temperature. Serve at room temperature or chilled.

Makes 6 servings. Per serving: 175 calories, 1.7 g total fat (12% saturated), 1 g protein, 42 g carbohydrate, 2.8 g fiber, 0 mg cholesterol, 108 mg sodium

roasted garlic ranch dressing

Use this as you would any creamy salad dressing. It can be made several days in advance and refrigerated until serving time.

- 1 BULB GARLIC (3 OUNCES)
- 2 TEASPOONS GRATED LEMON ZEST
- 1 TABLESPOON FRESH LEMON JUICE
- 1 TABLESPOON OLIVE OIL
- 1 TEASPOON ONION POWDER
- ½ TEASPOON SALT
- ⅛ TEASPOON CAYENNE PEPPER
- 1 CUP UNSWEETENED SOY MILK

1 Preheat the oven to 400°F. Wrap the garlic bulb in foil and roast for 45 minutes or until the packet is soft to the touch.

2 Cut off the top of the garlic bulb and squeeze the garlic pulp into a medium bowl. Whisk in the lemon zest, lemon juice, oil, onion powder, salt, and cayenne until smooth. Whisk in the soy milk. Keep refrigerated until serving time.

Makes 4 servings. Per serving: 20 calories, 3.5 g total fat (14% saturated), 0 g protein, 1 g carbohydrate, 1.5 g fiber, 0 mg cholesterol, 157 mg sodium

◀ **savory cranberry chutney**

general index

recipe index

Prevent & Reverse Disease with a
PLANT-BASED DIET

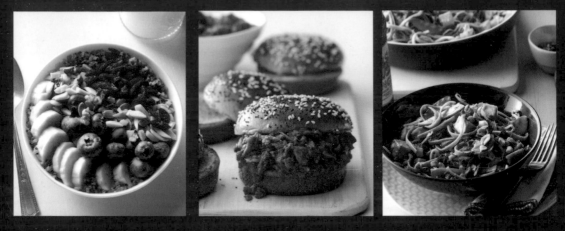

Have a cold? Plagued by heartburn? Just diagnosed with type 2 diabetes? Look in your fridge for help.

Study after study shows that eating more plant foods—not just fruits and veggies, but also grains, beans, nuts, and legumes—can save your life. It aids in weight loss, boosts your brain health, and reduces the risk of heart disease, cancer, and many other diseases. Plus, it's an environmentally friendly and economical way to eat.

Based on the latest scientific studies, *Plant-Based Health Basics* includes:

• almost 50 superstar foods, from apples to winter squash, with tips on maximizing their benefits and including them in your daily diet

• a specific food arsenal to manage and prevent more than 55 common ailments, from asthma to osteoporosis

• almost 90 delicious disease-combating recipes using easy-to-find ingredients

Whether you are completely vegan or just want to add a few more vegetables to your meals, this beautiful book is your complete guide to eating for wellness.

$19.99 US/$26.99 CAN
COOKING/Vegetarian

ISBN 978-1-62145-551-6